Identification and Treatment of Gynecological Cancers

Identification and Treatment of Gynecological Cancers

Editor: Isabella Dawson

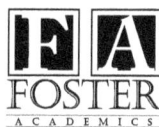

FA FOSTER
ACADEMICS

www.fosteracademics.com

www.fosteracademics.com

FA
FOSTER
ACADEMICS

Cataloging-in-Publication Data

Identification and treatment of gynecological cancers / edited by Isabella Dawson.
　　p. cm.
Includes bibliographical references and index.
ISBN 978-1-63242-741-0
1. Generative organs, Female--Cancer. 2. Generative organs, Female--Cancer--Diagnosis.
3. Generative organs, Female--Cancer--Treatment. I. Dawson, Isabella.
RC280.G5 I44 2019
616.994 65--dc23

Foster Academics,
118-35 Queens Blvd., Suite 400,
Forest Hills, NY 11375, USA

ISBN 978-1-63242-741-0 (Hardback)

Contents

Preface

The cancers originating in the ovaries, uterus, vagina, fallopian tubes, cervix and vulva are called gynecological cancers. Uterine cancer emerges in the uterine tissue. Its types include cervical cancer, endometrial cancer, gestational trophoblastic disease and uterine sarcoma. Vaginal cancer is malignant and forms in the tissue of the vagina. Squamous-cell carcinoma is the primary form of vaginal cancer. The other types of vaginal cancer are vaginal adenocarcinoma, vaginal germ cell tumor, clear cell adenocarcinoma, vaginal melanoma, etc. The diagnosis of such cancers is made on the basis of a pelvic exam, pap smear, physical exam and history, biopsy and colposcopy. High-dose-rate interstitial brachytherapy, external-beam radiation therapy and concurrent carboplatin plus paclitaxel are some nascent strategies for the management of advanced ovarian cancers. In cases where surgery is the recommended pathway for the treatment of cancers, genitoplasty may be performed to repair the damage and may include procedures such as vaginoplasty, labiaplasty, vaginal reconstruction, etc. This book explores all the important gynecological disorders in the present day scenario. It presents this complex subject in the most comprehensible language. For someone with an interest and eye for detail, it covers the most significant treatments and management strategies of such cancers.

This book is a result of research of several months to collate the most relevant data in the field.

When I was approached with the idea of this book and the proposal to edit it, I was overwhelmed. It gave me an opportunity to reach out to all those who share a common interest with me in this field. I had 3 main parameters for editing this text:

1. Accuracy – The data and information provided in this book should be up-to-date and valuable to the readers.

2. Structure – The data must be presented in a structured format for easy understanding and better grasping of the readers

3. Universal Approach – This book not only targets students but also experts and innovators in the field, thus my aim was to present topics which are of use to all

Thus, it took me a couple of months to finish the editing of this book.

Editor

Novel Systemic Treatments in High Grade Ovarian Cancer

Amit Samani, Charleen Chan and Jonathan Krell

Abstract

Most patients with ovarian cancer present at an advanced stage and are never cured. To improve outcomes a variety of novel systemic strategies are being developed. Traditional cytotoxic chemotherapy is being optimised, anti-angiogenic strategies are already in the clinic and several PARP inhibitors have gained regulatory approval. In addition, immunotherapy is showing promise and novel targeted strategies including against folate receptor alpha are also generating excitement. As our therapeutic choice increases, a challenge will be how to best utilize the options available. Here we discuss recently established and other emerging therapies with a focus on key concepts rather than detailed synopses of trial designs and outcomes.

Keywords: ovarian cancer, PARP inhibitors, immunotherapy, antiangiogenic therapy

1. Introduction

Over a quarter of a million women are diagnosed with epithelial ovarian cancer (EOC[1]) each year and it is responsible for around 140,000 deaths worldwide. There is no effective screening program so the majority present with advanced disease. Despite improved surgical technique most patients are never cured. Novel systemic treatments are needed both to prolong overall survival *with* the disease but also increase the fraction of patients in whom cure is achieved. A variety of distinct but complementary approaches are discussed here.

---

[1]In this chapter, EOC refers also to primary peritoneal and fallopian tube carcinoma. Definitions of platinum-sensitive, resistant and refractory are as per the relevant citation.

2. Chemotherapy in ovarian cancer

Despite the emergence of alternate antineoplastic strategies, chemotherapy remains the backbone of EOC treatment. Although EOC is chemosensitive, with most patients responding initially, the majority will eventually relapse and subsequent responses are poorer. Efforts are being made to try and enhance the efficacy of 'traditional' cytotoxic chemotherapy. These include manipulation of dosing schedules, efforts to understand resistance and discovery of novel agents. These strategies are discussed in this subsection.

2.1. Dose-dense chemotherapy

Dose densification refers to the administration of an agent more frequently than in the 'standard' regimen. It can imply dose intensification (i.e. increasing the net $mg/m^2/week$) but some authors use it to describe splitting the standard scheduled dose into weekly fragments while maintaining the same (rather than increased) dose intensity [1].

The rationale for dose-dense treatment stems from the Norton-Simon hypothesis (**Figure 1**).

The rationale for dose densification extends beyond the Norton-Simon hypothesis. Firstly, the pharmacokinetics of a dose-dense approach may reduce toxicity. For example, paclitaxel-induced myelosuppression is dependent on the time during which the plasma level exceeds 50 nM [3]. This is considerably shorter for 80 mg/m^2 weekly compared to 240 mg/m^2 q3w [4]. Secondly, weekly paclitaxel may confer an additional anti-angiogenic effect compared to q3w scheduling [5].

Weekly paclitaxel was initially studied in the recurrent setting. Notably in one trial patients resistant to the q3w regimen achieved an objective response rate (ORR) of 25% with the weekly regimen possibly due to the additional anti-angiogenic effect of this schedule [6].

Weekly paclitaxel has also been studied in the adjuvant setting (**Table 1**).

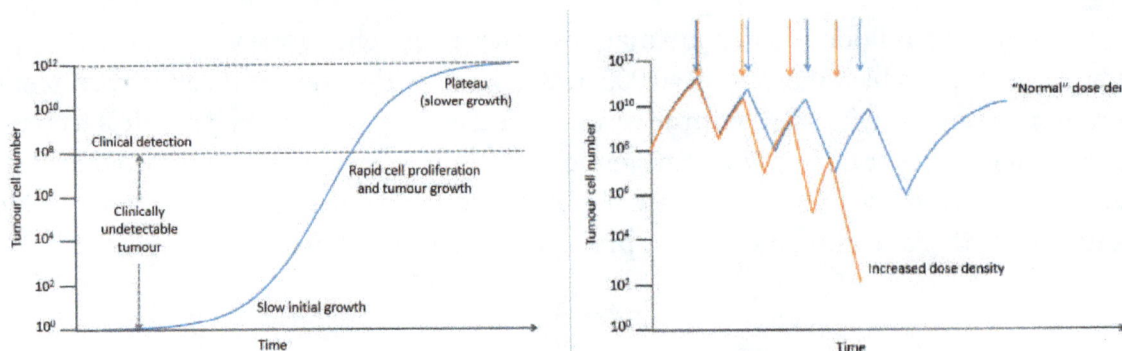

Figure 1. The Norton-Simon hypothesis assumes a Gompertzian model of tumour growth (left). This was combined with their observation that after treatment, smaller tumours regress faster than larger ones. Crucial to their mathematical model is the fact that 'log-kill' is not constant for a given dose of therapy but instead depends on tumour size, being greater for smaller tumours. Their model predicts that a dose-dense approach is more likely to eradicate a tumour [2].

Study	Eligibility	Treatment	Efficacy (months)	Safety (grade ≥ 3, P < 0.001)
JGOG 3016 [10]	Stage II-IV	Carbo q3w + either taxol q3w **or** weekly[1]	PFS 28.2 vs. 17.5 OS 100.5 vs. 62.2	Anaemia 69% vs. 44% Discontinuation due to tox. 60% vs. 43%
GOG 0262 [11]	Incompletely resected III or IV	As above + uncontrolled bevacizumab[2]	PFS 14.7 vs. 14.0 (not significant)	Anaemia 36% vs. 16% Neutropenia 72% vs. 83%
MITO-7 [12]	Stage IC-IV	Carobplatin/paclitaxel either q3w **or** weekly[3]	PFS 18.3 vs. 17.3 (not significant)	Neutropenia 42% vs. 50% Thrombocytopenia 1% vs. 7%

[1]Carboplatin AUC 6, paclitaxel 180 mg/m^2 (q3w) or 80 mg/m^2 (weekly).
[2]Carboplatin AUC 6, paclitaxel 175 mg/m^2 (q3w) or 80 mg/m^2 (weekly). 84% of patients received bevacizumab.
[3]Carboplatin AUC 6, 175 mg/m^2 (q3w) or carboplatin AUC 2, paclitaxel 60 mg/m^2 (weekly).

Table 1. Comparison of phase III trials testing weekly paclitaxel in the adjuvant setting. All values given as weekly vs. q3w.

In JGOG 3016 patients derived both PFS and OS benefit from the dose-dense approach, whereas in GOG 0262, there was no PFS difference in the intention to treat (ITT) population [7–9]. The two trials, however, had key differences. Patients in GOG 0262 were allowed bevacizumab (BEV) in an uncontrolled fashion. Since weekly paclitaxel has an anti-angiogenic effect, this may have been negated by the addition of BEV in 85% of the trial population. Consistent with this, in those who didn't receive BEV, weekly paclitaxel improved PFS (14.2 vs. 10.3 months). Pharmacogenomic differences in the two trial populations may also have been important. There are consequently unanswered questions about dose-dense chemotherapy which may be answered by two phase III trials yet to report. In the 3-arm ICON 8 trial (NCT01654146), q3w carboplatin/paclitaxel is compared to 2 dose-dense regimens without BEV. In ICON 8B (NCT01654146), bevacizumab use is allowed but is controlled and pre-specified.

2.2. Understanding resistance to facilitate chemosensitization

EOC is initially chemosensitive so efforts to understand resistance could improve outcomes. Acquired resistance is secondary to diverse mechanisms which includes alterations to DNA repair and/or response to DNA damage. Mk-1775 is an anti-Wee1 tyrosine kinase inhibitor (TKI) that may sensitize cells to chemotherapy by abrogating the G2 checkpoint (crucial in P53 deficient cells) causing premature entry into mitosis [10]. It has shown promising results in several phase II trials [11]. In a different approach, the 2-arm PiSARRO trial (NCT02098343) involves the addition of APR-246 (capable of restoring mutant P53 to wild-type confirmation) to platinum-based therapy with the aim of restoring the apoptotic-response to chemotherapy-induced DNA damage. There are many other pre-clinical and early clinical efforts aiming to reverse chemoresistance including efforts to target primary resistance by targeting cancer stem cells and epithelial to mesenchymal transition [12].

2.3. Novel chemotherapeutic agents

Lurbinectedin is a recently discovered marine-derived antineoplastic agent that has a multi-modal mechanism of action similar to trabectedin. It showed promising results in a phase II trial in platinum-resistant EOC and is being investigated in a phase III trial against either PLD or topotecan [13]. It has also shown *in vitro* synergy with cisplatin raising hopes of clinical application to reverse platinum resistance [14]. Trabectedin itself is undergoing phase III testing in patients with platinum partially-sensitive disease (NCT01379989).

3. Antiangiogenic strategies in ovarian cancer

Key mediators of physiological angiogenesis include products of the vascular endothelial growth factor (VEGF) gene family including VEGF-A (often abbreviated to VEGF), VEGF-B, C and D and placental growth factor. The receptor family includes VEGFR-1, 2 and 3. Different combinations of ligand-receptor interaction result in diverse outcomes such as promotion of survival, proliferation of endothelium, increased permeability and lymphangiogenesis. The binding of VEGF-A to VEGFR-2 is most important in endothelial proliferation and the regulation of permeability [15].

In physiology VEGF is important for the cyclical angiogenesis that takes place in the female reproductive tract [16]. Many tumour cell lines overexpress VEGF and in one series over 97% of human ovarian lines had overexpression [17]. Clinically, expression levels have been found to be an independent prognostic factor in several studies [18] and have also been found to correlate with peritoneal dissemination and ascites formation [19].

Given the role of VEGF in physiology as well as pre-clinical and observational data supporting a role for VEGF in cancer, several VEGF-directed therapies exist.

3.1. Bevacizumab

Bevacizumab (BEV) is a humanized monoclonal antibody able to bind all VEGF-A isoforms [20]. It is the most extensively studied of the antiangiogenic agents in EOC. Two phase III studies (GOG-218 and ICON7) tested adjuvant BEV. In GOG-218 [21] patients received 6 cycles of carboplatin/paclitaxel q3w and either 1) placebo (cycles 2–22), 2) BEV induction (cycles 2–6) then placebo maintenance (7–22) or 3) BEV induction (cycles 2–6) then maintenance (7–22). BEV was given at 15 mg/kg. The median PFS was 14.1 months in the BEV throughout arm compared to 11.2 months in the induction-only arm and 10.3 months for the control. Overall survival was not significantly different. 22.9% developed grade ≥ 2 hypertension in the BEV throughout arm vs. 7.2% in the control arm. In ICON7 [22], high-risk patients were given carboplatin/paclitaxel q3w with either placebo or bevacizumab (7.5 mg/kg) for cycles 2–18. Median PFS was 19.0 months in the BEV arm vs. 17.3 months (HR 0.81, $p < 0.01$). Among patients with incompletely resected IIIC or IV disease the median PFS was 15.9 vs. 10.5 months in the control arm. Bleeding (39 vs. 11%), hypertension (18 vs. 2%), thromboembolism (7 vs. 3%) and GI perforations (10 vs. 3 patients) were higher with BEV. Mean global QoL score was higher, at 54 weeks, in the control arm (76.1 vs. 69.7 points - EORTC questionnaire) [23]. Recent exploratory analysis of a 'high-risk' subgroup revealed significantly increased OS (restricted means) in the BEV group of 39.3 vs. 34.5 months [24].

There were similarities and differences between these trials. Both suggested greater benefit in a subpopulation with higher stage and suboptimal debulking. They also agreed that QoL was not improved with BEV. Conversely, different doses and durations of treatment were used and overall survival data also differed, perhaps confounded by the 40% crossover in GOG 218. BEV received regulatory approval from the EMA using 15 mg/kg [25] although ESMO guidelines supported the 7.5 mg/kg dose used in ICON7, which is also prescribed in the UK currently [26]. Analysis of both trials showed greatest separation of the PFS curves at the end of BEV treatment (12 or 15 months), raising questions about extending maintenance duration. This is being investigated in the phase III BOOST study (NCT01462890).

Bev has also been studied for recurrence. In AURELIA [27], patients with platinum-resistant disease and ≤2 prior lines of chemotherapy were given single agent investigator-choice chemotherapy either alone or with BEV continued until progression/toxicity. Median PFS was higher in the BEV arm, 6.7 vs. 3.4 months with an ORR of 27.3 vs. 11.1%. Of the 113 patients with baseline ascites 17% required paracentesis in the control arm vs. 2% in the BEV arm and PROMs for GI symptoms were better with BEV [28]. OS was not significantly different in the context of 40% crossover but a recent exploratory analysis suggestive a survival advantage in those who received BEV during or after the study [29]. Adverse events were consistent with previous studies. BEV has been granted FDA and EMA approval for this indication.

In the OCEANS study [30], the addition of BEV to carboplatin/gemcitabine in patients with platinum-sensitive disease resulted in a median PFS of 12.4 months vs. 8.4 months. OS was not significantly (38% crossover). Hypertension, proteinuria and non-CNS bleeding were significantly more common in the BEV arm. BEV was also tested in the platinum-sensitive setting with carboplatin/paclitaxel, in the factorial GOG-213 trial [31]. Median OS with BEV was 42.2 months compared to 37.3 months without (p = 0.056). BEV has EMA regulatory approval in this setting.

3.2. VEGFR tyrosine kinase inhibitor (TKI) therapy

Whereas BEV binds directly to VEGF, VEGFR TKIs affect signalling via competitive inhibition of the intracellular kinase domain. They have the advantage of being orally bioavailable and multitargeted. Conversely, plasma concentration is unpredictable and off-target effects narrow the therapeutic window.

Cediranib inhibits VEGR-1,2 and 3 and c-Kit. ICON 6 [32] randomised patients with recurrent platinum-sensitive disease to chemotherapy plus: placebo concurrently + maintenance (Arm A), cediranib concurrently + placebo maintenance (Arm B) or cediranib concurrently + maintenance (Arm C). Median PFS was 11 months in Arm C vs. 8.7 months in Arm A (p < 0.0001). Recent OS data [33] by restricted means showed 34.2 months vs. 29.4 months in Arms C and A respectively (95% CI for the difference: −0.1-9.8). During chemotherapy grade ≥ 3 fatigue (16 vs. 8%), diarrhoea (10 vs. 2%), hypertension (12 vs. 3%), febrile neutropenia (7 vs. 3%) and thrombosis (3 vs. 1%) were higher with cediranib. 48% discontinued treatment due to toxic effects in Arm C compared to 17% in Arm A and 37% in B. Although recent analysis showed no detriment in

QOL at 1 year [34], filing for regulatory approval for cediranib had been previously withdrawn. Nonetheless cediranib maintenance is undergoing investigation in ICON9 (see below).

Pazopanib inhibits VEGR1,2 and 3, c-Kit and PDGFR. The AGO-OVAR 16 study [35] evaluated first-line maintenance pazopanib. PFS was 17.9 months for pazopanib compared to 12.3 months for control. Grade 3/4 adverse events were significantly higher for pazopanib including hypertension (30.8%), neutropenia (9.9%) and diarrhoea (8.2%). Discontinuation due to AEs occurred in 33% in the pazopanib arm compared to 5.6% in the placebo arm. Regulatory approval filing was withdrawn due to perceived imbalance in benefit–risk ratio.

Other VEGFR TKIs have been studied in ovarian cancer [35]. Nintedanib was given in the first-line setting with chemotherapy and then maintenance. Again, a PFS benefit was seen but no significant OS advantage [36]. Other multitargeted VEGFR TKIs such as sunitinib and sorafenib have also been studied with similar outcomes. As a class the TKIs appear to have some effect however their multi-targeted nature and unpredictable bioavailability means that their perceived risk:benefit ratio has not led to any regulatory approvals as yet.

3.3. Other antiangiogenic strategies

The Ang-Tie pathway is distinct from the VEGF axis, involved in vascular remodelling. Trebananib is peptide-Fc fusion protein that binds Angiopoietin 1 and 2 and prevents interaction with Tie on endothelium. Although promising results were seen in phase II [37], a phase III trial (TRINOVA-2) [38] failed to meet its PFS endpoint and a third terminated early for futility (NCT01493505).

3.4. Combination therapy

Vascular disrupting agents (VDAs), in contrast to inhibiting formation of new vessels, target existing tumour vasculature. The VDA's combretastatin and fosbretabulin disrupt the endothelial cytoskeleton (by binding tubulin) aiming to cause endothelial detachment and eventual vessel obstruction. Tumour vasculature lacks pericytes and smooth muscle making them selectively susceptible. Fosbretabulin is being examined for synergy with bevacizumab and chemotherapy in platinum-resistant disease in a phase II/III trial (NCT02641639).

There is pre-clinical rationale for the combination of VEGF-targeted therapy with poly (ADP-ribose) polymerase inhibitors (PARPi); anti-VEGF induced hypoxia can impair DNA repair and sensitize otherwise insensitive cells to PARPi. In a phase II trial of olaparib and cediranib [39] PFS with the combination was prolonged (17.7 vs. 9.0 months) and, consistent with pre-clinical rationale, the difference was most marked in BRCA wild-type patients. Grade 3/4 toxicity however was 70% with the combination vs. 7% for olaparib monotherapy. The combination is currently undergoing phase III testing (ICON 9). The combination of bevacizumab and olaparib in first-line maintenance is also being studied (NCT02477644).

Combining VEGF blockade and immunotherapy also has pre-clinical rationale (see below). Combinations of anti-angiogenesis and chemotherapy have been discussed in the paragraphs above. Of note, an early phase trial of pazopanib with carboplatin/paclitaxel was terminated early because of toxicity (GI perforations and myelotoxicity).

3.5. Predictive biomarkers in anti-angiogenic therapy

Given the relatively modest median PFS benefits and lack of OS benefit in some trials combined with toxicity and economic considerations, biomarkers for patient selection are needed. None have yet been validated for routine use although many have been suggested. Studies have been retrospective and focussed on different markers including gene-expression signatures, serum and tissue proteomic biomarkers. There have been some intriguing results including a 63-gene signature that identifies an immune subgroup that may be harmed by bevacizumab treatment [40]. Prospective validation is needed for this and other candidate markers.

4. PARP inhibitor therapy

DNA constantly undergoes single and double-strand breaks (SSBs/DSBs). SSBs are repaired predominantly by base excision repair (BER). PARPs are nuclear proteins with diverse functions including in BER and chromatin remodelling. PARP-1 is the most abundant member which upon binding to SSBs activates its ADP-ribosyltransferase catalytic domain allowing PARylation and recruitment of DNA repair effectors [41]. DSBs are mostly repaired by homologous recombination (HR) or non-homologous end joining (NHEJ), the latter being error-prone [42]. HR involves a number of key proteins including BRCA1, BRCA2, RAD51 and PALB2. A detailed discussion is beyond the scope of this chapter but the process of HR is reviewed here [43]

4.1. Homologous recombination repair in ovarian cancer

The Australian Ovarian Cancer Study Group screened 1001 patients with stage I-IV ovarian cancer for point mutations or large deletions in BRCA genes. 14.4% of patients overall had a germline mutation (including 17.1% with serous histology) [44]. A similar frequency was found in The Cancer Genome Atlas (TCGA) [45] although globally the prevalence varies between ethnic groups. In addition to germline mutations, BRCA genes can be somatically mutated, epigenetically silenced or the protein inactivated through post-translational mechanisms, e.g. EMSY amplification [46]. Various series have found somatic mutations of BRCA in 3–6% of EOC [47]. In contrast to somatic mutations, epigenetic silencing by promoter methylation is a dynamic process and may be harder to quantify. Studies report prevalence in the region of 5–30% of ovarian cancers.

However, BRCA1 and 2 are just two of many proteins involved in HR. TCGA undertook exomic analysis of 316 ovarian cancers as well as studies of promoter methylation, RNA expression and copy number changes [45]. Pathway analysis demonstrated that 51% of tumours had either mutations or silencing of components in the HR pathways. (**Figure 2**).

4.2. PARP inhibitors in ovarian cancer

HR deficiency (HRD) in EOC provides a target that can be exploited therapeutically. It was noted that cells with non-functioning PARP develop increased nuclear foci of Rad51 implying an increased burden of lesions being repaired by HR in these cells [48]. Farmer et al. [49] tested

HR gene mutation frequency

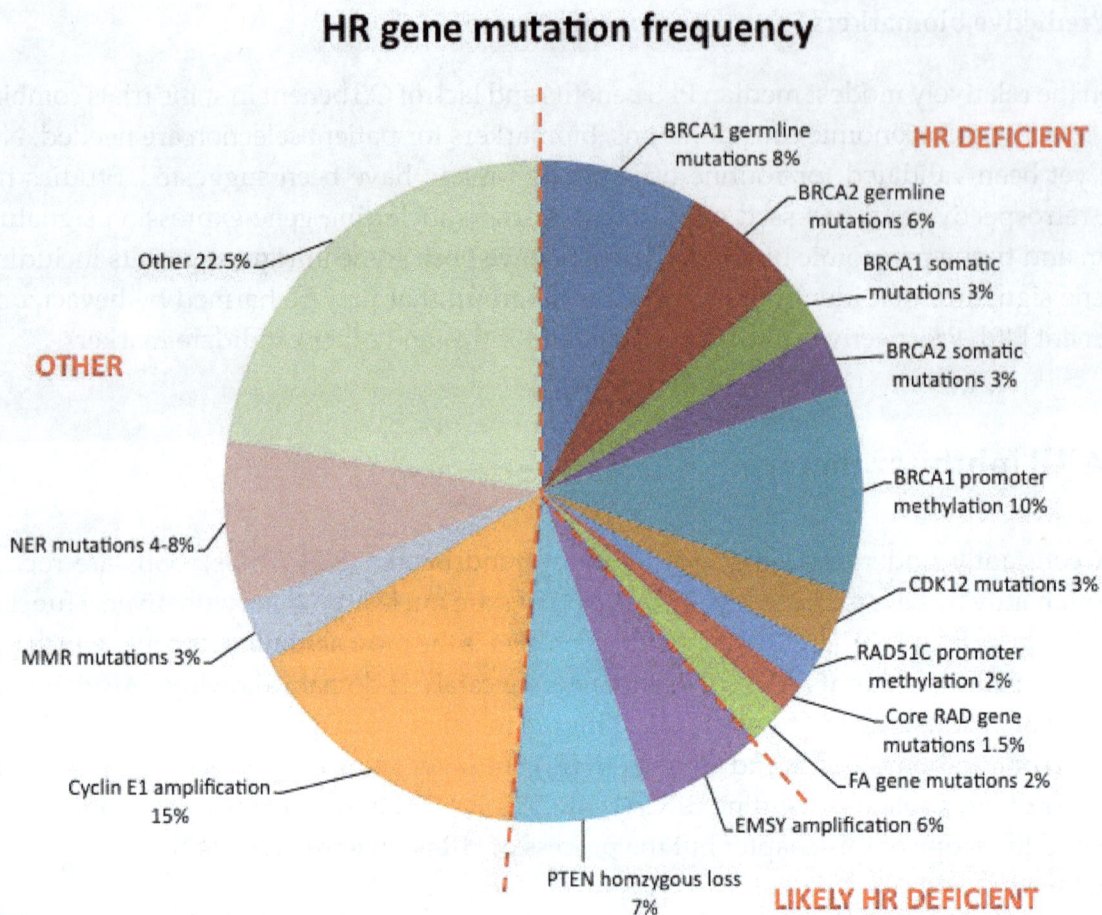

Figure 2. Distribution of HR gene mutations in EOC. Adapted from Ref. [47].

the hypothesis that BRCA 1/2 dysfunction would hypersensitize cells to PARP inhibition and were able to demonstrate this in BRCA deficient cell lines. This example of 'synthetic lethality' whereby either defect alone is tolerable but the combination is fatal has been exploited in the generation of a family of drugs, the PARP inhibitors. (**Figure 3**).

Following this, further work began on designing a PARP inhibitor (PARPi) suitable for clinical use. Early agents mimicked the substrate-enzyme interaction between NAD^+ and the catalytic domain of PARP1/2 and further optimization led to the design of Compound 47, that would be developed as Olaparib [50]. Since Olaparib, several agents have been developed (discussed later) designed to inhibit PARP 1/2 catalytic activity.

In addition to catalytic inhibition, a distinct antitumour mechanism of PARPi, 'PARP-trapping' has been described. Trapped PARP-DNA complexes were more cytotoxic than unrepaired SSBs in PARP deficient cells and different PARP inhibitors had different PARP-trapping potency which was not correlated with their catalytic inhibitory properties [51].

4.3. Olaparib

Olaparib is an orally bioavailable small molecule with a nicotinamide moiety that competes with NAD^+ for binding to PARP. The MTD for olaparib was established from early phase

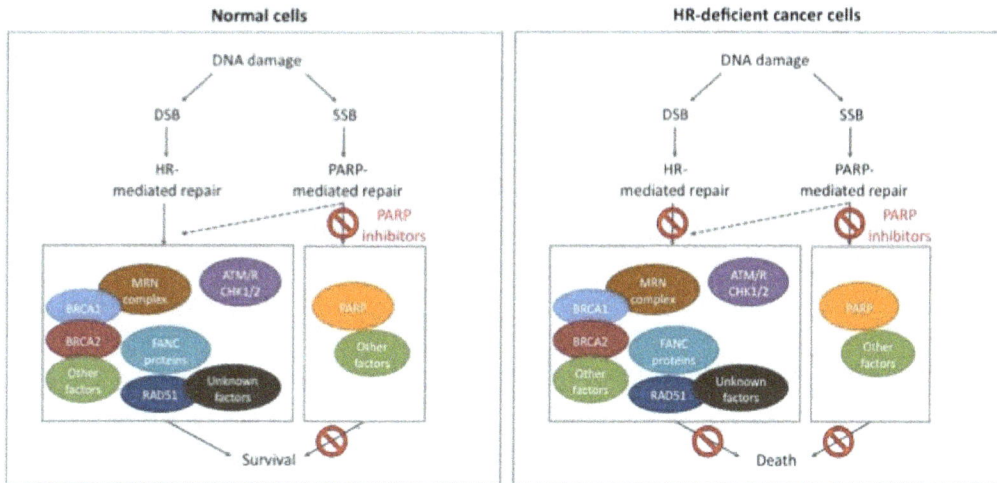

Figure 3. Schematic of synthetic lethality of PARP inhibition in HR deficient cells.

trials at 400 mg BD. Objective responses were seen mainly in patients with germline BRCA mutations (gBRCAm) [52] Further support for the efficacy of olaparib in in the gBRCAm population came from a proof-of-concept phase II where the ORR in the 400 mg BD cohort was 33% including some complete responses (CRs) [53]. Of note, one heavily pre-treated patient developed acute myeloid leukaemia (AML) 9 months after cessation.

A further phase II study gave 193 heavily pre-treated EOC platinum-resistant/unsuitable patients with gBRCA mutations olaparib at a dose of 400 mg BD [54]. The ORR was 31%. AEs were similar to those seen in earlier trials with a grade 3/4 rate of 54% including anaemia (17%) and fatigue (6%). Two patients developed leukaemia and one myelodysplastic syndrome, all were heavily pre-treated (25, 26 and 34 cycles each). These results (along with other applicant-submitted data) earnt olaparib FDA approval as monotherapy for patients with gBRCA mutations after three prior lines. The recent phase III SOLO3 study randomised patients with gBRCA mutations who have received at least 2 prior lines of platinum-based therapy and who are deemed at least partially platinum-sensitive to either Olaparib 300 mg BD or single agent chemotherapy of investigators choice [55]. Results are awaited. While the previous formulation of Olaparib required 16 capsules a day, the current tablet formulation requires only four raising hopes that some of the gastrointestinal toxicity will be mitigated.

In the aforementioned studies olaparib was given as monotherapy for treatment of 'active' disease. In contrast, Study 19 randomised patients with recurrent platinum-sensitive cancer with at least 2 prior lines to *maintenance* olaparib or placebo post-chemotherapy [56]. In a predefined subset analysis of patients with known germline or somatic BRCA mutation (most retrospectively determined), median PFS in the gBRCAm group was 11.3 vs. 4.3 months with Olaparib and placebo respectively (HR 0.18). OS was not significantly different (23% crossover). The findings led to EMA approval. SOLO2 was a phase III double-blind placebo-controlled study in patients with recurrent platinum-sensitive EOC who had received at least 2 prior chemotherapy lines. Patients either got maintenance olaparib 300 mg BD or placebo. Investigator-assessed median PFS was 19.1 vs. 5.5 months (HR 0.30). Median PFS2 was also improved from not reached vs. 18.4 months (HR 0.5) and OS data are immature. Although nausea (76% vs. 33%) and vomitting (37% vs. 19%) were higher in the olaparib arms, grade 3/4 events were infrequent (2.6% for both). Grade 3/4 anaemia occurred in 20%. Patient-reported outcomes showed no detriment for olaparib [57].

The phase III SOLO1 has completed accrual and randomised patients with BRCAm following first-line platinum-based chemotherapy to either Olaparib 300 mg BD or placebo.

4.4. Niraparib

Niraparib is a potent PARP1 and PARP2 inhibitor whose pharmacokinetics allows once daily dosing. A phase I dose escalation trial established the MTD as 300 mg/day. Dose-limiting toxicities included fatigue, reversible pneumonitis (in the context of recent chest wall irradiation) and reversible grade 4 thrombocytopenia. Of the 20 patients with gBRCA mutations and evaluable tumours the ORR (at doses between 80 and 400 mg) was 40% [58].

The pivotal phase III NOVA trial enrolled patients with platinum-sensitive disease who had received at least two prior lines of chemotherapy and who had measurable disease of <2 cm post-treatment [59]. Patients were randomised to niraparib 300 mg or placebo as maintenance till PD or unacceptable toxicity. Patients were stratified into gBRCA mutations vs. those without. Those without gBRCA mutations were further stratified into those with or without a positive HRD score (see below) and a predefined cut-off. PFS in the gBRCA mutated group was 21 vs. 5.5 months in the niraparib and control arms respectively (HR 0.30) and 12.9 vs. 3.8 months (HR 0.45) in the HRD positive cohort.

QUADRA is an ongoing single-arm phase II trial in patients pre-treated with 3–4 lines of chemotherapy and who were platinum sensitive at first recurrence regardless of BRCA mutation status. Patients who entered the trial underwent testing for homologous recombination deficiency (HRD) using a validated commercial assay. This assesses tumour samples for three SNP array-based 'signatures' of genomic instability (loss of heterozygosity, telomeric allelic imbalance and large scale transition) to derive an overall 'HRD score' that should predict sensitivity to PARP inhibition [NCT02354586].

PRIMA is an ongoing phase III of niraparib maintenance after 1st line chemotherapy. Unlike SOLO1, patients are enrolled on the basis of HRD score rather than gBRCA mutation status.

4.5. Rucaparib

Rucaparib is another orally bioavailable PARPi with both catalytic inhibitory and PARP-trapping activity, the potency of the latter being equivalent to olaparib [60].

Rucaparib was granted accelerated FDA approval largely based on composite data from 2 phase II studies. 106 patients with gBRCA mutations who had received at least 2 prior lines of chemotherapy received continuous rucaparib at 600 mg BD [61]. The confirmed ORR by RECIST was 54%. Toxicity at ≥ grade 3 included anaemia (27%), fatigue (15%), transient AST/ALT elevation (13%), vomiting (6%) and nausea (4%).

Part 1 of the ARIEL2 trial (from which the gBRCA mutation data was pooled in the above analysis) enrolled 206 patients who had been received at least 1 prior platinum containing chemotherapy regimen and who had progressed after at least 6 months after their most recent course [62]. Patients were prospectively divided into three subgroups based on their HRD status: 1) germline or somatic BRCA mutations 2) BRCA wild-type and LOH-high 3) BRCA wild-type and LOH-low. LOH was assessed using a next generation sequencing assay and a cut-off of 14% was assigned using microarray and survival data from TCGA. Based on this pre-specified score, PFS was 12.8 months, 5.7 months and 5.2 months in the BRCA mutated, BRCA wild-type/LOH-high and BRCA wild-type/LOH-low subgroups. Although median PFS was similar in the latter groups, the HR for PFS was significantly in favour of the LOH-high subgroup (0.62 95% CI 0.42–0.90), and ORR by RECIST (29% vs. 10%) and 1 year survival (28% vs. 10%) were also better for the LOH-high subgroup. Of note, LOH exists on a continuum and exploratory post-hoc analysis revealed that a cut-off of 16% provided better discrimination between the two subgroups [63]. Also importantly, there were patients in the LOH-negative group with very good partial and even complete responses (by ca125). In this single arm phase II study, it is not possible to exclude the possibility that LOH-high tumours simply have a better prognosis and that LOH is a prognostic rather than predictive marker. In order to address this question (in a maintenance setting at least) the NGS assay is being prospectively applied in the phase III Ariel 3 study which is investigating maintenance rucaparib in platinum-sensitive ovarian cancer. The phase III Ariel 4 study is will compare rucaparib as an active treatment vs. standard of care chemotherapy in platinum-sensitive disease after at least 2 prior lines.

4.6. Veliparib

Another orally bioavailable PARP inhibitor, veliparib is far less potent at PARP-trapping than the previously mentioned agents although it is a more potent catalytic inhibitor than niraparib and has been shown to cross the blood–brain barrier [51]. In a phase I trial 40% of the 28 BRCAm positive evaluable patients had an ORR at the MTD (400 mg BD). Commonest toxicities were nausea, vomiting and lymphopenia and 2 patients had grade 2 seizures [NCT01472783].

In a phase II trial in patients with gBRCAm who had been treated with 3 or fewer prior regimens (median 2) and of whom 60% were platinum resistant, the ORR was 26% (35% in the platinum-sensitive cohort). Grade 3 fatigue, nausea and neutropenia occurred in 6%, 4% and 2% respectively with no other grade 3 toxicities. Veliparib is currently being explored in phase III trial concurrently with carboplatin/paclitaxel and then continued as maintenance (NCT02470585, see below).

4.7. Talazoparib

Talazoparib is a novel PARPi that traps PARP approximately 100-fold more efficiently than olaparib and rucaparib and exhibits cytotoxicity at nanomolar (compared to micromolar) concentrations) [60]. At an MTD of 1 mg/kg, 5/12 patients with BRCAm ovarian cancer achieved an ORR with a 24% and 18% rate of G3 anaemia and thrombocytopenia respectively [64]. Given its unique potency for trapping, there is hope that it may have efficacy as a second line agent for patients who have progressed on a previous PARPi [65].

4.8. Combination therapy with PARP inhibitors

PARPi were originally developed as potential chemo/radiosensitizers. There is obvious rationale in combining PARPi with other agents, especially in tumours that are HR proficient. When combining PARPi with chemotherapy, rational combination necessitates consideration of the mechanism of action of the chemotherapy plus the relative catalytic inhibitory/trapping properties of the PARPi. For example, PARPi combination with topo-1 inhibitors is synergistic primarily because of catalytic PARP inhibition whereas synergy with alkylating agents relies on trapping too [66]. Several PARPi/chemotherapy combinations are in trials, reviewed here [67]. Synergistic toxicity (e.g. myelotoxicity) will have to be borne in mind. PARPi/VEGFR targeting combinations have previously been discussed. Other targeted combinations include PI3K/MTOR pathway inhibitors, HSP90 and CHK1/2 inhibitors [67]. Finally, talazoparib had immunomodulatory effects in a pre-clinical mouse model; studies looking at immunotherapy with PARPi are underway (NCT0257172).

4.9. Resistance to PARP inhibitors

Several putative mechanisms of resistance have been described. These include a secondary mutation in BRCA which either restores the correct open reading frame (i.e. where the original mutation caused a frameshift) or which fully reverts the original mutation to wild-type. This also causes platinum resistance and in one study of platinum resistance in BRCAm patients, 46% had acquired a secondary BRCA mutation [68]. Other mechanisms include upregulation of P-glycoprotein and loss of 53BP1 (which usually promotes NHEJ and prevents HR). Knowledge of the specific resistance mechanism may have clinical relevance as some (e.g. secondary mutations) cause platinum resistance too whereas others do not. Also, 53BP1 loss causes resistance in BRCA1 but not BRAC2 deficient tumours.

5. Immunotherapy in ovarian cancer

In 2003 Zhang and colleagues showed that the presence or absence of tumour-infiltrating lymphocytes (TILs) in EOC is an independent prognostic factor (in multivariate analysis) for PFS and OS. Of 174 patients, those with TILs had a median overall survival of 50.3 months compared to 18.0 months in the 72 patients without [69]. Tumour-associated antigens discovered in EOC include mesothelin, Her2, NY-ESO and ca125 amongst others [70].

Around 50% of EOC has genomic/epigenetic changes in genes implicated in HRD [45]. Therefore there is a subset of EOC with a higher mutational burden possibly more likely to benefit from immunotherapy. Analysis of TCGA data showed a significantly higher predicted neoantigen load in HRD vs. HR proficient tumours [71]. In addition, BRCA1/2 status and neoantigen load were independent predictors of OS in multivariate analysis and BRCA mutated tumours had an increased TIL burden and PD-L1 expression. Lastly, tumour burden/volume is an important factor in predicting the response to immunotherapy [72]. Ovarian cancer is unusual as patients presenting *de novo* with bulky disease can be treated with radical surgery to no residual disease. Although the majority relapse, there is a window of time where disease remains undetectable. Given the data that exists on enhanced effectiveness of immunotherapy in patients with a low overall tumour burden, this may present a window of opportunity to maximise effectiveness of this therapeutic approach.

5.1. Checkpoint blockade

Co-inhibitory checkpoints usually act to minimize collateral tissue damage during immune-activation. Upregulation of these checkpoints can subvert anti-tumour immunity. The binding of CTLA-4 to B7.1/B7.2 is one such inhibitory interaction that can be prevented by the anti CTLA-4 monoclonal antibody ipilimumab.

In a phase I study including 2 patients with ovarian cancer, one patient had a 43% reduction in ca125 levels while the other developed a plateau in ca125 levels despite rapidly rising levels before treatment [73]. In a follow-up study of 9 patients one developed a radiologic PR with complete resolution of mesenteric lymphadenopathy. Three others achieved radiographic and ca125-defined stable disease of 2, 4 and >6 months duration. In a phase II study of 40 patients with recurrent platinum-sensitive EOC (NCT01611558), 50% developed at least G3 toxicity and the ORR was 10.9% by RECIST. A phase II trial testing a combination of nivolumab and ipilimumab for recurrent ovarian cancer is currently underway (NCT02498600).

A trial using another CTLA4 antagonist, tremelimumab, is currently enrolling patients for phase I trials in combination with olaparib (NCT02571725, NCT02485990).

Another inhibitory checkpoint interaction is between PD-1 (on T-cells) and PD-L1 (that may be upregulated on tumour cells and their microenvironment). Avelumab, a fully humanised IgG1 anti-PD-L1 antibody, was tested in a phase Ib trial in 124 patients with platinum resistant/refractory disease after a median of 4 lines of therapy [73, 74]. The drug was well tolerated with a grade 3/4 adverse event rate of 6.4%. ORR in this heavily pre-treated population was 9.7% and the relationship between germline BRCA status and probability of response is being investigated. Avelumab is currently being tested in two randomised phase III trials. The three-arm JAVELIN Ovarian 200 study (NCT02580058)I is recruiting patients with their first platinum resistant/refractory relapse and randomising to either Avelumab or PLD alone or in combination. In JAVELIN Ovarian 100 (NCT02718417) patients with previously untreated III/IV ovarian cancer are randomised to carboplatin and paclitaxel followed by placebo or avelumab maintenance or carboplatin and paclitaxel with concurrent *and* maintenance avelumab.

Atezolizumab is also a fully humanized IgG1 anti-PD-L1 antibody. In the phase III ATALANTE trial (NCT02891824) patients with platinum-sensitive relapse are being randomised to platinum-based chemotherapy with concurrent and maintenance bevacizumab + placebo (control arm) or bevacizumab + avelumab (experimental arm). The combination of bevacizumab and avelumab is a rational one based on evidence that endogenous VEGF signalling has a variety of immunomodulatory effects. VEGF-A has been postulated to suppress dendritic cell maturation, increase the presence of immunosuppressive CD34+ haematopoetic progenitor cells in the tumour microenvironment and inhibit T-cell maturation [75]. Another trial combining atezolizumab with bevacizumab (NCT02839707) in a phase II/III setting is randomising platinum resistant patients between 3 arms each containing PLD with either bevacizumab alone (control), atezolizumab alone or bevacizumab and atezolizumab.

Instead of targeting PD-L1, pembrolizumab is a humanized anti PD-1 antibody. Keynote-028 included 26 EOC patients. 1 patient had a CR and 2 had PR by RECIST. The median duration of response was not reached (range 24.9+ to 26.5+) [76]. There are currently several ongoing phase I/II trials with pembrolizumab both as monotherapy and in combination with chemotherapy, niraparib and various small molecule inhibitors in the frontline and recurrent settings (NCT02865811, NCT02520154, NCT02440425, NCT02674061).

Nivolumab, a PD-1 blocking antibody, was given to 20 patients with platinum resistant EOC. 40% of patients developed G3/4 toxicity (lymphopenia, anaemia, hypoalbuminaemia, maculopapular rash, fever, ALT increase). Three patients (15%) had an OR including 2 CRs. One of these was in a patient with clear cell carcinoma (often chemoresistant) and this response was ongoing at the time of study reporting [77]. As with the pembrolizumab data, although the ORR was modest, there was evidence of durable responses in both studies. Nivolumab is being studied in several ongoing trials including in combination with ipilimumab for (NCT02498600), in combination with bevacizumab (NCT02873962) and with a vaccine against the tumour-associated antigen WT1 (NCT02737787).

5.2. Adoptive T-cell therapy

Adoptive T-cell therapy (ATT) involves the direct administration of various types of anti-tumour T-cells to the patient. Given the prognostic value of TILs (see above), TIL-based ATT seems logical. In one study, 13 patients who had no residual disease after surgery and adjuvant therapy were treated with TIL infusion. A matched control group was followed up concurrently [78]. In this small study 3 year OS was 100% in the TIL group vs. 67.5% in the control group. TIL-based trials are ongoing (NCT02482090, NCT01883297). Another ATT approach involves using chimeric antigen receptor (CAR) T-cells that have been engineered to express a CAR with an extracellular single chain variable fragment incorporating immunoglobulin heavy and light chains capable of targeting any extracellular target (not just those complexed with MHC). There are currently over 20 trials registered on ClinicaTrials.gov testing CAR-T-cell-based therapy in ovarian cancer against targets including Her2, mesothelin, folate receptor-α (FRα) and NY-ESO-1.

5.3. Other approaches

The field of immunotherapy is advancing rapidly and various other approaches are in early phase trials. Vaccine based therapy has yielded objective responses demonstrating proof-of-concept, for example using a dendritic cell whole-tumour based approach [79]. Although clinical trials for vaccines have been disappointing, various techniques for optimisation are leading to renewed enthusiasm [80]. Another approach used a tri-functional antibody, catumaxomab, which binds to epithelial cell adhesion molecule (EpCAM), CD3 (found on T-cells) and has an Fc portion that is recognised by various cells including macrophages. This allows immune cells to colocalize with tumour and cause cytotoxicity. EpCAM positive cells are found in 70–100% of malignant effusions and in a phase II study intraperitoneal (IP) administration of catumaxomab significantly improved the puncture free interval in heavily pre-treated patients [81]. It was given EMA approval for IP administration but the manufacturer withdrew this for commercial reasons in July 2017. One of the problems of 'targeted' immune therapy such as this is toxicity with systemic administration. Consequently, IP administration may be the only viable route with some therapies.

5.4. Combinations

Combination immune therapy PARP inhibitors, VEGF therapy and chemotherapy have already been mentioned. In addition, checkpoint inhibition has recently been combined with epacadostat, an inhibitor of 2,3-dioxygenase (IDO). IDO activation in tumours is associated with immune escape via T-cell dysfunction. Combining epacadostat and pembrolizumab has shown efficacy in patients with EOC although randomised trials are needed to ascertain the effect of epacadostat over and above pembolizumab monotherapy [82].

6. Other novel agents

The aforementioned systemic strategies are of most relevance because they are either already in (or close to) the clinic. There are however various other strategies being explored, some of which have already been trialled in clinical studies. One approach involves targeting folate receptor and, specifically, the α isoform (FRα). This receptor is absent from normal ovarian epithelium but expressed on the majority of EOC [83]. The receptor has been targeted by various classes of therapy including folate-drug conjugates, small molecule FRα inhibitors, monoclonal antibodies, vaccines and oncolytic viruses. The phase III trial of vintafolide (folate conjugated with a derivative of vinblastine) in combination with PLD (NCT01170650) was discontinued for futility. Further trials of folate-drug conjugates are ongoing [84]. Farletuzumab, a monoclonal antibody that causes antibody and complement- dependant cellular cytotoxicity is being investigated in combination with platinum-based chemotherapy in patients with relapsed EOC and low ca125 following promising sub-group analysis from a previous phase III trial (NCT02289950). Phase I results for ONX-0801, a FRα-targeted thymidylate synthase inhibitor that accumulates in EOC cells generated a PR in 5/11 patients at the MTD with 4/4 FRα expressing tumours showing response [85].

Aside from FRα targeting therapy, there are multiple other targeted strategies in EOC in pre-clinical and early clinical phases. Cell cycle targeting with WEE-1 inhibition has been discussed but other strategies including CHK1/2 inhibition with prexasertib (which yielded a PR in 5/13 patients in cohort 1 of a recent phase II trial [86]) are being explored. PI3k/AKT/mTOR, Her2 and molecules in the apoptotic machinery are amongst a plethora of other avenues being explored. As our understanding of the molecular basis of EOC progresses, future therapies are likely to employ biomarker or other selection criteria within trial protocols. For example, clear cell ovarian carcinoma is known to harbour mutations in the PI3K/AKT/mTOR pathway and the GOG-0268 trial of temsirolimus in addition to carboplatin/paclitaxel as first-line therapy was restricted to the clear cell population for this reason. Beyond the 'traditional' histological subtyping of EOC, analysis of TCGA data and recent advances in bioinformatics as led different groups to propose various molecular classifications of high grade serous EOC. Once such classification proposes four subtypes; mesenchymal, immunoreactive, differentiated and proliferative. Prospectively defined subgroup analysis of future trials using such novel molecular classifications may allow us to tailor therapy to maximise efficacy.

7. Conclusion

Several distinct strategies have been discussed. PARP inhibition have probably had the biggest clinical impact however mature OS data is awaited from many trials and further work is required to understand resistance and the potential role of combination therapy and sequencing of PARPi. Anti-angiogenic strategies have had a modest impact overall but research into patient selection may identify a subset who have more marked benefit. Similarly, with immunotherapy, the majority of patients do not show objective response but a subset has durable benefit. It seems, therefore that future success will depend on improved patient selection for trials, possibly through continued progress in understanding the molecular landscape of EOC. While progress has been made, there is a long way to go and the next few years should see continued incremental benefit in this difficult to treat disease.

Author details

Amit Samani[1,2]*, Charleen Chan[1] and Jonathan Krell[1,2]

*Address all correspondence to: amit.samani@nhs.net

1 Department of Medical Oncology, Hammersmith Hospital, London, United Kingdom

2 Department of Surgery and Cancer, Imperial College, London, United Kingdom

References

[1] Vasey P. "Dose dense" chemotherapy in ovarian cancer. International Journal of Gynecological Cancer. 2005;**15**:226-232. DOI: 10.1111/j.1525-1438.2005.00438.x

[2] Simon R, Norton L, et al. The Norton–Simon hypothesis: Designing more effective and less toxic chemotherapeutic regimens. Nature Clinical Practice. Oncology. 2006;**3**(8):406-407. DOI: 10.1038/ncponc0560

[3] Gianni L, Kearns CM, Giani A, Capri G, Viganó L, Lacatelli A, et al. Nonlinear pharmacokinetics and metabolism of paclitaxel and its pharmacokinetic/pharmacodynamic relationships in humans. Journal of Clinical Oncology. 1995;**13**(1):180-190. DOI: 10.1200/JCO.1995.13.1.180

[4] Marchetti P, Urien S, Cappellini GA, Ronzino G, Ficorella C. Weekly administration of paclitaxel: theoretical and clinical basis. Critical Reviews in Oncology/Hematology. 2002;**44**(suppl):S3-13

[5] Bocci G, Di Paolo A, Danesi R. The pharmacological bases of the antiangiogenic activity of paclitaxel. Angiogenesis 2013;**16**(3):481-492. DOI: 10.1007/s10456-013-9334-0

[6] Baird RD, Tan DS, Kaye SB. Weekly paclitaxel in the treatment of recurrent ovarian cance. Nature Reviews. Clinical Oncology. 2010;**7**(10):575-582. DOI: 10.1038/nrclinonc.2010.120

[7] Katsumata N, Yasuda M, Isonishi S, Takahashi F, Michimae H, Kimura E. Long-term results of dose-dense paclitaxel and carboplatin versus conventional paclitaxel and carboplatin for treatment of advanced epithelial ovarian, fallopian tube, or primary peritoneal cancer (JGOG 3016): A randomised, controlled, open-label trial. The Lancet Oncology. 2013;**14**(10):1020-1026. DOI: 10.1016/S1470-2045(13)70363-2

[8] Chan JK, Brady MF, Penson RT, Huang H, Birrer MJ, Walker JL, et al. Weekly vs. every-3-week paclitaxel and carboplatin for ovarian cancer. The New England Journal of Medicine. 2016;**374**:738-748. DOI: 10.1056/NEJMoa1505067

[9] Pignata S, Scambia G, Katsaros D, Gallo C, Pujade-Lauraine E, De Placido S, et al. Carboplatin plus paclitaxel once a week versus every 3 weeks in patients with advanced ovarian cancer (MITO-7): A randomised, multicentre, open-label, phase 3 trial. The Lancet Oncology. 2014;**15**(4):396-405. DOI: http://dx.doi.org/10.1016/S1470-2045(14)70049-X

[10] Hirai H, Iwasawa Y, Okada M, Arai T, Nishibata T, Kobayashi M, et al. Small-molecule inhibition of Wee1 kinase by MK-1775 selectively sensitizes p53-deficient tumor cells to DNA-damaging agents. Molecular Cancer Therapeutics. 2009;**8**(11):2992-3000. DOI: 10.1158/1535-7163

[11] Brasseur K, Gévry N, Asselin E. Chemoresistance and targeted therapies in ovarian and endometrial cancers. Oncotarget. 2017;**8**(3):4008-4042

[12] Deng J, Wang L, Chen H, Hao J, Ni J, Chang L, et al. Targeting epithelial-mesenchymal transition and cancer stem cells for chemoresistant ovarian cancer. Oncotarget. 2016;**7**(34):55771-55788

[13] Gaillard S, Ghamande SA, Pardo B, Lorusso D, Vergote I, Papai Z. CORAIL trial: Randomized phase III study of lurbinectedin (PM01183) versus pegylated liposomal doxorubicin (PLD) or topotecan (T) in patients with platinum-resistant ovarian cancer. Journal of Clinical Oncology 2016;**34**(15_suppl). DOI: 10.1200/JCO.2016.34.15_suppl.TPS5597

[14] Nuñez GS, Guillén MJ, Martínez-Leal JF, Avilés P, Galmarini CM. 1211/26-Lurbinectedin reverses platinum dependent IRF1 overexpression and nuclear localization, partially responsible for resistance to platinum drugs in ovarian cancer. AACR Annual Meeting. 2017

[15] Chung A, Lee J, Ferrar N. Targeting the tumour vasculature: insights from physiological angiogenesis. Nature Reviews. Cancer. 2010;**10**(7):505-514. DOI: 10.1038/nrc2868

[16] Fraser HM, Lunn SF. Angiogenesis and its control in the female reproductive system. British Medical Bulletin. 2000;**56**(3):787-797

[17] Yamamoto S, Konishi I, Mandai M, Kuroda H, Komatsu T, Nanbu K, et al. Expression of vascular endothelial growth factor (VEGF) in epithelial ovarian neoplasms. British Journal of Cancer. 1997;**76**(9):1221-1227

[18] Bandiera E, Franceschini R, Specchia C, Bignotti E, Trevisiol C, Gion M, et al. Prognostic significance of vascular endothelial growth factor serum determination in women with ovarian cancer. Obstetrics and Gynecology. 2012. DOI: 10.5402/2012/245756

[19] Herr D, Sallmann A, Bekes I, Konrad R, Holzheu I, Kreienberg R, Wulff C. VEGF induces ascites in ovarian cancer patients via increasing peritoneal permeability by down-regulation of Claudin 5. Gynecologic Oncology. 2012;**127**(1):210-216. DOI: 10.1016/j.ygyno.2012.05.002

[20] Presta LG, Chen H, O'Connor SJ, Chisholm V, Meng YG, Krummen L, Winkler M, et al. Humanization of an anti-vascular endothelial growth factor monoclonal antibody for the therapy of solid tumors and other disorders. Cancer Research. 1997;**57**(20):4593-4599

[21] Burger RA, Brady MF, Bookman MA, Fleming GF, Monk BJ, Huang H, et al. Incorporation of bevacizumab in the primary treatment of ovarian cancer. The New England Journal of Medicine. 2011;**365**(26):2473-2483. DOI: 10.1056/NEJMoa1104390

[22] Perren TJ, Swart AM, Pfisterer J, Ledermann JA, Pujade-Lauraine E, Kristensen G, et al. A phase 3 trial of bevacizumab in ovarian cancer. The New England Journal of Medicine. 2011;**365**(26):2484-2496. DOI: 10.1056/NEJMoa1103799

[23] Stark D, Nankivell M, Pujade-Lauraine E, Kristensen G, Elit L, Stockler M, et al. Standard chemotherapy with or without bevacizumab in advanced ovarian cancer: Quality-of-life outcomes from the International Collaboration on Ovarian Neoplasms (ICON7) phase 3 randomised trial. The Lancet Oncology. 2013;**14**(3):236-243. DOI: 10.1016/S1470-2045(12) 70567-3

[24] Oza AM, Cook AD, Pfisterer J, Embleton A, Ledermann JA, Pujade-Lauraine E, et al. Standard chemotherapy with or without bevacizumab for women with newly diagnosed ovarian cancer (ICON7): Overall survival results of a phase 3 randomised trial. The Lancet Oncology. 2015;**16**(8):928-936. DOI: 10.1016/S1470-2045(15)00086-8

[25] EMA. Avastin [Internet]. [Updated: 21-02-2017]. Available from: http://www.ema.europa.eu/ema/index.jsp?curl=pages/medicines/human/medicines/000582/human_med_000663.jsp&mid=WC0b01ac058001d124 [Accessed: 18-06-2017]

[26] Ledermann JA, Raja FA, Fotopoulou C, Gonzalez-Martin A, Colombo N, Sessa C. Newly diagnosed and relapsed epithelial ovarian carcinoma: ESMO Clinical Practice Guidelines for diagnosis, treatment and follow-up. Annals of Oncology. 2013;24(suppl_6):24-32. DOI: https://doi.org/10.1093/annonc/mdt333

[27] Pujade-Lauraine E, Hilpert F, Weber B, Reuss A, Poveda A, Kristensen G. Bevacizumab combined with chemotherapy for platinum-resistant recurrent ovarian cancer: The AURELIA open-label randomized phase III trial. Journal of Clinical Oncology. 2014; 32(13):1302-1308. DOI: 10.1200/JCO.2013.51.4489

[28] Stockler M, Hilpert F, Friedlander M, King MT, Wenzel L, Lee CK, et al. Patient-reported outcome results from the open-label phase III AURELIA trial evaluating bevacizumab-containing therapy for platinum-resistant ovarian cancer. Journal of Clinical Oncology. 2014;32(13):1309-1316. DOI: 10.1200/JCO.2013.51.4240

[29] Bamias A, Gibbs E, Khoon LC, Davies L, Dimopoulos M, Zagouri F, et al. Bevacizumab with or after chemotherapy for platinum-resistant recurrent ovarian cancer: exploratory analyses of the AURELIA trial. Annals of Oncology. 2017;28(8):1842-1848. DOI: https://doi.org/10.1093/annonc/mdx228

[30] Aghajanian C, Blank SV, Goff BA, Judson PL, Teneriello MG, Husain A, et al. OCEANS: A randomized, double-blind, placebo-controlled phase III trial of chemotherapy with or without bevacizumab in patients with platinum-sensitive recurrent epithelial ovarian, primary peritoneal, or fallopian tube cancer. Journal of Clinical Oncology. 2012;30(17): 2039-2045. DOI: 10.1200/JCO.2012.42.0505

[31] Coleman RL, Brady MF, Herzog TJ, Sabbatini P, Armstrong DK, Walker JL, et al. A phase III randomized controlled clinical trial of carboplatin and paclitaxel alone or in combination with bevacizumab followed by bevacizumab and secondary cytoreductive surgery in platinum-sensitive, recurrent ovarian, peritoneal primary and fallopian tube cancer (Gynecologic Oncology Group 0213). In: Society of Gynecologic Oncology's Annual Meeting; 28-03-2015; Chicago. Online: 2015

[32] Ledermann JA, Embleton AC, Raja F, Perren TJ, Jayson GC, Rustin GJS, et al. Cediranib in patients with relapsed platinum-sensitive ovarian cancer (ICON6): A randomised, double-blind, placebo-controlled phase 3 trial. Lancet. 2016;387(10023):1066-1074. DOI: 10.1016/S0140-6736(15)01167-8

[33] Ledermann JA, Embleton AC, Perren T, Jayson GC, Rustin GJS, Kaye SB, et al. Overall survival results of ICON6: A trial of chemotherapy and cediranib in relapsed ovarian cancer. In: ASCO Annual Meeting; June 2; Chicago. 2017. p. Abstract 5506

[34] Stark DP, Cook A, Brown JM, Brundage MD, Embleton AC, Kaplan RS. Quality of life with cediranib in relapsed ovarian cancer: The ICON6 phase 3 randomized clinical trial. Cancer. 2017;123(14):2752-2761. DOI: 10.1002/cncr.30657

[35] du Bois A, Floquet A, Kim JW, Rau J, del Campo JM, Friedlander M, et al. Incorporation of pazopanib in maintenance therapy of ovarian cancer. Journal of Clinical Oncology 2014;32(30):3374-3382. DOI: 10.1200/JCO.2014.55.7348

[36] du Bois A, Kristensen G, Ray-Coquard I, Reuss A, Pignata S, Colombo, N et al. Standard first-line chemotherapy with or without nintedanib for advanced ovarian cancer (AGO-OVAR 12): A randomised, double-blind, placebo-controlled phase 3 trial. The Lancel Oncology 2016;**17**(1):78-89. DOI: 10.1016/S1470-2045(15)00366-6

[37] Monk BJ, Poveda A, Vergote I, Raspagliesi F, Fujiwara K, Bae DS, et al. Final results of a phase 3 study of trebananib plus weekly paclitaxel in recurrent ovarian cancer (TRINOVA-1): Long-term survival, impact of ascites, and progression-free survival. Gynecologic Oncology. 2016;**143**(1):27-34. DOI: 10.1016/j.ygyno.2016.07.112-34

[38] Marth C, Vergote I, Scambia G, Oberaigner W, Clamp A, Berger R, et al. ENGOT-ov-6/TRINOVA-2: Randomised, double-blind, phase 3 study of pegylated liposomal doxorubicin plus trebananib or placebo in women with recurrent partially platinum-sensitive or resistant ovarian cancer. European Journal of Cancer. 2017;**70**:111-121. DOI: 10.1016/j.ejca.2016.09.004

[39] Liu JF, Barry WT, Birrer M, et al. Combination cediranib and olaparib versus olaparib alone for women with recurrent platinum-sensitive ovarian cancer: A randomised phase 2 study. The Lancet Oncology. 2014;**15**(11):1207-1214. DOI: 10.1016/S1470-2045(14)70391-2

[40] Mitamura T, Gourley C, Sood A. Prediction and failure of anti-angiogenesis. Gynecologic Oncology. 2016;**141**(1):80-85. DOI: 10.1016/j.ygyno.2015.12.033-5

[41] Satoh MS, Lindahl T. Role of poly(ADP-ribose) formation in DNA repair. Nature. 1992;**356**(6367):356-358. DOI: 10.1038/356356a0

[42] Valerie K, Povirk LF. Regulation and mechanisms of mammalian double-strand break repair. Oncogene. 2003;**22**(37):5792-5812. DOI: 10.1038/sj.onc.1206679

[43] Mehta A, Haber JE. Sources of DNA double-strand breaks and models of recombinational DNA repair. Cold Spring Harbor Perspectives in Biology. 2014;**6**(9):a016428. DOI: 10.1101/cshperspect.a016428

[44] Alsop K, Fereday S, Meldrum C, de Fazio A, Emmanuel C, George J, et al. BRCA mutation frequency and patterns of treatment response in BRCA mutation-positive women with ovarian cancer: a report from the Australian Ovarian Cancer Study Group. Journal of Clinical Oncology. 2012;**30**(21):2654-2663. DOI: 10.1200/JCO.2011.39.8545

[45] Bell D, Berchuck A, Birrer M, Chien J, Cramer D, Dao F, et al. Integrated genomic analyses of ovarian carcinoma. Nature. 2011;**474**(7353):609-615. DOI: 10.1038/nature10166

[46] Moschetta M, George A, Kaye SB, Banerjee S. BRCA somatic mutations and epigenetic BRCA modifications in serous ovarian cancer. Annals of Oncology. 2016;**27**(8):1449-1455. DOI: https://doi.org/10.1093/annonc/mdw142

[47] Konstantinopoulos PA, Ceccaldi R, Shapiro GI, D'Andrea AD. Homologous recombination deficiency: exploiting the fundamental vulnerability of ovarian cancer. Cancer Discovery 2015;**5**(11):3570-3576. DOI: 10.1200/JCO.2009.27.2997

[48] Schultz N, Lopez E, Saleh-Gohari N, Helleday T. Poly(ADP-ribose) polymerase (PARP-1) has a controlling role in homologous recombination. Nucleic Acids Research. 2003;31(17): 4959-4964. DOI: 10.1093/nar/gkg703

[49] Farmer H, McCabe N, Lord CJ, Tutt A, Johnson D, Richardson TB, et al. Targeting the DNA repair defect in BRCA mutant cells as a therapeutic strategy. Nature. 2005;434:917-921. DOI: 10.1038/nature03445

[50] Menear KA, Adcock C, Boulte R, Cockcroft X, Copsey L, Cranston A, et al. 4-[3-(4-Cyclopropanecarbonylpiperazine-1-carbonyl)-4-fluorobenzyl]-2H–phthalazin-1-one: A novel bioavailable inhibitor of poly(ADP-ribose) polymerase-1. Journal of Medical Chemistry. 2008;51(20):6581-6591. DOI: 10.1021/jm8001263

[51] Murai J, Huang SY, Das BB, Renaud A, Zhang Y, Doroshow JH, et al. Trapping of PARP1 and PARP2 by clinical PARP inhibitors. Cancer Research. 2012;72(21):5588-5599. DOI: 10.1158/0008-5472.CAN-12-2753

[52] Fong PC, Yap TA, Boss DS, Carden CP, Mergui-Roelvink M, Gourley C, et al. Poly(ADP)-ribose polymerase inhibition: frequent durable responses in BRCA carrier ovarian cancer correlating with platinum-free interval. Journal of Clinical Oncology. 2010;28(15):2512-2519. DOI: 10.1200/JCO.2009.26.9589

[53] Audeh MW, Carmichael J, Penson RT, Friedlander M, Powell B, Bell-McGuinn KM. Oral poly(ADP-ribose) polymerase inhibitor olaparib in patients with BRCA1 or BRCA2 mutations and recurrent ovarian cancer: a proof-of-concept trial. Lancet. 2010;376(9737):245-251. DOI: 10.1016/S0140-6736(10)60893-8

[54] Kaufman B, Shapira-Frommer R, Schmutzler RK, Audeh MW, Friedlander M, Balmaña J, et al. Olaparib Monotherapy in Patients With Advanced Cancer and a Germline BRCA1/2. Journal of Clinical Oncology. 2015;33(3):244-250. DOI: 10.1200/JCO.2014.56.2728

[55] Pujade-Lauraine E, Ledermann JA, Selle F, Gebski V, Penson RT, Oza AM. SOLO3: A randomized phase III trial of olaparib versuschemotherapy in platinum-sensitive relapsed ovarian cancer patients with a germline BRCA1/2mutation (gBRCAm). The Lancet Oncology. 2016;34(15_suppl):5598. DOI: 10.1016/S1470-2045(17)30469-2

[56] Ledermann J, Harter P, Gourley C, Friedlander M, Vergote I, Rustin G. Olaparib maintenance therapy in patients with platinumsensitive relapsed serous ovarian cancer: A preplanned retrospective analysis of outcomes by BRCA status in a randomised phase 2 trial. The Lancet Oncology. 2014;15(8):852-861. DOI: 10.1016/S1470-2045(14)70228-1

[57] Pujade-Lauraine E, Ledermann JA, Penson RT, Oza AM, Korach J, Juzarski T. Late Breaking Abstract. Treatment with olaparib monotherapy in the maintenance setting significantly improves progression-free survival in patients with platinum-sensitive relapsed ovarian cancer: Results from the phase III SOLO2 study. Gynecologic Oncology. 2017;145(1_suppl):219-220. DOI: https://doi.org/10.1016/j.ygyno.2017.03.505

[58] Sandhu SK, Schelman WR, Wilding G, Moreno V, Baird RD, Miranda S. The poly(ADP-ribose) polymerase inhibitor niraparib (MK4827) in BRCA mutation carriers and patients

with sporadic cancer: A phase 1 dose-escalation trial. The Lancet Oncology. 2013;**14**(9):882-892. DOI: 10.1016/S1470-2045(13)70240-7

[59] Mirza MR, Monk BJ, Herrstedt J, Oza AM, Mahner S, Redondo A. Niraparib maintenance therapy in platinum-sensitive, recurrent ovarian cancer. The New England Journal of Medicine. 2016;**375**(22):2154-2164

[60] Murai J, Huang SY, Renaud A, Zhang Y, Ji J, Takeda S. Stereospecific PARP trapping by BMN 673 and comparison with olaparib and rucaparib. Molecular Cancer Therapeutics. 2014;**13**(2):433-443. DOI: 10.1158/1535-7163.MCT-13-0803

[61] Kristeleit RS, Shapira-Frommer R, Oaknin A, Balmaña J, Ray-Coquard IL, Domchek S. Clinical activity of the poly(ADP-ribose) polymerase (PARP) inhibitor rucaparib in patients (pts) with high-grade ovarian carcinoma (HGOC) and a BRCA mutation (BRCAmut): Analysis of pooled data from Study 10 (parts 1, 2a, and 3) and ARIEL2 (parts 1 and 2). Annals of Oncology. 2016;**27**(6):8560. DOI: https://doi.org/10.1093/annonc/mdw374.03

[62] Swisher EM, Lin KK, Oza AM, Scott CL, Giordano H, Sun J. Rucaparib in relapsed, platinum-sensitive high-grade ovarian carcinoma (ARIEL2 Part 1): An international, multicentre, open-label, phase 2 trial. The Lancet Oncology. 2017;**18**(1):75-87. DOI: 10.1016/S1470-2045(16)30559-9

[63] Coleman RL, Swisher EM, Oza AM, Scott CL, Giordano H, Lin K. Refinement of pre-specified cutoff for genomic loss of heterozygosity (LOH) in ARIEL2 part 1: A phase II study of rucaparib in patients (pts) with high grade ovarian carcinoma (HGOC). Journal of Clinical Oncology. 2016;**34**(15_suppl):5540

[64] de Bono J, Ramanathan RK, Mina L, Chugh R, Glaspy J, Rafii S. Phase I, dose-escalation, two-part trial of the parp inhibitor talazoparib in patients with advanced germline BRCA1/2 mutations and selected sporadic cancers. Cancer Discovery. 2017;**7**(6):620-629. DOI: 10.1158/2159-8290

[65] Konecny GE, Kristeleit RS. PARP inhibitors for BRCA1/2-mutated and sporadic ovarian cancer: current practice and future directions. British Journal of Cancer. 2016;**115**(10):1157-1173. DOI: 10.1038/bjc.2016.311

[66] Murai J, Zhang Y, Morris J, et al. Rationale for poly(ADP-ribose)polymerase (PARP) inhibitors in combination therapy with camptothecins or temozolomide based on PARP trapping versus catalytic inhibition. The Journal of Pharmacology and Experimental Therapeutics. 2014;**349**:408-416

[67] Drean A, Lord CJ, Ashworth A. PARP inhibitor combination therapy. Critical Reviews in Oncology/Hematology. 2016;**108**:73-85. DOI: https://doi.org/10.1016/j.critrevonc.2016.10.010

[68] Norquist B, Wurz KA, Pennil CC, Garcia R, Gross J, Sakai W, et al. Secondary somatic mutations restoring BRCA1/2 predict chemotherapy resistance in hereditary ovarian carcinomas. Journal of Clinical Oncology. 2011;**29**(22):3008-3015. DOI: 10.1200/JCO.2010.34.2980

[69] Zhang L, Conejo-Garcia JR, Katsaros D, Gimotty PA, Massobrio M, Regnani G, et al. Intratumoral T cells, recurrence, and survival in epithelial ovarian cancer. The New England Journal of Medicine. 2003;**348**(3):203-213

[70] Coukos G, Tanyi J, Kandalaft LE. Opportunities in immunotherapy of ovarian cancer. Annals of Oncology. 2016 Apr;**27**(Suppl 1):i11-i15. DOI: 10.1093/annonc/mdw084

[71] Strickland KC, Howitt BE, Shukla SA, Rodig S, Ritterhouse LL, Liu JF, et al. Association and prognostic significance of BRCA1/2-mutation status with neoantigen load, number of tumor-infiltrating lymphocytes and expression of PD-1/PD-L1 in high grade serous ovarian cancer. Oncotarget. 2016;**7**(12):13587-13598. DOI: 10.18632/oncotarget.7277

[72] Huang A, Postow M, Orlowski R, Mick R, Bengsch B, Manne S, et al. T-cell invigoration to tumour burden ratio associated with anti-PD-1 response. Nature. 2017;**545**:60-65. DOI: 10.1038/nature22079

[73] Hodi FS, Mihm MC, Soffer RJ, Haluska FG, Butler M, Seiden MV, et al. Biologic activity of cytotoxic T lymphocyte-associated antigen 4 antibody blockade in previously vaccinated metastatic melanoma and ovarian carcinoma patients. Proceedings of the National Academy of Sciences. 2003;**100**(8):4712-4717

[74] Disis M, Patel M, Pant S, Hamilton E, Lockhart A, Kelly K, et al. Avelumab (MSB0010718C; anti-PD-L1) in patients wiht recurrent/refractory ovarian cancer from the JAVELIN Solid Tumour phase 1b trial: Safety and clinical activity. In: J Clin Onc. 2016

[75] Elamin YY, Rafee S, Toomey S, Hennessy BT. Immune effects of bevacizumab: Killing two birds with one stone. Cancer Microenvironment. 2015;**8**(1):15-21. DOI: 10.1007/s12307-014-0160.8

[76] Varga A, Piha-Paul S, Ott P, Mehnert J, Berton-Rigaud D, Morosky A. et al. Pembrolizumab in patients (pts) with PD-L1–positive (PD-L1+) advanced ovarian cancer: Updated analysis of KEYNOTE-028. In: ASCO Annual Meeting; 2017; Chicago

[77] Hamanishi J, Mandai M, Ikeda T, et al. Safety and antitumor activity of anti–PD-1 antibody, nivolumab, in patients with platinum-resistant ovarian cancer. Journal of Clinical Oncology. 2015;**33**(34):4015-22. DOI: 10.1200/JCO.2015.62.3397

[78] Fujita K, Ikarashi H, Takakuwa K, Kodama S, Tokunaga A, Takahashi T, et al. Prolonged disease-free period in patients with advanced epithelial ovarian cancer after adoptive transfer of tumour-infiltrating lymphocytes. Clinical Cancer Research. 1995;**1**(5):501-507

[79] Chiang CL, Kandalaft LE, Tanyi J, Hagemann AR, Motz GT, Svoronos N, et al. A dendritic cell vaccine pulsed with autologous hypochlorous acid-oxidized ovarian cancer lysate primes effective broad antitumor immunity: From bench to bedside. Clinical Cancer Research. 2013;**19**(17):4801-4815. DOI: 10.1158/1078-0432.CCR-13-1185

[80] Ojalvo LS, Nichols PE, Jelovac D, Emens LA. Emerging immunotherapies in ovarian cancer. Discovery Medicine. 2015;**20**(109):97-109

[81] Berek JS, Edwards RP, Parker LP, DeMars LR, Herzog TJ, Lentz SS, et al. Catumaxomab for the treatment of malignant ascites in patients with chemotherapy-refractory ovarian cancer: A phase II study. International Journal of Gynecological Cancer. 2014;**24**(9):1583-1589. DOI: 10.1097/IGC.0000000000000286

[82] Spira AI, Hamid O, Bauer TM, Borges VF, Wasser JS, Smith DC, et al. Efficacy/safety of epacadostat plus pembrolizumab in triple-negative breast cancer and ovarian cancer: Phase I/II ECHO-202 study. Journal of Clinical Oncology. 1103;**35**(15_suppl):2017

[83] Kalli KR, Oberg AL, Keeney GL, Christianson TJ, Low PS, Knutson KL, et al. Folate receptor alpha as a tumor target in epithelial ovarian cancer. Gynecologic Oncology. 2008;**108**(3):619-626. DOI: j.ygyno.2007.11.020

[84] Cheung A, Bax HJ, Josephs DH, Ilieva KM, Pellizzari G, et al. Targeting folate receptor alpha for cancer treatment. Oncotarget. 2016;**7**(32):52553-52574. DOI: doi.org/10.18632/oncotarget.9651

[85] Banerji U, Garces A, Michalarea V, Ruddle R, Raynaud F, Riisnaes R, et al. An investigator-initiated phase I study of ONX-0801, a first-in-class alpha folate receptor targeted, small molecule thymidylate synthase inhibitor in solid tumors. Journal of clinical oncology. 2017;**35**(15_suppl):2503

[86] Lee J-M, Karzai FH, Zimmer A, Annunziata CM, Lipkowitz S, Parker B, et al. A phase II study of the cell cycle checkpoint kinases 1 and 2 inhibitor (LY2606368; Prexasertib monomesylate monohydrate) in sporadic high-grade serous ovarian cancer (HGSOC) and germline BRCA mutation-associated ovarian cancer (gBRCAm+ OvCa). Annals of Oncology. 2016;**27**(suppl_6):8550. DOI: 10.1093/annonc/mdw374.02

2

Great Role in Gynecological Cancer Prophylaxis of a Unique Health Check-Up Institute, Ningen Dock in Japan

Atsushi Imai, Hiroyuki Kajikawa, Chinatsu Koiwai,
Satsoshi Ichigo and Hiroshi Takagi

Abstract

In Japan, there are unique facilities (namely Ningen Dock) for health check-up that provide asymptomatic participants with a health examination, including cancer screening activities, at their own expense. The most advanced examination equipment and examinations do not only provide high accuracy, but they also reduce stress on the body of the client. Usage of the medical equipment and diagnostic techniques allows us for successful detection of many diseases in their early stages of development. This early detection leads to quicker response for the disease. On the other hand, gynecological cancer screening is a relatively simple, low cost, and noninvasive method. In this chapter, we introduce a major role of Ningen Dock in gynecological malignancy prophylaxis. Ningen Dock attendances are associated with extremely low positive gynecology cancer screening incidence (0.03%). The level of knowledge and attitude toward screening may be related to multiple factors such as ethnicity, place of residence, income, and social-economic status. Not paying attention to cancer screening may be the risk factors for non-attendance to health check-up. These findings are of importance for improving the gynecological cancer screening practices of the lower screening attendance in Japan.

Keywords: health check-up, Ningen Dock, gynecological cancer, attitude toward screening, cancer screening, cervical cancer

1. Introduction

Health and medical check-ups aim to discover problems that may be harmful to the future health of the examinees, providing proposals for health promotion support solutions. Health check-ups focus on comprehensive assessments regarding the whole body even without disorders, while medical examinations include a specific disease or organ. In many countries, including Japan, a series of systemic routine health examinations and preventive medicine development in response to client needs undergo on a voluntary basis.

In Japan, there are unique facilities (namely Ningen Dock) for health check-up that provide asymptomatic participants with a health examination, including cancer screening activities, at their own expense [1]. Japan is indeed a country in the world with the most advanced medical devices. For example, about half of the CT scans and about one-third of the MRI scans are owned by medical facilities in Japan [2]. The most advanced examination equipment and examinations do not only provide high accuracy, but they also reduce stress on the body of the client. Usage of the medical equipment and diagnostic techniques allows us for successful detection of many diseases in their early stages of development. This early detection leads to quicker response for the disease.

The "OMOTENASHI" services provided by staffs, including nurses, technologists, and doctors, is supporting the popularity. With the careful client support underpinned by the Japanese culture of hospitality, the Ningen Dock in Japan is popular in neighboring countries. The number of people from another country is rapidly increasing, to visit Japan, to receive the medical services of Ningen Dock. These situations prompted us to introduce a major role of Ningen Dock in gynecological malignancy prophylaxis.

2. Gynecological examination flow

In general, there are three Ningen Dock programs, a half-day course, one-day course, and two-day course. Depending on the selection of the course, different diagnostic and procedural options are available. The cost is not covered by the social insurance. Asymptomatic women, aged from 18 until ~90 undergo medical evaluations, including a medical history, physical examination, blood sampling, urine sampling, and radiological imaging, as part of a routine health check-up and cancer screening (see **Table 1**). The popular plan for women is a gynecological cancer screening. Gynecologic examinations include uterine cytology (Papanicolaou test), transvaginal ultrasonography, and pelvic examination by a gynecologist.

Cervical and endometrial smears are performed using a speculum and/or brush. The cytology findings divided into seven groups: high-grade squamous intraepithelial lesions (HSIL), low-grade squamous intraepithelial lesions (LSIL), atypical squamous cells of undetermined significance (ASC-US), squamous cell carcinoma, atypical glandular cells (AGC), cervical adenocarcinoma, and normal. The cytological findings of endometrium are classified into four categories: suspected endometrial carcinoma, atypical endometrial cell, benign endometrial abnormality, and normal endometrium. When inadequate for classification, smears were again taken from examinees, and their smear samples are retrospectively reviewed if needed.

Abnormal cytologic and/or ultrasonographic findings introduce all examinees to the medical facilities for further managements. Even though no additional information are provided regarding their detailed examination outcomes, the present findings obtained from asymptomatic women may indicate annual gynecologic check-up and adequate follow-up programs

Basic examination (1-day course)	
Life Habits Check	Investigation of lifestyle through medical questionnaire, physical check-up, and advice on how to prevent the development of diseases and how to treat them.
Lungs	Chest X-ray to screening pulmonary disorders such as lung cancer, tuberculosis, and emphysema.
Heart	Screening for high blood pressure and cardiac disorder by electrocardiogram.
Digestive organs	Upper GI tests, abdominal ultrasonography, blood tests, and stool analysis to screen gastrointestinal diseases such as cancer, ulcer, polyp, and dysfunction of liver and pancreas by investigating esophagus, stomach, duodenum, liver, pancreas, and gallbladder.
Eyes	Screening for cataract, glaucoma, and visual change by fundus photography and intraocular pressure measurement.
Breast	X-ray and ultrasonography
Gynecology	Screening for gynecological disorders such as uterine cancer and ovarian tumors through pelvic examination, cervical cytology and ultrasonography. Tumor markers (CA125, CA72-4, CA19-1, and SCC) are optional.
Others	Screening tests for hearing, infections such as hepatitis virus and syphilis and determining blood type.
Optional	
This course is arranged for those who want to take an opportunity to refresh and receive the screening in a more relaxed manner. The courses contain optional examinations that can be added upon the request.	

Table 1. Test items of Ningen dock.

against symptom-free population, and this can cause remarkable reduction in the probability of malignant disease. The study sample is derived from the representative population of high-income and high-attitude toward health maintenance, providing most of our observations as important implications in terms of public health.

If anything abnormal is found, the participants are provided the most appropriate advice, by determining whether follow-up observations would be sufficient, or if medical treatment is required, what kind of medical treatment should be provided, and what facility would be appropriate for a particular treatment.

3. Incidence of positive gynecological cancers in examinees of Ningen Dock

Table 2 shows the cytologic and ultrasonographic findings of all subjects who visited the Ningen Dock in our institute between 2002 and 2016 [3, 4]. Of the cytology from cervix, 140 cases (0.8%)

were found as abnormal. Among them, 127 cases were classified as low-grade cervical smear abnormalities: LSIL and HSIL were seen in 105 cases, ASC-US was seen in 22. Suspected malignancy of squamous cell was detected in five cases within this study period, while case of cervical adenocarcinoma was not found. No cytological abnormality categories were clustered in any specific age group. Endometrial smear showed hyperplasia suspicious in 2.7% cases.

Uterine enlargement was the most frequently detected gynecologic finding, with a peak reaching approximately 25% in 40–49 years age group. The uterine abnormalities had a tendency to decrease in those aged over 60 years. Ovarian tumor (including solid and cystic enlargement) was detected in 5.2–8.0% of those in the age groups of 30–49 years, while those aged over 60 years had less frequency. In 91.3% participants, no gynecologic abnormality was detected.

The abnormal cytologic findings, including dysplastic changes and cervical cancer, are observed to be very low compared with other studies performed in developed countries (3.4–9%) [5–10]. Our findings based on 2011–2016 Ningen Dock records are similar to those of the former observations, and most of participants (95.6%) revealed no gynecological cytology

Age group (years)	No. (%)	Cytology					Uterine tumor and abnormalities	Ovary tumor and abnormalities	Others*
		Cervix				EM			
		LSIL	HSIL	ASC-US	SCC	Other than normal			
<19	12 (<0.1)	1 (<0.1)	0	0	0	0	0	2 (0.1)	0
20–29	794 (4.8)	9 (0.6)	0	5 (0.3)	1 (<0.1)	0	6 (0.4)	18 (1.3)	13 (0.9)
30–39	3172 (19.2)	26 (1.8)	4 (0.3)	3 (0.2)	0	1 (<0.1)	80 (5.6)	74 (5.2)	68 (4.7)
40–49	6217 (37.6)	37 (2.6)	6 (0.4)	3 (0.2)	1 (<0.1)	2 (0.1)	361 (25.2)	114 (8.0)	139 (9.7)
50–59	4615 (27.9)	22 (1.5)	4 (0.3)	9 (0.6)	2 (0.1)	35 (2.4)	164 (11.4)	42 (2.9)	95 (6.6)
60–69	1464 (8.9)	4 (0.3)	0	2 (0.1)	1 (<0.1)	0	44 (30.7)	8 (0.6)	16 (1.1)
70–79	228 (1.4)	0	0	0	0	0	5 (0.3)	1 (<0.1)	6 (0.4)
> 80	18 (<0.1)	0	0	0	0	0	0	0	0
Total	16,520 (100)	99 (0.6)	14 (<0.1)	22 (0.1)	5 (<0.1)	37 (0.2) 1433 (8.7)	660 (4.0)	259 (1.6)	337 (2.0)

Between January 2002 and December 2016, 16,520 asymptomatic women, aged 18–85, visited the Ningen Dock in Matsunami General Hospital for their gynecological health check-up. *Including vaginosis, leukoplakie, Bartholin cyst, posthysterectomy, cervical polyp, and prolaps/ptosis. LSIL, low-grade squamous intraepithelial lesion; HSIL, high-grade squamous intraepithelial lesion; ASC-US, atypical squamous cells of undetermined significance; SCC, cervical squamous cell carcinoma; AGC, atypical glandular cells; EM; endometrium. Modified from our previous reports [3, 4].

Table 2. Gynecologic findings of participants distributed by age group.

and ultrasonographic abnormalities. Gynecologic cancer is detected in 0.03%, all of which were at the early stages (so-called CIN3). The very low incident is in good agreement with the primary report in some Ningen Docks [1, 11].

HPV stands for human papilloma virus, which is a group of more than 200 viruses. Most people will get a HPV infection during their lifetime, usually from sexual activity. Most of these infections do not need treatment, but they can cause genital warts. In some, however, HPV infection causes changes in the cervix that can develop into cervical cancer. HPV can infect the cells on the surface of the cervix and damage them, causing their appearance to change and lead to abnormalities in these cells over a number of years. These abnormalities are known as cervical intraepithelial neoplasia (CIN). These changes are classified according to their severity. The mean time between the virus infection and invasive cancer takes about 15 years, and within 2–4 years of detection 15.5–25.5% of low-grade epithelial lesions that become high-grade lesions. In some cases, these more severe changes can develop into cervical cancer. The progression of mild and severe changes to cancer takes many years so these abnormalities are known as precancerous [12–14]. HPV infection is most common in people in their late teens and early 20s [15, 16]. A study in Jordan, one of the most conservative and religious country, found that 0.8% of 1176 women aged 18–70 years are classified as ASC-US and 0.2% as LSIL. In our unique system Ningen Dock in Japan, symptom-free women undergo medical check-up at their own expense. Their educational tradition and high concern on sex-transmitted infection, such as HPV, may restrict the likelihood of multiple sexual partners. This may be the most plausible explanation for extremely low incidence of dysplastic changes and cervical cancer found in our study group of women.

As uterine enlargement, uterine myoma with or without adenomyosis are found in 20–25% of reproductive-age women, indicating that they are one of the most frequent women's lower abdominal tumor [17–19]. The women with myoma do not necessarily complain of symptoms, and even large ones may go undetected by the patient, particularly if she is obese. Myoma-linked symptoms (abdominal distention, vaginal bleeding, constipation, and peritoneal irritation) depend on their location, size, and state of presentation; symptoms are present in 35–50% of patients with myomas. Ovarian tumors, cystic or solid, also seldom cause symptoms. Although the ovarian enlargement is frequently undetected by the patients, the diagnosis of these tumors is not usually difficult by ultrasonographic examination at physical check-up. Our subjects showed lower frequency of uterine enlargement and ovarian tumors.

Many previous trials demonstrated a reduction in the average overall mortality among ovarian cancer patients screened with an annual sequential, multimodal strategy that tracked biomarkers CA125 over time, where increasing serum CA125 levels prompted ultrasound [20–23]. A critical factor which could contribute to false negatives is that many aggressive ovarian cancers are believed to arise from epithelial cells on the fimbriae of the fallopian tube, which are not readily imaged. In addition, because, only a fraction of metastatic tumors may reach an imaging device-detectable size before they metastasize, annual screening with imaging diagnosis may fail to detect a large fraction of early stage ovarian cancers [24, 25]. The ability to detect ovarian carcinomas before they metastasize is critical and future efforts toward improving screening should focus on identifying unique features specific to aggressive, early stage tumors, as well as improving imaging sensitivity to allow for detection of tubal lesions. So far, multimodal screening strategy in which blood-based assay is positive, and subsequent imaging examination may prove useful in detecting early stage cases [20–22, 25].

4. Gynecological cancer screening intervals

In many countries, undergoing cancer screening is not mandatory but voluntary. Many women are advised to annual gynecological screening for more than a decade. Recently, recommendations of many developed countries include one Pap smear every 3 years after two annual negative results from the age of 18 until 69 years [26]. According to the current American Cancer Society guidelines, adequate negative prior screening and no history of CIN 2 of higher recommend that cervical smear test stops at age 65 [27]. On the other hand, annual screening continues among women of 65 years of age and older, even among those with less than a 5-year life expectancy due to poor health [28]. Likely, as clinical practice continues to change around the screening pelvic examination, consequent changes in utilization of reproductive health services among young adolescence to postmenopausal.

First care visit volume is a key step for continuous use of an extended screening interval, with women who report to first gynecologic care visit during the last year being over 10 times more likely to report current use of a 3-year screening interval than those with three or more visits. It is not possible to separate which come first of less-frequent care seeking and an extended gynecological cancers (including uterine and ovarian malignancies) screening interval. Clearly, some women are screened on 3-year intervals by default; however, others who purposefully follow an extended screening interval may have no perceived need to seek care during a given year.

The continuous screening preference of Japanese women may reflect long-held beliefs about the importance of annual cervical smear examinations and pelvic ultrasonographic examination with limited awareness of the potential harms associated with this practice. The level of knowledge and attitude toward screening are related to multiple factors such as ethnicity, place of residence, income, and social-economic status [29]. From an examiner perspective, annual gynecologic cancer screening has facilitated regular contact with examinees. In general, women are invited by their gynecologists for the examination. The cytologic screening time interval depends on the doctor's personal judgment [30]. If he feels that the test will benefit their patients, the likelihood of performing the test increases. Some systemic review found a positive correlation of educational level, financial status, and an awareness of the mortality rates associated gynecological cancer with gynecological cancer attendance [26, 31, 32]. The level of knowledge and attitude toward health check-up are related to multiple factors such as ethnicity, place of residence, income, and social-economic status [33–37].

5. Discussion

Uterine cancer, in particular cervical cancer, is preventable. More than half of the women diagnosed with cervical cancer have not attended screening in the past 3 years. A community-based screening strategy is one of the greatest success stories in cancer prevention, and widespread screening reduces the cervical cancer incidence worldwide [38–42]. The mean time between the virus infection and invasive cancer takes about 15 years, and within 2–4 years of detection 15.5–25.5% of low-grade epithelial lesions become high-grade lesions. In some cases, these more severe changes can develop into cervical cancer [5–10]. A routine screening test includes cytology smear test used for the detection of early cervical abnormalities (precancerous dysplastic changes) of the uterine cervix [5–10]. The screening is a relatively simple, low cost, and noninvasive method. Concurrent transvaginal ultrasonography for detection of ovarian and uterine tumors, the cervical and endometrial cytology smear tests attenuate the probability of developing gynecological malignant diseases.

Ningen Dock check-ups provide an occasion to realize preventive medicine. An important aim of gynecological health check-up is to provide support in improving the risk factors that accelerate the risk of outbreak of a malignant disease at an early stage, before subjective symptoms become apparent. Additionally, meticulous educational guidance is provided to match individual living patterns, education level, and ways of thinking. Ningen Dock can also conceive of time in the future when more appropriate and effective educational advice could be continuously provided according to a participant cultural background and lifestyle habits, via collaboration with health-related public services.

Qualitative evaluation of Ningen Dock Facilities consists of documentation and an inspection. These are administration of the facility, satisfaction and safety of examinees, and quality of check-up and follow-up [1]. Recently, the usefulness of Ningen Dock has greatly increased not only in the primary, but also in the secondary prevention of non-communicable diseases due to advances in diagnostic medical technology and therapeutic medicine. However, one of the problems is that relatively large numbers of Ningen Dock examinees who require a second, more detailed examination do not have the examination that has been recommended. For instance, only 61% of the Ningen Dock examinees who required total colon fiberscope as a second, detailed examination due to a positive fecal occult blood test underwent it. Similar tendencies were recognized for almost all Ningen Dock examinations [11]. The reason why Ningen Dock examinees who need second, more detailed examinations do not have them may be that most of them do not understand the importance of such examinations for the early detection of non-communicable diseases and their risk factors because we do not adequately explain the need for more detailed examinations to examinees. Therefore, better education of examinees may be urgently needed in order to further increase the usefulness of Ningen Dock.

In Japan, there are also free physical check-up programs of cancer screening, by which asymptomatic participants undergo a medical examination at public expense. Takagi et al. [43] reported similar data using records of the public expense-covered free examination, and suggested that active gynecologic check-up and adequate follow-up programs even against symptom-free population can reduce in the probability of malignant disease development. Their findings from representative population of high-attitude toward screening, but non-high income, may give new insight into the terms of public health.

The present data are from subject to the limitations of any analysis of self-covered health check-up survey data from participants of Ningen Dock in Japan. Although data are weighted to reflect the Japanese population, the extent to which results are generalizable is no known. Future studies, extended to non-Asian, should attempt to oversample racial minorities and include a detailed assessment of gynecologic cancer screening history and follow-up treatment.

Women attitudes and beliefs related to screening frequency may differ if they reflected truly informed preference and may be related to less screening. The present chapter introduced the extremely low positive gynecology cancer screening incidence in Ningen Dock participants, providing the active strategy in the gynecological cancer screening practices of the lower screening attendance in Japan. However, strategies may be needed to encourage examiners to adopt recommended screening intervals and to educate women about the reasoning behind less-than-annual testing, including explicit discussions about the meaningless and potential harms associated with excess screening.

Disclosure statement

The authors declare no conflict of interest.

Author's contribution

AI designed the study and drafted the manuscript. AI managed all data and performed the analyses. All authors participated in the gynecological examinations at Ningen Dock and commented on various drafts and approved the final version of the manuscript.

Author details

Atsushi Imai*, Hiroyuki Kajikawa, Chinatsu Koiwai, Satsoshi Ichigo and Hiroshi Takagi

*Address all correspondence to: aimai@matsunami-hsp.or.jp

Department of Obstetrics and Gynecology, Mastunami General Hospital, Gifu, Japan

References

[1] Hinohara S. Automated multiphasic health testing and services and Ningen Dock in Japan. Ningen Dock International. 2015;**2**:61-64

[2] OECD Health Statistics [Internet]. 2016. Available from: http://www.oecd.org/els/health-systems/health-data.htm. [Accessed: June 6, 2017]

[3] Imai A, Matsunami K, Takagi H, Ichigo S. Trend of incidence in positive cervical smears from 2002-2010 in Ningen Dock, a special Japanese health check-up system. Ningen Dock. 2012;**26**:923-926

[4] Kiowai C, Ichigo S, Takagi H, Kajikawa H, Imai A. Lower incidence of positive gynecological cancers in examinees of a unique health check-up institute, Ningen Dock in Japan, 2011-2016. Open Journal of Obstetrics and Gynecology. 2017;**7**:545-557. DOI: 10.4236/ojog.2017.75057

[5] Anttila A, Ronco G, Clifford G, Bray F, Hakama M, Arbyn M, et al. Cervical cancer screening programmes and policies in 18 European countries. British Journal of Cancer. 2004;**91**:935-941. DOI: 10.1038/sj.bjc.6602069

[6] Bray F, Loos A, McCarron P, Weiderpass E, Arbyn M, Møller H, et al. Trends in cervical squamous cell carcinoma incidence in 13 European countries: Changing risk and the effects of screening. Cancer Epidemiology, Biomarkers and Prevention. 2005;**14**:677-686. DOI: 10.1158/1055-9965.EPI-04-0569

[7] Greenlee R, Hill-Harmon M, Murray T, Thun M. Cancer statistics, 2001. CA: A Cancer Journal for Clinicians. 2001;**51**:15-136. DOI: 10.3322/canjclin.51.1.15

[8] Hakama M, Coleman M, Alexe D, Auvinen A. Cancer screening: Evidence and practice in Europe 2008. European Journal of Cancer. 2008;**44**:1404-1413. DOI: 10.1016/j.ejca.2008.02.013

[9] Johannesson G, Geirsson G, Day N, Tulinius H. Screening for cancer of the uterine cervix in Iceland 1965-1978. Acta Obstetricia et Gynecologica Scandinavica. 1982;**61**:199-203. DOI: 10.3109/00016348209156556

[10] Mount S, Papillo J. A study of 10,296 pediatric and adolescent Papanicolaou smear diagnoses in northern New England. Pediatrics. 1999;**103**:539-545. DOI: 10.1542/peds.103.3.539

[11] Hirohara S. The annual report of totaling of questionnaires to accredited Ningen Dock facilities nationwide in Japan. Ningen Dock. 2009;**23**:199-207

[12] Muñoz N, Bosch F, de Sanjosé S, Herrero R, Castellsagué X, Shah K, et al. Epidemiologic classification of human papillomavirus types associated with cervical cancer. New England Journal of Medicine. 2003;**348**:518-527. DOI:10.1056/NEJMoa021641

[13] Rocha-Zavaleta L, Yescas G, Cru zR, Cruz-Talonia F. Human papillomavirus infection and cervical ectopy. International Journal of Gynaecology and Obstetrics. 2004;**85**:259-266. DOI: 10.1016/j.ijgo.2003.10.002

[14] Tachezy R, Saláková M, Hamsíková E, Kanka J, Havránková A, Vonka V. Prospective study on cervical neoplasia: Presence of HPV DNA in cytological smears precedes the development of cervical neoplastic lesions. Sex Transmited Infection. 2003;**79**:191-196. DOI: 10.1136/sti.79.3.191

[15] Baseman J, Koutsky L. The epidemiology of human papillomavirus infections. Journal of Clinical Virology. 2005;**32**(Suppl 1):S16-S24. DOI: 10.1016/j.jcv.2004.12.008

[16] Clavel C, Masure M, Bory J, Putaud I, Mangeonjean C, Lorenzato M. Human papillomavirus testing in primary screening for the detection of high-grade cervical lesions: A study of 7932 women. British Jounal of Cancer. 2001;**84**:1616-1623. DOI: 10.1054/bjoc.2001.1845

[17] Levy B. Modern management of uterine fibroids. Acta Obstetricia et Gynecologica Scandinavica. 2008;**87**:812-823. DOI: 10.1080/00016340802146912

[18] Parker W. Uterine myomas: Management. Fertility and Sterility. 2007;**88**:255-271. DOI: 10.1016/j.fertnstert.2007.06.044

[19] Sankaran S, Manyonda I. Medical management of fibroids. Best Practice & Research. Clinical Obstetrics & Gynaecology. 2008;**22**:655-676. DOI: 10.1016/j.bpobgyn.2008.03.001

[20] Mathieu K, Bedi D, Thrower S, Qayyum A, Bast RJ. Screening for ovarian cancer: Imaging challenges and opportunities for improvement. Ultrasound in Obstetrics and Gynecology. 2017. DOI: 10.1002/uog.17557 [Epub ahead of print]

[21] Lambert P, Galloway K, Altman A, Nachtigal M, Turner D. Ovarian cancer in Manitoba: Trends in incidence and survival, 1992-2011. Current Oncology. 2017;**24**:e78-e84. DOI: 10.3747/co.24.3312

[22] Bakour S, Emovon E, Nevin J, Ewies A. Is routine adnexal scanning for postmenopausal bleeding of value? Observational study of 2101 women. Journal of Obstetrics and Gynaecology. 2017;**37**:779-782. DOI: 10.1080/01443615.2017.1306031

[23] Yuan Q, Song J, Yang W, Wang H, Huo Q, Yang J, et al. The effect of CA125 on metastasis of ovarian cancer: Old marker new function. Oncotarget. 2017;**8**:50015-50022. DOI: 10.18632/oncotarget.18388

[24] Andrews L, Mutch D. Hereditary ovarian cancer and risk reduction. Best Practice & Research. Clinical Obstetrics & Gynaecology. 2017;**41**:31-48. DOI: 10.18632/oncotarget.18388

[25] Eddie S, Quartuccio S, Zhu J, Shepherd J, Kothari R, Kim J, et al. Three-dimensional modeling of the human fallopian tube fimbriae. Gynecologic Oncology. 2015;**136**:348-354. DOI: 10.1016/j.ygyno.2014.12.015

[26] Richard A, Rohrmann S, Schmid S, Tirri B, Huang D, Güth U, et al. Lifestyle and health-related predictors of cervical cancer screening attendance in a Swiss population-based study. Cancer Epidemiology. 2015;**39**:870-876. DOI: 10.1016/j.canep.2015.09.009

[27] Smith R, Manassaram-Baptiste D, Brooks D, Doroshenk M, Fedewa S, Saslow D, et al. Cancer screening in the United States, 2015: A review of current American cancer society guidelines and current issues in cancer screening. CA: A Cancer Journal for Clinicians. 2015;**65**:30-54. DOI: 10.3322/caac.21261

[28] Royce T, Hendrix L, Stokes W, Allen I, Chen R. Cancer screening rates in individuals with different life expectancies. JAMA Internal Medicine. 2014;**174**:1558-1565. DOI: 10.1001/jamainternmed.2014.3895

[29] Kuppermann M, Sawaya G. Shared decision-making: easy to evoke, challenging to implement. JAMA Internal Medicine. 2015;**175**:167-168. DOI: 10.1001/jamainternmed.2014.4606

[30] O'Connor M, Murphy J, Martin C, O'Leary J, Sharp L. (CERVIVA) ICSC. Motivators for women to attend cervical screening: The influential role of GPs. Family Practice. 2014;**31**:475-482. DOI: 10.1093/fampra/cmu029

[31] Limmer K, LoBiondo-Wood G, Dains J. Predictors of cervical cancer screening adherence in the United States: A systematic review. Journal of the Advanced Practitioner in Oncology. 2014;**5**:31-41

[32] Kamberi F, Theodhosi G, Ndreu V, Sinaj E, Stramarko Y, Kamberi L. Nurses, healthy women and preventive gynecological examinations—Vlora City scenario, Albania. Asian Pacific Journal of Cancer Prevention. 2016;**17**:311-314

[33] Dietrich A, Tobin J, Cassells A, Robinson C, Greene M, Sox C, et al. Telephone care management to improve cancer screening among low-income women: A randomized, controlled trial. Annals of Internal Medicine. 2006;**144**:563-571

[34] Lawson H, Henson R, Bobo J, Kaeser M. Implementing recommendations for the early detection of breast and cervical cancer among low-income women. MMWR Recommendationa and Reports. 2000;**49**(RR-2):37-55

[35] Ng E, Wilkins R, Fung M, Berthelot J. Cervical cancer mortality by neighbourhood income in urban Canada from 1971 to 1996. Canadian Association Medical Journal. 2004;**170**:1545-1549

[36] Schoenberg N, Hopenhayn C, Christian A, Knight E, Rubio A. An in-depth and updated perspective on determinants of cervical cancer screening among central Appalachian women. Women & Health. 2005;**42**:89-105

[37] Yabroff K, Lawrence W, King J, Mangan P, Washington K, Yi B, et al. Geographic disparities in cervical cancer mortality: What are the roles of risk factor prevalence, screening, and use of recommended treatment? The Journal of Rural Health. 2005;**21**:149-157

[38] Mitchell S, Pedersen H, Sekikubo M, Biryabarema C, Byamugisha J, Mwesigwa D, et al. Strategies for community education prior to clinical trial recruitment for a cervical cancer screening intervention in Uganda. Frontiers in Oncology. 2016;**6**:90. DOI: 10.3389/fonc.2016.00090

[39] Teixeira L. From gynaecology offices to screening campaigns: A brief history of cervical cancer prevention in Brazil. História, Ciências, Saúde - Manguinhos. 2015;**22**:221-239. DOI: 10.1590/S0104-59702015000100013

[40] Vinekar K, Vahratian A, Hall K, West B, Caldwell A, Bell J, et al. Cervical cancer screening, pelvic examinations, and contraceptive use among adolescent and young adult females. The Journal of Adolescent Health. 2015;**57**:169-173. DOI: 10.1016/j.jadohealth.2015.04.001

[41] Emanuel E, Wendler D, Killen J, Grady C. What makes clinical research in developing countries ethical? The benchmarks of ethical research. Jounal of Infectious Diseases. 2004;**189**:930-937. DOI: 10.1086/381709

[42] Dal-Ré R, Ndebele P, Higgs E, Sewankambo N, Wendler D. Protections for clinical trials in low and middle income countries need strengthening not weakening. British Medical Journal. 2014;**349**:g4254. DOI: 10.1136/bmj.g4254

[43] Takagi H, Ichigo S, Matsunami K, Imai A. Evaluation of a public expense-covered gynecologic screening program in Japan 2005-2009. Open Journal of Obstetrics and Gynecology. 2011;**1**:21-24. DOI: 10.4236/ojog.2011.12005

3

Ovarian Cancer Genetics: Subtypes and Risk Factors

Jeff Hirst, Jennifer Crow and Andrew Godwin

Abstract

The genetics of ovarian cancer are a complex, ever evolving concept that presents hurdles in classification, diagnosis, and treatment in the clinic. Instead of common driver mutations, genomic instability is one of the hallmarks of ovarian cancer. While ovarian cancer is stratified into different clinical subtypes, there still exists extensive genetic and progressive diversity within each subtype. In high-grade serous ovarian cancer, the most common subtype, *TP53* is mutated in over 90% of all patients while the next most common mutation is less than 20%. However, next-generation sequencing and biological statistics have shown that mutations within DNA repair pathways, including *BRCA1* and *BRCA2*, are common in about 50% of all high-grade serous patients leading to the development of a breakthrough therapy of poly ADP ribose polymerase (PARP) inhibitors. This is just one example of how a better understanding of the complex genetic background of ovarian cancer can improve clinical treatment. A thorough review of ovarian cancer genetics and the effect it has on disease development, diagnosis, progression, and treatment will enhance the understanding of how to better research and treat ovarian cancer.

Keywords: genetics, subtypes, pathogenesis, *BRCA1*, *BRCA2*, *TP53*, risk factors

1. Introduction

Ovarian cancer is a generic term used to classify cancers involving the ovaries though they can arise from many different cell types within the Müllerian compartment. Ovarian cancer presents as a distinct subset of cancers with a wide variety of genomic variation (*e.g.*, somatic *TP53* mutations, germline *BRCA1/2* mutations, copy number gains in *BRAF*, *CCNE1*, *TERC*, *TERT*, and copy number loss of *RB1* and/or *PTEN*) as demonstrated through a Pan-Cancer analysis using The Cancer Genome Atlas (TGCA) database (**Figure 1**). The pathogenesis and the debate of cellular origins of ovarian cancer will be discussed in Section 4.

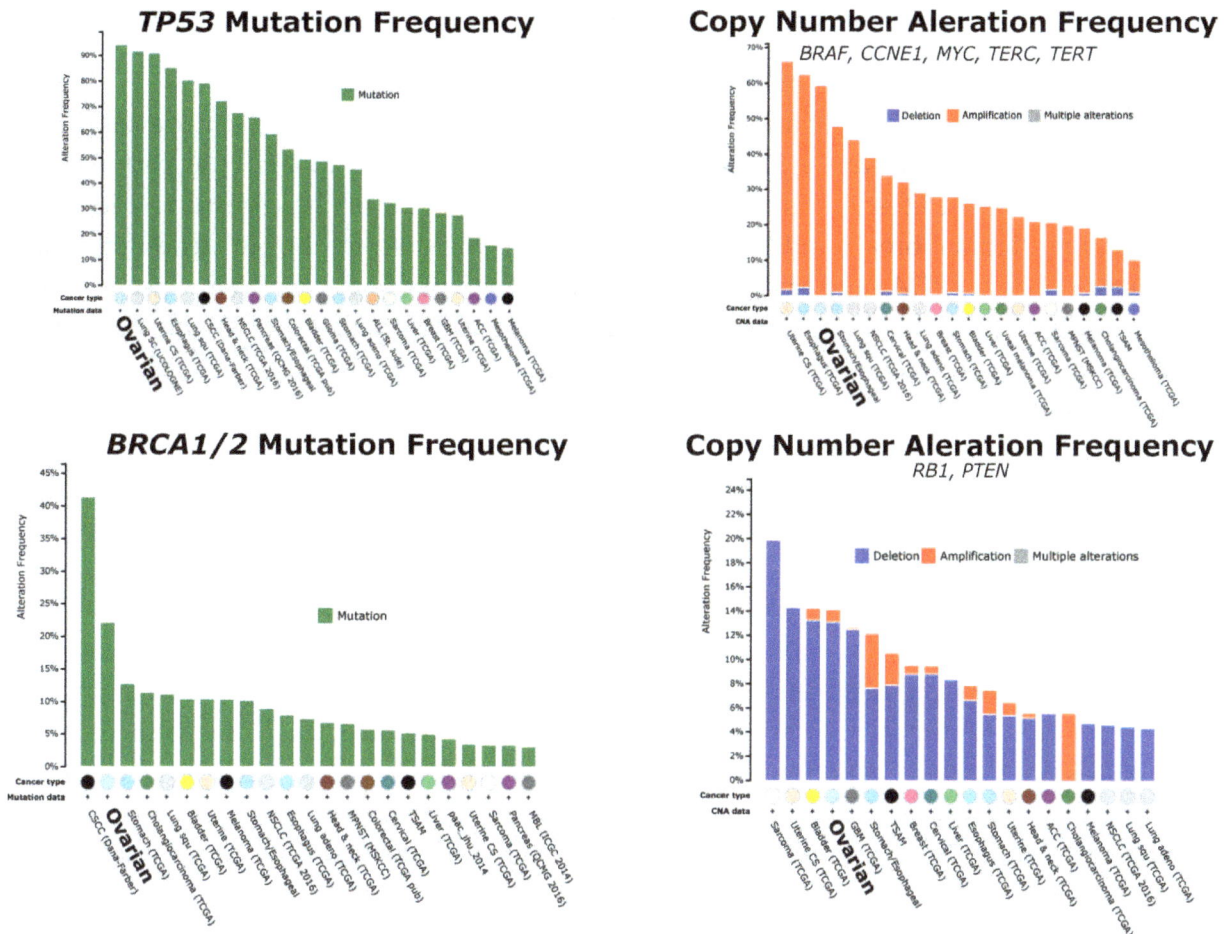

Figure 1. Common genetic alterations in ovarian cancer represented across pan-Cancer analysis from the TCGA. Bar graphs depict % of cases with mutations (green), amplification (red), and/or deletion of commonly dysregulated genes across a panel of cancers in the TCGA.

Ovarian cancer is a pathological and genetically diverse disease that presents many hurdles towards clinical detection and treatment. These clinical barriers have prevented significant improvement in patient survival for the past three decades. The heterogeneity of ovarian cancer is one of the driving factors limiting clinical progress. In this chapter, we will discuss the diversity of ovarian cancers and how these genetic factors effect clinical detection, progression, and treatment. A better understanding of the genetic differences in ovarian cancer will open up new areas for research and treatment.

Ovarian cancer can be classified into subclasses based on pathological and genetic observations. Each subclass has distinct genetic alterations, disease pathogenesis, tumor progression, and survival outcomes in response to therapy. Not only does each subclass behave differently, heterogeneity within specific subclasses presents challenges in regards to treatment options, drug resistance, and overall clinical response. Genetic diversity has greatly limited the development of targeted therapies, which have been successful in other cancers, such as *HER2* amplified breast cancers (trastuzumab, Herceptin®), *BCR-ABL* fusion in chronic myelogenous leukemia (CML) or *KIT* mutant gastrointestinal stromal tumor (imatinib mesylate, Gleevec®), and *BRAF* V600E mutant melanoma, vemurafenib (Zelboraf®). However, understanding genetic vulnerabilities such as deficiencies in homologous DNA repair prompted the development of poly

ADP ribose polymerase (PARP) inhibitors, a breakthrough in the treatment of specific ovarian cancer patients.

Finally, we will discuss genetic and lifestyle factors that can contribute to the development or progression of ovarian cancer. Since ovarian cancer is difficult to detect at early stages, knowing genetic and lifestyle risk factors for the development of the disease is critical. In fact, studying familial breast and ovarian cancer led to the discovery of inherited mutation in either *BRCA1* or *BRCA2* and improved detection of patients at risk for both cancers. While germline *BRCA1/2* mutations are two of the highest risk factors for developing ovarian, other genetic and lifestyle factors have been shown to influence the risk of disease development. A more thorough understanding of the risks of ovarian cancer is needed to stratify the chances of developing ovarian cancer for each patient.

2. Classification of ovarian cancer

Ovarian cancers of epithelial cell origin account for more than 85% of all ovarian tumors when compared to tumors that arise from germ, epidermoid, stromal, and border cells [1]. Since EOCs are the most common and deadly form of ovarian cancer, we will refer to EOC as ovarian cancer for the remainder of this chapter and primarily discuss ovarian cancers of epithelial origin [2, 3]. Typically, EOC is classified into five different histological subtypes: high-grade serous (HGS), low-grade serous (LGS), endometrioid, clear cell and mucinous [3, 4] (**Table 1**). Low-grade and high-grade disease can typically be distinguished based on the extent of nuclear atypia and mitosis [5]. Low-grade tumors are slower growing, more genetically stable and do not respond to chemotherapy as well as the faster growing, gnomically instable high-grade tumors [6–8]. High-grade serous carcinomas are the most common ovarian cancer subtype (more than 70%) followed by endometrioid, clear cell and low-grade serous [9]. Mixed ovarian cancers that represent more than one subtype are more rare, accounting for less than 1% of all ovarian cancers [10, 11]. Globally, each subtype follows a similar distribution of incidence outside of Asia, where clear cell and endometrioid tumors are more frequent compared to other locations [12]. Each subtype behaves as a discrete disease with differences in presentation, progression, mutation profile, association with hereditary cancer syndromes, and response to chemotherapy (**Table 1**) [13]. The 10-year survival for each subtype can be influenced by each of these factors and ranges from mucinous (87%), endometrioid (59.7%), clear cell (58.7%), to serous (24.4%) [14, 15].

Each subtype has distinct histological protein expression patterns, mutations and even epigenetic signatures. Further classification based on molecular profiles may provide insights into improving therapy selection [16, 17]. Recent studies have helped to further stratify the genomic differences between each subtype where 12 different loci contribute to the susceptibility of serous (3q28, 4q32.3, 8q21.11, 10q24.33, 18q11.2, 22q12.1, 2q13, 8q24.1 and 12q24.31), mucinous (3q22.3 and 9q31.1) and endometrioid (5q12.3) subtypes of ovarian cancer [18]. Molecular classification has been shown to stratify low-grade diseases into separate clusters, whereas high-grade diseases have less genetic separation [19–21], indicating early pathogenesis of the disease might be the best time to molecularly phenotype or develop targeted therapies.

Sub Type	Mutations	Clinical Prognosis	Frequency
High-grade serous	*TP53, BRCA1, BRCA2, CDK12*	Often diagnosed at late stage and chromosomally unstable.	~65%
Low-grade serous	*BRAF, KRAS, NRAS, ERBB2*	Often diagnosed in younger patients, less aggressive, gnomically stable.	~5%
Endometrioid	*PTEN, CTNNB1, PPP2R1α,* MMR deficient	Favorable prognosis and response to chemotherapy.	~20%
Clear cell carcinoma	*PIK3CA, KRAS, PTEN, ARID1A*	Low response to chemotherapy and intermediate prognosis.	~5%
Mucinous	*KRAS, HER-2* amplification	Low response to chemotherapy.	~5%

Table 1. Subtypes of ovarian cancer.

Within each subclass ovarian cancers are diagnosed and staged after primary cytoreductive surgery which attempts to remove any visible mass within the peritoneal cavity. The International Federation of Gynecology and Obstetrics (FIGO) have established guidelines for the staging of ovarian cancer. These guidelines are established based on disease localization from ovaries only (Stage I), pelvic extension (Stage II), peritoneum spread (Stage III), to distant metastases (Stage IV). While the 5-year relative survival for localized disease is over 90%, the majority of patients are diagnosed with regional (15%) or distant (60%) disease where the 5-year survival is 73% and 28.9% respectively [22]. While molecular characterization of each stage is still progressing, some data suggest there is a stepwise progressing in gene expression that could be exploited for enhanced staging [23].

In the next sections of this chapter we will discuss each subtype of ovarian cancer. We will focus primarily of specific genomic alterations, clinical pathogenesis, and responses to therapy.

2.1. High-grade serous tumors

High-grade serous tumors account for both the majority of ovarian cancer diagnoses and deaths [5, 9]. HGS tumors show a broad range of histological phenotypes with papillary, micropapillary, glandular, cribriform and trabecular structures involving columnar cells with pink cytoplasm [24, 25]. HGS is a separate disease from its LGS counterpart (and not different grades of the same neoplasm) and is identified by high mitotic index and high-grade nuclear features [5, 26] (**Figure 2**). HGS disease can be identified from other malignancies such as uterine cancer and endometrioid cancer through positive staining in WT-1, p53, and p16 [27–31]. The majority of HGS tumors are diagnosed at late stages when a complete resection of the tumor is difficult. In fact, less than 5% of HGS cancers are diagnosed at a Stage 1 (when the tumor is confined to the ovaries). Finally, while extremely rare, there is some evidence to support the progression of LGS or borderline tumors into high-grade disease. These cases have been identified through concurrent mutations in *KRAS* and *TP53* in both a borderline lesion and HGS carcinoma [32]. This progression could be due to a secondary mutation of *TP53* in borderline or low-grade tumors [33].

HGS tumors are associated with genomic instability [2, 34] since almost all (>95%) high-grade serous cancers have somatic *TP53* mutations and over half have homologous DNA repair

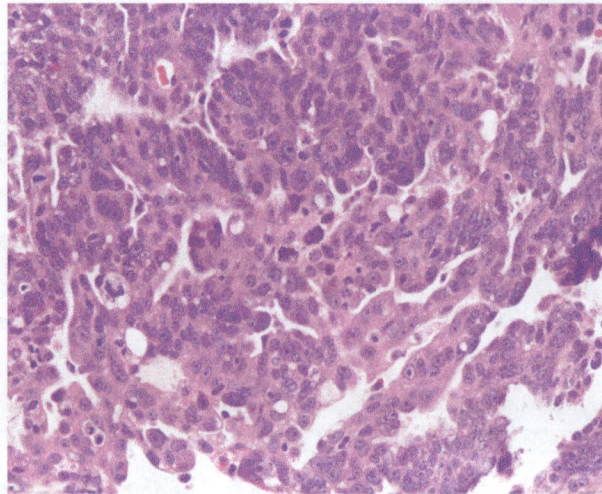

Figure 2. Representative H&E staining of high-grade serous ovarian carcinoma.

pathway deficiencies mainly represented by defects in BRCA1, BRCA2, or related proteins [35–38]. Many of these genomic alterations are similar to basal-like breast cancer, opening the opportunity for comparative studies [39]. In fact, when compared to other cancers HGS ovarian cancer had the most genomic instability when comparing copy number alterations to mutation rates [40]. Other genetic alterations that have been identified in HGS disease include cyclin E1 (*CCNE1*) amplifications. *CCNE1* amplification in HGS disease is associated with poor prognosis and platinum resistance [41]. Likewise, HGS genomic instability leads to inactivation of tumor suppressor genes through gene breakage [42]. Loss of expression of *PTEN* in tumor specific cells is predictive of poor patient survival in ovarian cancer [43].

To provide an example of this, we utilized data available through TCGA to demonstrate genetic aberrations within 34 common cell cycle control genes from 316 HGS ovarian cases with complete mutation, copy number alteration, and mRNA data [44] (**Figure 3**). While some alterations were fairly consistent across patient samples (such as up-regulation or amplification of *MYC* in ~30% of cases, down-regulation of *RBL2* in ~25% of cases, and up-regulation or amplification of *CCNE1* in ~20% of cases) the remaining 31 queried genes had between 3 and 29% alteration rates of which there was little discernable pattern. As a comparison, *TP53* is shown to be altered in most of the cases.

Examples such as this demonstrate just how difficult high-grade EOC is to treat with single molecularly-targeted therapies [45, 46]. However, one of the major breakthroughs for the treatment of ovarian cancer has been the development and FDA approval of PARP inhibitors, olaparib (Lynparza), rucaparib (Rubraca), and niraparib (Zejula). Specifically, in BRCA deficient or other homologous repair deficient cells, PARP inhibitors induce the error prone DNA repair pathway non-homologous end joining [47]. Therefore, PARP inhibitors were investigated for efficacy in ovarian cancer due to the high number of patients with BRCA and/or homologous recombination (HR) deficient tumors [48]. Rucaparib, an oral PARP-1, –2 and –3 inhibitor, has been approved for treatment in patients with *BRCA* mutations (somatic or germline) who have received at least two prior chemotherapy treatments [49, 50]. Another PARP inhibitor, niraparib, was approved in early 2017 for the maintenance treatment of adult patients with recurrent epithelial ovarian, fallopian tube, or primary peritoneal cancer, regardless of the *BRCA* mutation status. However, in the Phase III trial of niraparib, the progression

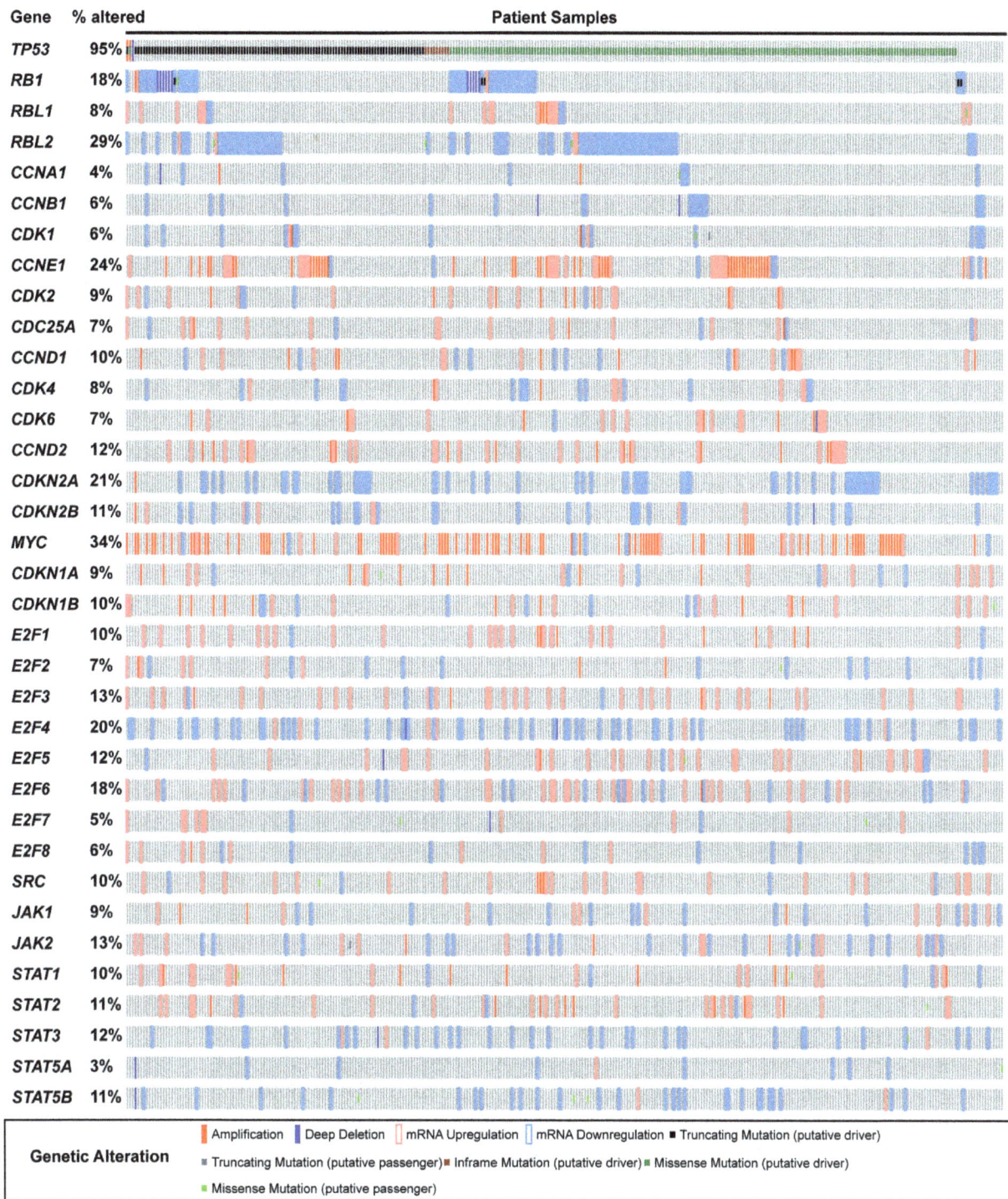

Figure 3. Genetic Dysregulation in high grade serous ovarian cancer. Data from the TCGA showing mutation, copy number alteration, and mRNA dysregulation of 34 cell cycle control genes and *TP53* alteration status (as a comparison) within 316 cases of high grade serous ovarian cancer demonstrates the overall heterogeneity of the disease.

free survival (PFS) was superior only for germline *BRCA* mutant patients when compared to standard of care (22 months vs. 9 months) versus *BRCA* competent patients compared to standard of care (9.3 months vs. 3.9 months) [51], indicating better activity in the BRCA deficient tumors. To address this limitation, our laboratory has shown that alisertib (MLN8237) can inhibit DNA double strand break repair as well as BRCA expression which sensitizes resistant cells to PARP inhibitors [52]. Using therapies to mimic different genetic phenotypes such as BRCAness has promising clinical application for ovarian cancer in trying to identify target therapies in a genetically diverse disease. Both of these therapies show that and understanding of the dynamic genes expressed in ovarian cancer can be used to mimic more sensitive disease (synthetic lethality) and improve therapy efficacy in the laboratory.

To add to this hurdle, while HGS tumors are initially responsive to platinum-chemotherapy, most patients' tumors recur which are resistant to standard chemotherapy, thus limiting treatment options for these women. The deficiencies in DNA repair pathways associate with widespread copy number alterations and make HGS cancer initially sensitive to platinum-based chemotherapy (and PARP inhibitors) but develop therapy resistance. Specifically the genomic instability can drive changes that reverse the initial sensitivity to PARP inhibitors through reversion of BRCA1/2 mutants to wild-type function [42, 53]. Similar to PARP inhibitors, patients with *BRCA* mutations are initially more sensitive to chemotherapy; however, reversion of the *BRCA1/2* mutations promotes cisplatin resistance [53, 54]. Further, specific expression of many different genes such as *ABC1* [55–59], *ABC2* [60, 61], and *GSH1* [62, 63] correlate to disease progression and drug resistance. The expression of mesenchymal genes such as *SNAIL*, *SLUG*, and *TWIST* through the epithelial to mesenchymal transitions (EMT) promotes chemotherapy resistance [64, 65]. EMT is a dynamic cellular process that can be transferred from on cell to the next through many cellular pathways including extracellular vesicles [66, 67]. Since EMT is a dynamic process, therapies that reverse the process and promote the expression of epithelial genes are an intriguing area for drug development to reverse cell growth into more sensitive phenotypes [68]. The relative success of PARP inhibitors and lack of clinical efficacy of more specific targeted therapies shows the value of identifying and exploiting the underlining molecular vulnerabilities of ovarian cancer.

2.2. Low-grade serous and borderline tumors

Low-grade serous (LGS) account for approximately 10% serous tumors. LGS tumors are more common in younger patients with an average age at diagnosis of 55.5 years compared to 62.6 years for their high-grade counterpart. LGS ovarian cancer is more commonly diagnosed at early stages, with bilateral involvement, and without invasive potential [69]. Patients with non-invasive tumors have a significantly higher 7-year survival (95.3%) compared to those with invasive tumors (66%) [70, 71]. LGS tumors appear with extensive papillary features and psammoma bodies, uniform round to oval nuclei, evenly distrusted chromosomes, and ~10 mitoses/HPF (**Figure 4**).

When compared to high-grade disease, LGS tumors are typically slower growing and have more frequent mutations in *KRAS, BRAF,* and *ERBB2,* and tend to lack *TP53* mutations [72–74]. Mutations in *KRAS, BRAF,* and *ERBB2* in LGS tumors are mutually exclusive. However, each gene mutation are signatures of activated mitogen-activated protein kinase (MAPK) pathways. MAPK activation is higher in LGS compared to HSG and correlates with paclitaxel sensitivity and an improved 5-year survival [75]. Along with having functional p53, LGS tumors have a more stable genome with less rearrangements, mutations, and tumor heterogeneity [76]. However, due to more competent DNA repair pathways, LGS tumors do not respond

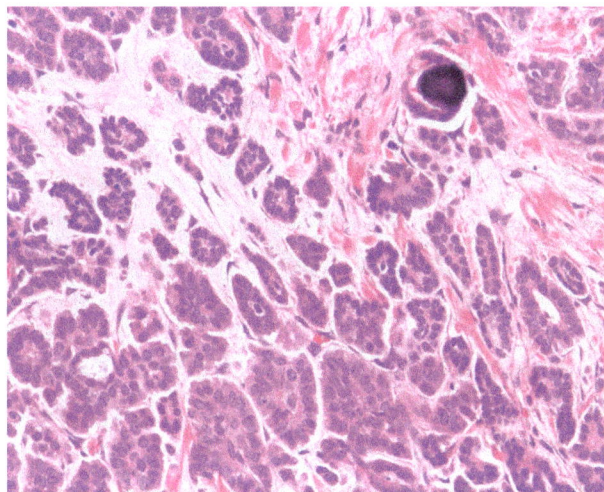

Figure 4. Representative H&E staining of low-grade serous ovarian carcinoma.

to front-line chemotherapy as well as HGS tumors [77]. Consequently, a patient with optimal debulking surgery with minimal residual tumor is the best predictor of survival [78]. The involvement of MAPK regulation of cell cycle is thought to be strongly associated with LGS chemoresistance [75], but in turn provides a potential subpopulation for targeted therapeutic development [79]. Selumetinib, a MEK1/2 inhibitor, showed some activity in recurrent LSG, leading to further investigation of MAPK pathway inhibitors for the treatment of LSG [80].

LGS tumors are thought to be borderline tumors formed step-wise from the ovarian surface [73]. Borderline tumors are epithelial tumors that appear to represent and intermediates step between benign cystadenomas and adenocarcinomas with histological features such as cellular atypia without stromal invasion. Progression of LGS tumors from borderline tumors is also thought be from recurrence of undetected borderline tumors [81–83]. While borderline tumors can be diagnosed as either serous or endometrioid the majority of such cases are diagnosed as serous tumors [26]. Borderline tumors account for ~15% of all ovarian cancer diagnoses with a large percent of cases diagnoses at early stage (~75%) and a high rate of overall survival [84]. Diagnosis at an early age (mean age of ~45 years) and minimal invasive disease are primary factors for the favorable survival [26]. While rare, invasive borderline tumors (Stages II-IV) account for the majority of deaths in borderline tumor patients [85]. Borderline tumors have a similar activation of MAPK compared to LGS tumors [75], but a higher frequency in *BRAF* mutations [86]. *BRAF* mutations are more common in early stage tumors as well as in late stage tumors that do not recur in the patient [87]. However, it is possible many LGS progress independent of borderline tumors and the pathogenesis of LGS requires further elucidation [88].

2.3. Endometrioid tumors

Endometrioid tumors account for about 10–20% of all ovarian cancers. Their morphology is described as having a smooth outer surface with solid, cystic areas inside while the pathological phenotype involves high amounts of proliferative cells that resemble squamous or endometrioid differentiations with secretory cell features. Tumors contain cystic spaces lined by gastrointestinal-type mucinous epithelium with stratification and may form filiform papillae with at least minimal stromal support. Histologic review find that endometrioid tumors possess nuclei that are slightly larger than cystadenomas; mitotic activity is present; goblet cells and sometimes Paneth cells (most commonly found in the small intestine) are present, but stromal invasion is absent [89, 90] (**Figure 5**). Endometrioid ovarian tumors are histologically similar to endometrial neoplasms. In fact, approximately one third of all endometrioid cases experience synchronous endometrial carcinoma or endometrial hyperplasia. This is not surprising given that endometrioid tumors are believed to arise from endometrial precursor cells and/or transformed endometrioses, possibly from back flow during menstruation that implants onto the ovarian surface epithelium [91–95].

The 5-year survival rate for endometrioid tumors is between 40 and 80%, and the 10-year survival is promising at~60%. This is mostly due to early stage presentation of the disease; however, there is no survival difference when matched with serous patients of the same age and stage of diagnosis [96, 97]. Likewise, with serous tumors, endometrioid tumors can be both high- and low-grade with similar growth patterns distinguishing the two [98]. High-grade endometrioid tumors are very similar to HGS tumors in terms of genome instability and response to chemotherapy [99]. The primary treatment regimen consists of surgical debulking followed by platinum-based chemotherapy. Mutation profiles of endometrioid tumors reveal frequent activating mutations in *CTNNB1* and *PIK3CA* [100, 101], as well as *ARID1A* (which helped link their origin to endometriosis) [102]. *PTEN* is altered in ~20% of endometrioid tumors, and to a lesser extent *KRAS* and *BRAF* [103, 104]. Given this mutational profile, it has been hypothesized that a subset of endometrioid tumors may be responsive to mTOR inhibitors; however, results of Phase I and II trials have shown minimal increases in overall response rate [105]. Ongoing studies emphasize a need for better molecular screening to identify individuals who could potentially benefit from a limited number of targeted therapies.

2.4. Mucinous ovarian cancer

Mucinous ovarian cancer (MOC) are primarily unilateral, can be very large (mean size of 10 cm and can range up to 48 cm) [106–108], and are diagnosed at early stages (most are stage I or II). Invasive disease accounts for less than 10% of all MOC cases [108, 109]. Mucinous ovarian tumors are rare when compared to other subtypes with reports of the overall incidence ranging from

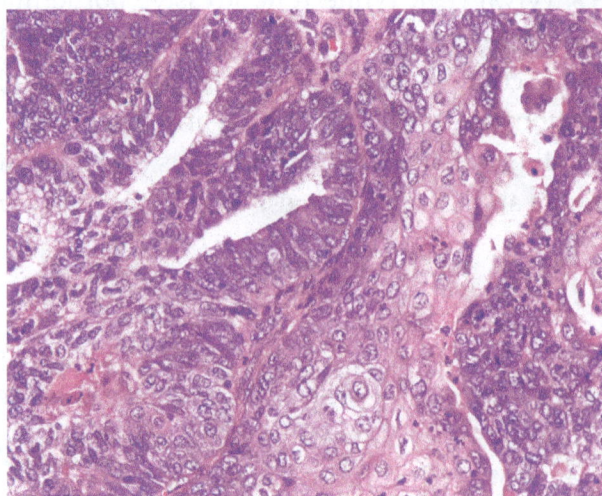

Figure 5. Representative H&E staining of endometrioid ovarian cancer.

~12% [110] to as low as 3% [3, 111]. Patients with invasive disease (FIGO Stage III or IV) have higher risk of death and shorter survival than patients with early disease (FIGO Stage I or II) [112]. The pathological definition of MOC dictates intracytoplasmic mucin is mandatory, although many mucinous tumors lack obvious apical mucin in large parts of tumor, thereby imparting an endometrioid appearance. Mucinous tumors are often heterogeneous contain endocervical-like or intestinal-like cells with gastric superficial/foveolar and pyloric cells, enterochromaffin cells, argyrophil cells, and Paneth cells (**Figure 6**). While cytokeratin 7 and 20 staining is used to define MOC pathologically, it is limited in distinguishing primary ovarian tumors from secondary metastases of gastrointestinal tumors [113, 114]. Secondary pathological markers such as SATB2, CDX2, and PAX8 have potential to help diagnose MOCs [115–117].

While the overall survival for mucinous ovarian disease is high due to the majority of cases being diagnosed at early stage, invasive disease has a worse clinical outcome [118] and low response rates to chemotherapy due to the high expression of genes involved in drug resistance, including the ABC transporters [119]. Mucinous disease is mostly thought to originate from the gastrointestinal tract [120], though the molecular mechanisms of the disease are still not fully elucidated. *KRAS* mutations, which are found in other ovarian cancer subtypes, are the most common genetic alterations found in MOC [29, 121, 122], followed by *HER2* amplifications [123]. Other mutations such as *BRAF*, *TP53*, and *CDKN2A* have been reported in MOC [124].

Extensive clinical studies of MOC are difficult to perform due to low number of cases and complex diagnosis and lead to early trial terminations such as GOG241 [125]. Small trials have shown that *HER2* amplifications in recurrent MOC are a potential therapeutic target with trastuzumab [126]. While most ovarian cancer trials of HER2 inhibitors have shown limited efficacy, the prevalence of *HER2* amplifications in MOC disease to other subtypes makes it a prospect for preselection if enough patients can be recruited [127].

2.5. Ovarian clear cell carcinoma

Ovarian clear cell carcinoma (CCC) accounts for approximately 5% of all ovarian cancer patients in the United States; however, it is more common in Asian women (~11%) than in African American

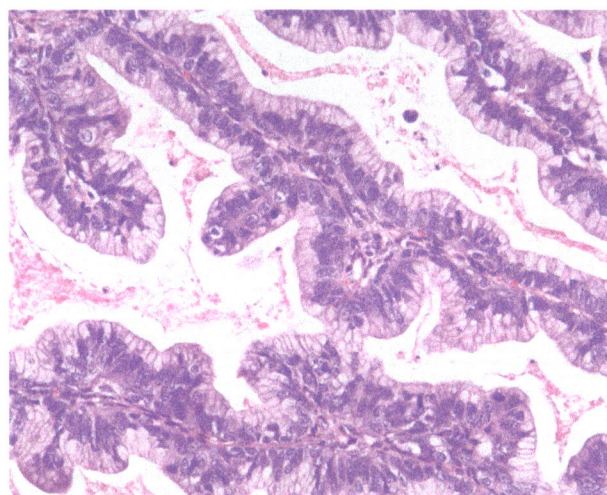

Figure 6. Representative H&E staining of mucinous ovarian cancer.

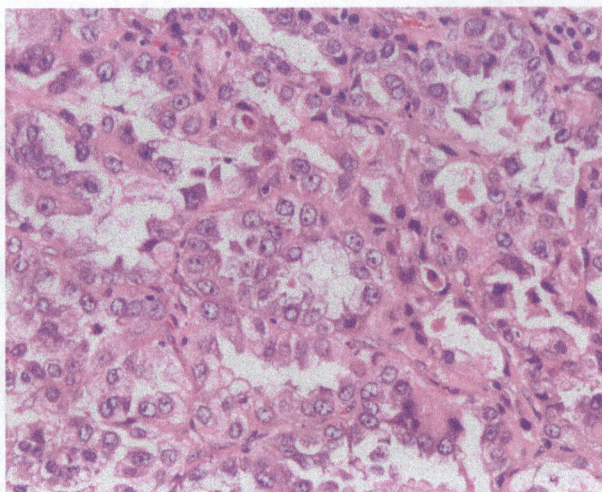

Figure 7. Representative H&E staining of ovarian clear cell carcinoma.

(~3%) or Caucasian (~5%) women [3, 128, 129]. CCCs are generally large (can grow over 15 cm), unilateral tumors that display only papillary, tubulocystic, and solid architectures with hobnail cells containing clear cytoplasm (**Figure 7**). While the pathogenesis of CCC is unknown, gene expression studies indicate clear cell ovarian cancer does not cluster with other ovarian cancers and more closely resembles lung cancers, endometriosis, and renal cell carcinoma [99, 130–132]. In terms of molecular mechanisms, CCCs are complex at the genomic level and can have mutations in *ARID1A*, *PIK3CA*, *KRAS* and *PTEN* [133, 134]: *ARID1A* is mutated in ~50% and *PIK3CA* mutated in ~33% of patient tumor samples [102, 135]. In contrast, CCCs are usually wild-type for *TP53* and have a lower frequency of *BRCA1* and *BRCA2* mutations [136, 137].

Clinically, CCCs are typically diagnosed at an early stage; however, they are less responsive to front-line platinum-based chemotherapy, especially at later FIGO stages. When compared to matched serous disease, early stage CCC (I-II) had a better overall survival than serous, but late stage CCC (III-IV) had a worse prognosis than both serous [138] and endometrioid adenocarcinoma [137]. Interestingly, some evidence suggests that drug response can be correlated to *CD44*-10v isoform expression [139]. Like endometrioid, clinical trials aimed at treating CCC include mTOR inhibitors, including a Phase II trial investigating the addition of temsirolimus to standard first-line chemotherapy (NCT01196429). Additionally, CCC is characterized by overexpression of the pro-inflammatory cytokine IL-6, which could prove to be an alternative therapeutic target [140].

3. Ovarian cancer pathogenesis

EOCs were, for years, believed to arise primarily from the ovarian surface epithelium. However, two novel hypotheses for the pathogenesis of HGS ovarian cancer have been proposed. In the first mechanism, genetic alterations occurring within the normal ovarian surface epithelium or inclusion cysts which either proceed via a high-grade pathway with no perceivable intermediate histology or a low-grade pathway encompassing several, benign and non-invasive steps (**Figure 8**). This first hypothesis was established in the 1970s and proposed that ovarian surface epithelial cells underwent repeated stress through multiple rounds of ovulation, leading to inflammation, DNA damage, and the initiation of tumorigenesis [141]. This hypothesis was in part supported by evidence on the decreased risk of ovarian cancer with the use of oral contraceptives, which inhibit complete ovulation [142, 143]. Other evidence supported the correlation between the number of lifetime ovulation cycles and the increase in ovarian cancer incidence [144]. Likewise, ovarian cancers are rare in other primates which have fewer ovulations cycles than humans [145]. However, ovarian tumors are more common in hens which have been induced to frequently ovulate [146, 147]. To further study the incessant ovulation theory, additional animal models will clearly be needed. In fact, Godwin and colleagues were some of the first investigators to establish ovarian surface epithelial cultures from rat and human ovaries and use model incessant ovulation *in vitro* as a mechanism for transformation and tumorigenesis [148–161]. Inactivation of p53 and Rb1 in mouse ovarian surface cells also led to tumorigenic transformation [162].

The second theory, which has gain much traction over the past decade, describes a progression model in which ovarian cancer precursors develop in the fimbria from occult serous tubal intraepithelial carcinoma (STIC), prior to metastasis to the ovary [163, 164]. Due to the aggressive nature of HGS tumors and the presence of early genomic instability, it is hypothesized that HGS ovarian tumors are instead metastatic lesions from the fallopian tube epithelial cells (**Figure 8**). To reduce the risk of HGS ovarian cancer in women *BRCA* mutation carriers it is beneficial to undergo a bilateral salpingo-oophorectomy (removal of both the ovaries along with the fallopian tubes) instead of just an oophorectomy (removal of only the ovaries) [165, 166]. The primary risk reduction for ovarian cancer following salpingo-oophorectomy was found to be serous disease [167]. Not only did these studies suggest a fallopian origin for serous disease, the use of salpingo-oophorectomy for preventative treatment for high-risk patients gave researchers and pathologist tissue to study and search for early ovarian cancer or precursor lesions. Microdissection of the fallopian tube epithelium following salpingo-oophorectomy from patients with a disposition to ovarian cancer showed lesions with *BRCA* and *TP53* alterations that resemble HGS tumors [168–171]. To follow-up, extensive evaluation of both the fallopian tube and ovarian surface from *BRCA* mutant patients also showed common precursor lesions in the fimbria and not the ovarian surface [164, 172–174]. In genetic mouse models, conditional inactivation of commonly mutated ovarian cancer genes (*BRCA1*, *TP53* and *RB1*) in ovarian surface epithelium cells leads to the formation of leiomyosarcomas and not HGSC following implantation into the mouse bursal sack [175]. Along with genetic alterations, fallopian lesions from *BRCA* patients showed gene expression profiles that mimicked HGS cancers [176]. Immortalization of human fallopian tube secretory epithelial cells (using hTERT and SV40 large T antigen) were transformed *in vivo* and *in vitro* by oncogenic *RAS* or *MYC* [177]. In contrast to ovarian surface epithelial cells, the inactivation of *Brca*, *Tp53* or *Pten* in *Pax8* over expressing mouse fallopian tubal secretory cells led to the development of HGSC [178]. Other genomic alterations common in HGS disease such as *CCNE1* amplification and other copy number alterations are also found in STIC lesions and might be an early step in the progression of HGS ovarian cancer [179, 180]. For example, *CCNE1* amplifications are common in both tubal lesions and HGS tumors, while centrosome amplification is more pronounced in HGS disease, indicating *CCNE1* copy number gain is an early step in tumorigenesis that later promotes centrosome amplification [181]. However, some evidence exists to show an independent clonal evolution between tubular lesions and

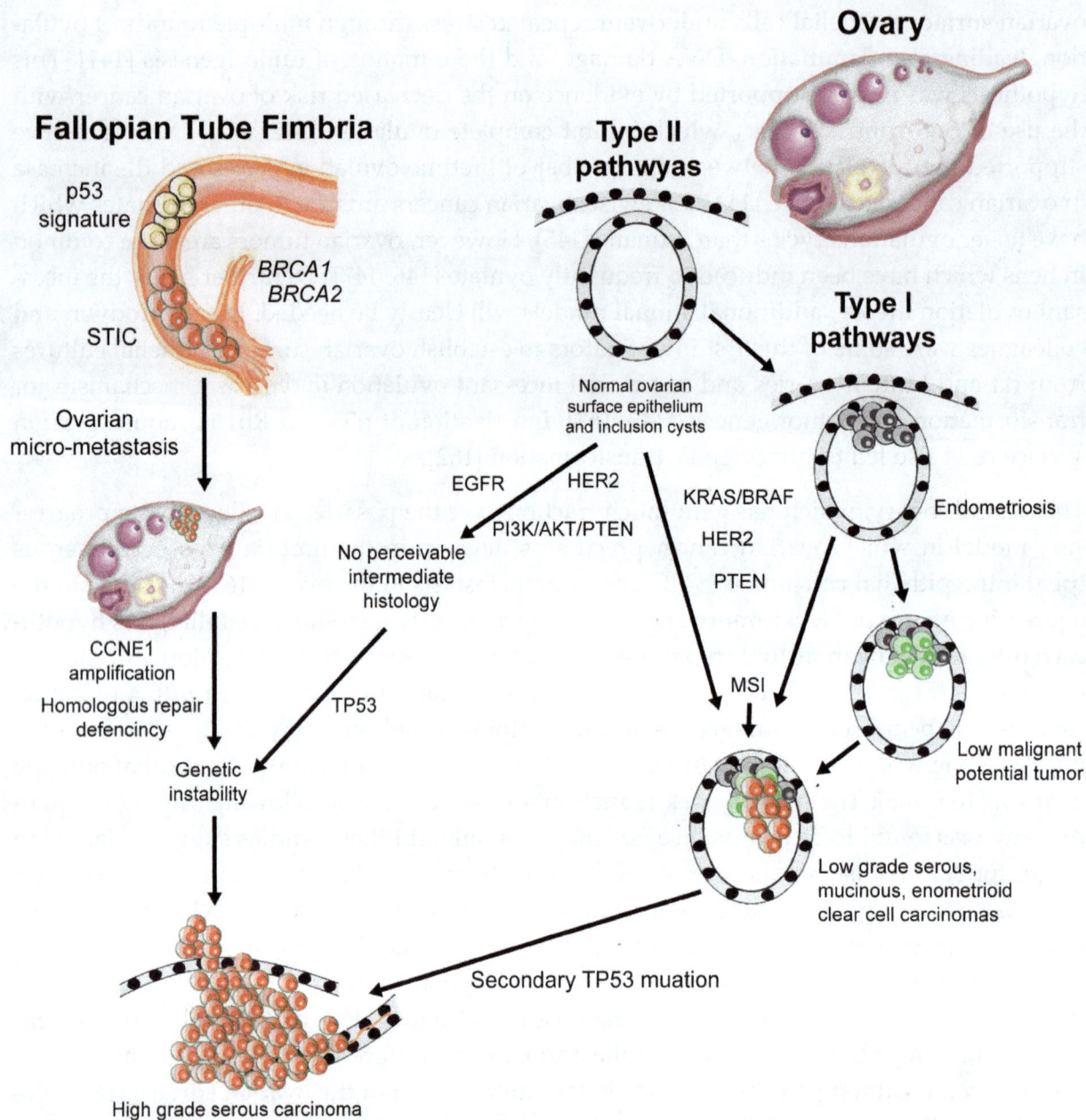

Figure 8. Pathogenesis pathways of ovarian cancer. Schematic representation of the prevailing theories behind ovarian cancer development.

the patient's synchronous carcinoma, indicating small number of fallopian tube lesions may be micrometastases from uterine endometrioid carcinomas [182].

Other studies suggest a different route of the pathogenesis of cancers, where somatic stem cells undergo oncogenic mutation and create cancer stem cells that populate tumors [183–187]. While this mechanism has been contested with evidence that cancer cell plasticity can induce a stem cell phenotype in cancer cells from differentiated tissue [188], understanding any stem cell niche in ovaries and fallopian tubes may provide insight into the pathogenesis of ovarian cancer. Both the ovarian surface epithelium and fallopian tube epithelium have stem cell niches with cells with regenerative properties that could serves as progenitor cells for ovarian cancer [189–191]. Some evidence supports there could be a stem cell niche within the junction between the ovarian surface the fallopian tube that helps repair the damage to the ovarian surface following follicle release [192]. Notch and Wnt, canonical stem cell pathways, have been shown to regulate differentiation in fallopian tube organoids and could contribute to fallopian tube repair [193]. Fallopian stem-like cells (CD44+ and PAX8+) can be isolated from distal end of the tube and are capable of clonal growth and self-renewal [194, 195]. Since these stem cell niches are located near the areas of ovarian and fallopian surface repair and precursor lesions they could be hotspots for the development of tumors from mutations in somatic stem cells. One recent study has shown that *SOX2* is overexpressed in the fallopian tubes of patients with HGS disease and in *BRCA1/BRCA2* mutation carries [196], indicating a possible stem cell precursor lesion. The role of stem cells in cancer and cancer progression will remain an influential area of research and can provide potential insight into ovarian cancer pathogenesis in the future.

Taken together, these data support that the pathogenesis of ovarian cancer is complex and thus contributes to the clinical difficulties in detecting the disease early. As our understanding of the genomic complexities of ovarian cancer continues to evolve and the cell type of origin is further defined, we should be able to use this information to improve detection at a time when disease can be cured and develop more precise therapies based on tumor profiling and precision medicine.

4. Ovarian cancer risk factors

4.1. Hereditary and genetic risk factors

Ovarian cancer risk is causally linked to both lifestyle and genetics. Firstly, hereditary ovarian cancer accounts for approximately 5–15% of all cases [197] and are often diagnosed at an earlier age than sporadic disease. Furthermore, hereditary ovarian cancer tends to be of the high-grade serous subtype [198]. Therefore, patients with a first or second-degree relative with ovarian cancer have an increased risk of developing the disease (**Figure 9**). Specifically, there is a 2.5% risk of ovarian cancer in woman who report a sister EOC and a 9% risk if their mother has been previously diagnosed [197]. Familial ovarian cancer was first observed in Lynch syndrome (a disease associated with familial cancer due to inherited mutations in DNA repair machinery) in the 1970s [199, 200]. Multiple group and genomic mapping studies of breast and/ or ovarian cancer-prone families ultimately led to the identification of inherited mutations in *BRCA1* [201] and later *BRCA2* [202, 203]. The prevalence of *BRCA1* or *BRCA2* mutations in the populations has been estimated from 0.1–0.3%, and 0.1–0.7%, respectively, in Caucasians with European origins [204–206]. *BRCA1* and *BRCA2* are mutated in the germline of approximately 9–13% patients with hereditary ovarian cancer [207–209]. For mutations in *BRCA1*, the estimated average risk of ovarian cancers ranges from 20 to 50% [210–214]. For *BRCA2*, average risk estimates range from 5 to 23% [210–214]. Mutation-specific cancer risks have been reported that suggest ovarian cancer cluster region (OCCR) exist in both *BRCA1* and *BRCA2* [211, 215]. The prevalence and spectrum of mutations in *BRCA1* and *BRCA2* have been reported in single populations with the majority of reports focused on Caucasians in Europe and North America. The Consortium of Investigators of Modifiers of *BRCA1* or *BRCA2* (CIMBA) has assembled data on more than 26,000 *BRCA1* and nearly 17,000 *BRCA2* female mutation carriers from 69 centers in 49 countries on six continents [216–222]. Ongoing studies by Tim Rebbeck and the

CIMBA consortium have comprehensively evaluated the characteristics of the over 1600 unique *BRCA1* and more than 1700 unique *BRCA2* deleterious (disease-associated) mutations found in the carriers [215]. The most common mutation types in these genes are frameshift mutations, followed by nonsense mutations. Therefore, understanding the type of mutations in *BRCA1* or *BRCA2* is important for risk assessment and determining medical management for patients. Most subtypes of ovarian cancer have been linked to *BRCA1* or *BRCA2* germline mutations but the development of HGS disease is the most common in these women carriers [223]. *BRCA1* and *BRCA2* mutations are more common in Ashkenazi Jewish women [206, 224, 225] due to the three common Jewish founder mutations *BRCA1* c.5266dup (5382insC) and *BRCA1* c.68_69del (185delAG) and *BRCA2* c.5946del (6174delT) which have long been used as a primary genetic screening test for women of Jewish descent. Other mutations that are relatively common in specific populations, referred to as founder mutations, can be used to in limited screening tests. For example, in Iceland, only two mutations have been reported: the common founder mutation *BRCA2* c.771_775del and the rarer *BRCA1* c.5074G > A [226]. Despite having a higher risk for developing ovarian cancer, *BRCA1/2* carriers have a better clinical outcome in terms of survival, with *BRCA2* carriers having a more favorable outcome than *BRCA1* carriers [54]. This

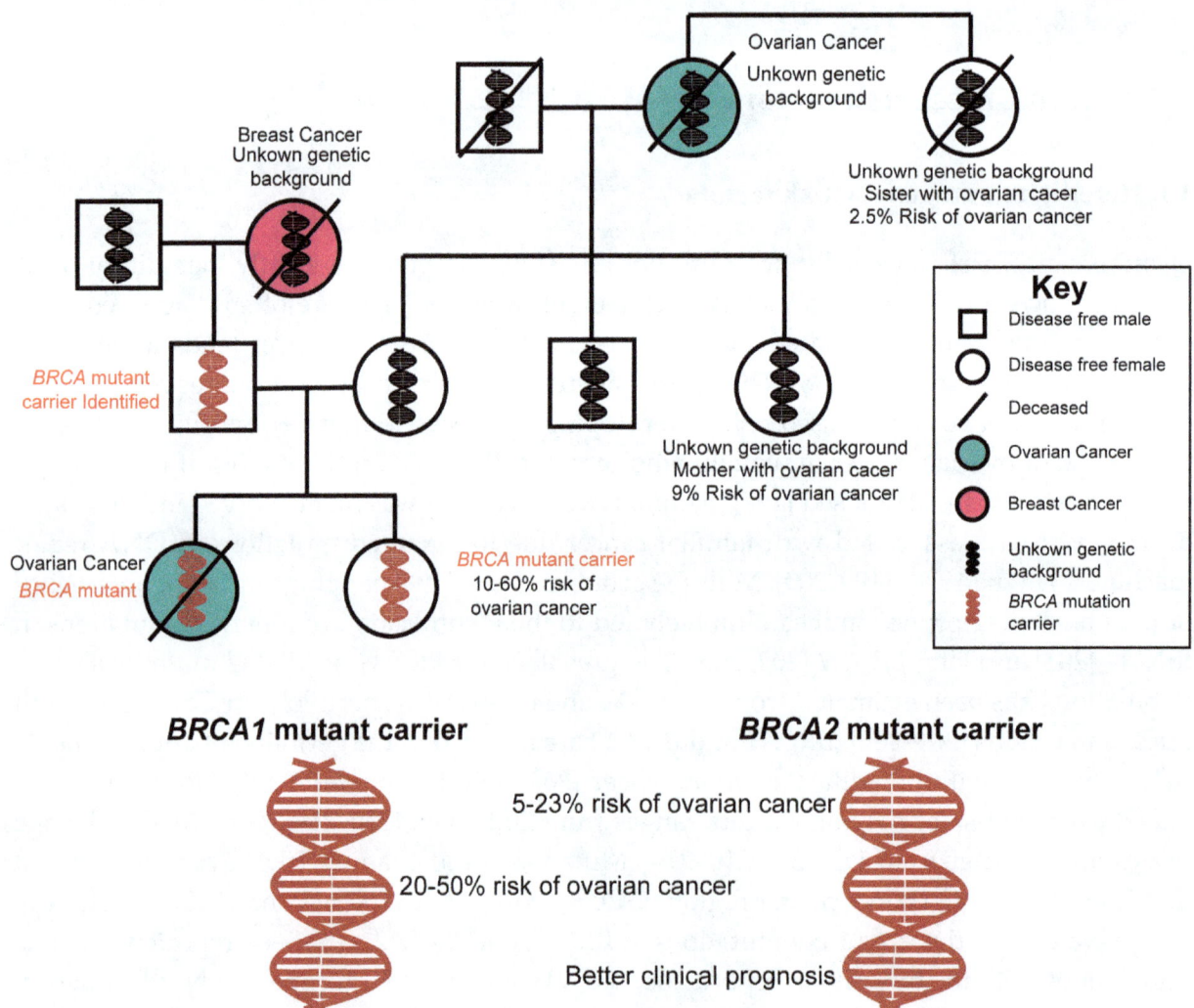

Figure 9. Hereditary ovarian cancer and BRCA mutations. Pedigree describing "BRCAness" and risk of ovarian cancer (top). The relative risk and prognosis for women with germline *BRCA1/2* mutations.

phenomenon is thought to be due to *BRCA2* carriers responding better to platinum-based chemotherapy [227]. However, the survival benefit decreases when examined over 10 years in HGS instead of 5 years [228]. Over time, this could be possible due to secondary intragenic mutations in *BRCA1* and *BRCA2* that restore the wild-type reading frame (conversion back to a functional BRCA) and losing favorable responses to chemotherapy [229].

As indicated, the location of the alteration within *BRCA1* or *BRCA2* may vary the risk of breast and ovarian cancer [215], but other studies including genome-wide association study (GWAS) have identified several single nucleotide polymorphisms (SNPs) associated with risk of ovarian cancer for women in the general population [230]. Four of these SNP, *i.e.,* rs10088218, rs2665390, rs717852, rs9303542, were associated with ovarian cancer risk in *BRCA2* carriers, while two loci (rs10088218 and rs2665390) were associated with ovarian cancer risk in *BRCA1* carriers [217]. Inherited variants in other loci along with *BRCA1* or *BRCA2* mutations can better predict the risk of either breast or ovarian cancer [220], indicating the need to better understand concurrent sequence variants in women with deleterious *BRCA1* or *BRCA2* mutations. Concurrent mutations in 1p36 (*WNT4*), 4q26 (*SYNPO2*), 9q34.2 (*ABO*), and 17q11.2 (*ATAD5*) increased risk of all EOC subtypes while 1q34.3 (*RSPO1*) and 6p22.1 (*GPX6*) mutations increased the risk of serous ovarian cancer in *BRCA* carriers [231]. *BRCA1* mutation carries can have reduced risk with concurrent sequence variants in *CASP8, i.e.,* the D302H polymorphism [232]. Other genetic markers of risk, such as a variant allele of *KRAS* at *rs61764370*, referred to as the *KRAS*-variant, which disrupts a *let-7* miRNA binding site in this oncogene, is associated with sporadic and familial ovarian cancer without *BRCA1/2* mutations [233]. *PALB2*, encoding for a BRCA2 interacting protein, has increased promoter hypermethylation which results in decreased *BRCA2* function and increased risk of ovarian cancer [234]. Recent data have shown that copy number variation in *BRCA1* or *BRCA2* mutation carriers can either increase the risk (*OR2A*) or decrease the risk (*CYP2A7*) of ovarian cancer [235]. A better understanding of secondary genetic alteration in *BRCA1/2* mutant carriers can help determine the best clinical approach for managing the risk of disease.

Genetic risk factors outside of *BRCA1* or *BRCA2* mutations are not as well defined but often take place in genes involved in genomic integrity, most commonly DNA mismatch repair (MMR). SNPs in the *TERT* locus (rs2242652 and rs10069690) were associated with decreased telomere length and increased breast and ovarian cancer risk in *BRCA* mutation carriers [236]. A study that sequenced 12 genes for germline mutations in patients with ovarian cancer found *BARD1, BRIP1, CHECK2, MREA11, MSH6, NMN, PALB2, RAD51C,* or *TP53* were mutated in 24% of the 360 patients enrolled [237]. Genes within the Fanconi anemia pathway are also associated with developing ovarian cancer, including *RAD51C, RAD51D,* and *BRIP1* [238, 239]. Other MMR genes have been associated with Lynch syndrome and ovarian cancer risk *MLH1, PMS2, MSH2,* and *MSH6* [240–242].

4.2. Lifestyle risk factors

Environment and lifestyle also play a risk for developing both hereditary and sporadic ovarian cancer by either increasing or decreasing the lifetime risk of developing ovarian cancer. Like many cancers, age is a risk factor for ovarian cancer with most cases being diagnosed after the age of 60 and the disease being extremely rare in patients under 40 years of age [243]. As previously discussed, surgical procedures such as tubal ligation, salpingectomy and unilateral or bilateral oophorectomy have varying degrees of success for the development of ovarian cancer by removal of the organs from which the cancer develops [244, 245]. In women with a *BRCA1* or *BRCA2* mutation, risk-reducing salpingo-oophorectomy (RRSO) decreased the lifetime risk of developing ovarian and breast cancer [165]. In a multicenter study, RRSO was associated with an 85% reduction in *BRCA1*-associated gynecologic cancer risk (hazard ratio [HR] = 0.15; 95% CI, 0.04 to 0.56), while protection against *BRCA2*-associated gynecologic cancer (HR = 0.00; 95% CI, not estimable) was suggested, its effect did not reached statistical significance [246]. The effects of RRSO can influence risk for each subtype given the nature of development from different tissues, hence why bilateral oophorectomy has a stronger influence on the development of HGS disease, since it is believed to develop from the fallopian tubes. Lifestyle factors which influence complete cycling during menstruation have some of the strongest effects on the risk of developing ovarian cancer. This hypothesis is attributed to incessant ovulation, in which the release of eggs from the ovary, the fusion on the fallopian tube and the rebuilding of the uterine wall all contribute to pathogenesis of ovarian cancer [141, 148]. One of the most common factors which can alter complete cycling is the use of oral contraceptives [243]. The increase in use of oral contraceptives could be attributed to the decrease in ovarian cancer in the last decade. The longer use of oral contraceptives has been shown to correlate to lower risk of developing ovarian cancer [247, 248]. The risk is reduced in both *BRCA* wild-type and mutant carriers [249] [250]. The risk of developing each subtype is decreased following oral contraceptive use, with the exception of clear cell carcinoma [251]. However, the associated side effects make it a poor treatment for prevention alone [252]. Another factor that can influence menstrual cycles and the risk of ovarian cancer is child birth [253], in specific the age at first birth and the number of births. In fact, it was discovered the risk of ovarian cancer decreases by approximately 10% for each 5-year increment in age at first birth [254]. Also, the number of births for a given women has additive decrease in the risk of ovarian cancer, decreasing by about 8% for each birth [255], while the age of each woman at the onset of menopause had a weak association [129, 256].

Other lifestyle factors can influence the risk of ovarian cancer, such as hormone replacement therapy, breast feeding, obesity and inflammation. Hormone replacement therapy increases the risk of developing ovarian cancer, depending on the therapy. For instance, the use of estrogen increases the risk of developing ovarian cancer by 22%, while the combination of estrogen and progesterone only has about a 10% chance of developing ovarian cancer [257–259]. A meta-analysis showed a similar risk for developing both HGS and endometrioid ovarian cancer in menopausal women [260]. Conversely, hormone replacement given for menopause symptoms may improve survival of ovarian cancer patients [261]. Another reproductive factor is breastfeeding, in *BRCA1* mutant carriers breastfeeding lead to a reduced the risk of developing ovarian cancer [129, 243]. Meta-analysis also suggests the duration of lifetime breastfeeding is additive in reducing the risk of developing ovarian cancer [262]. Like many other cancers, cigarette smoking and alcohol consumption have at least some association with increasing the risk of developing ovarian cancer. Specifically, smoking is associated with an increased risk of developing clear cell and endometrial ovarian cancer but not serous [263]. Smoking increased the risk of mucinous ovarian cancer, but cessation returns can reduce the risk over time [264] while heavy smoking (>10 packs per day) more than doubles the risk of developing ovarian cancer [265]. Alcohol consumption increased the risk of ovarian cancer, but seems to have an effect only in heavy drinkers. Consumption of more than 20 drinks per week is associated with increased risk [266] while with moderate use the risk is less pronounced or significant [267, 268]. Obesity is associated with less common subtypes of ovarian cancer and not HGS [269] and the lifetime risk decreases with recreation physical activity [270]. Finally, inflammation increases the risk of developing ovarian cancer [271] while the use of aspirin was shown to reduce risk of developing ovarian cancer from between 20 and 34% [272]. The use of other non-steroidal anti-inflammatory drugs (NSAIDs) showed a reduction in risk but was not significant.

5. Conclusion

Genetically, ovarian cancer is a heterogeneous and dynamic disease that presents several clinical and research challenges. While epithelial ovarian cancer is categorized pathologically into five basic subtypes, within each subtype exist genetic diversity that limits the development of target therapies. To add to this complexity, one of the hallmarks of serous ovarian cancer is genomic instability, which is driven by frequent *TP53* mutations and deficiencies in DNA repair pathways. While this genomic alterations have led to the development of breakthrough therapies (PARP inhibitors), they also contributes to the dynamic cell growth and frequent genomic alterations and gene expression changes which contribute to the adaptation to therapy. Likewise, the pathogenesis of ovarian cancer remains a debated field with the recent insights of progression of a subset of serous ovarian cancer from fallopian tube epithelial lesions. Progression from the fallopian tube means tumors detected on the ovarian surface are already metastatic disease, leading to quick progression and limited response to therapy. Overall, while many genetic and genomic abnormalities have been identified in ovarian cancer, additional discovers are needed to (1) improve early detection of the disease (at a time when current treatment might be curative), (2) further define molecular classifiers of response to therapy, and (3) develop therapies that will be more effective across or specific to the different molecular subtypes. Other than the very common *TP53* mutation in high-grade serous ovarian cancer (96% of cases), which to date is undruggable, and the previously mentioned *BRCA* mutations (approximately 10–12% of ovarian cancers), only a small overall percentage of tumors from patients with this malignancy will be found to possess a specific causative mutation that can be effectively targeted therapeutically. Therefore, implementation of genomic-based medicine remains a challenge for the management of women with ovarian cancer.

Acknowledgements

Pathology images for each ovarian cancer subtype generously provided by Dr. Rashna Madan from the University of Kansas Medical Center and the University of Kansas Cancer Center (Kansas City, KS).

Author details

Jeff Hirst[1]*, Jennifer Crow[1] and Andrew Godwin[1,2]

*Address all correspondence to: jhirst@kumc.edu

1 Department of Pathology and Laboratory Medicine, University of Kansas Medical Center, Kansas City, KS, USA

2 University of Kansas Cancer Center, University of Kansas Medical Center, Kansas City, KS, USA

References

[1] Sankaranarayanan R, Ferlay J. Worldwide burden of gynaecological cancer: The size of the problem. Best Practice & Research. Clinical Obstetrics & Gynaecology. 2006;**20**(2): 207-225

[2] Braicu EI et al. Role of histological type on surgical outcome and survival following radical primary tumour debulking of epithelial ovarian, fallopian tube and peritoneal cancers. British Journal of Cancer. 2011;**105**(12):1818-1824

[3] Seidman JD et al. The histologic type and stage distribution of ovarian carcinomas of surface epithelial origin. International Journal of Gynecological Pathology. 2004;**23**(1):41-44

[4] Gershenson DM. The heterogeneity of epithelial ovarian cancer: Getting it right. Cancer. 2010;**116**(6):1400-1402

[5] Malpica A et al. Grading ovarian serous carcinoma using a two-tier system. The American Journal of Surgical Pathology. 2004;**28**(4):496-504

[6] Iwabuchi H et al. Genetic analysis of benign, low-grade, and high-grade ovarian tumors. Cancer Research. 1995;**55**(24):6172-6180

[7] Oswald AJ, Gourley C. Low-grade epithelial ovarian cancer: A number of distinct clinical entities? Current Opinion in Oncology. 2015;**27**(5):412-419

[8] Groen RS, Gershenson DM, Fader AN. Updates and emerging therapies for rare epithelial ovarian cancers: One size no longer fits all. Gynecologic Oncology. 2015;**136**(2):373-383

[9] Kurman RJ. Origin and molecular pathogenesis of ovarian high-grade serous carcinoma. Annals of Oncology. 2013;**24**(Suppl 10):x16-x21

[10] Taylor J, McCluggage WG. Ovarian seromucinous carcinoma: Report of a series of a newly categorized and uncommon neoplasm. The American Journal of Surgical Pathology. 2015;**39**(7):983-992

[11] Mackenzie R et al. Morphological and molecular characteristics of mixed epithelial ovarian cancers. The American Journal of Surgical Pathology. 2015;**39**(11):1548

[12] Coburn SB et al. International patterns and trends in ovarian cancer incidence, overall and by histologic subtype. International Journal of Cancer. 2017;**140**(11):2451-2460

[13] Vaughan S et al. Rethinking ovarian cancer: Recommendations for improving outcomes. Nature Reviews. Cancer. 2011;**11**(10):719-725

[14] Cress RD et al. Characteristics of long-term survivors of epithelial ovarian cancer. Obstetrics and Gynecology. 2015;**126**(3):491-497

[15] Jung ES et al. Mucinous adenocarcinoma involving the ovary: Comparative evaluation of the classification algorithms using tumor size and laterality. Journal of Korean Medical Science. 2010;**25**(2):220-225

[16] Bentink S et al. Angiogenic mRNA and microRNA gene expression signature predicts a novel subtype of serous ovarian cancer. PLoS One. 2012;**7**(2):e30269

[17] Tothill RW et al. Novel molecular subtypes of serous and endometrioid ovarian cancer linked to clinical outcome. Clinical Cancer Research. 2008;**14**(16):5198-5208

[18] Phelan CM et al. Identification of 12 new susceptibility loci for different histotypes of epithelial ovarian cancer. Nature Genetics. 2017;**49**(5):680-691

[19] Winterhoff B et al. Molecular classification of high grade endometrioid and clear cell ovarian cancer using TCGA gene expression signatures. Gynecologic Oncology. 2016;**141**(1):95-100

[20] Madore J et al. Characterization of the molecular differences between ovarian endometrioid carcinoma and ovarian serous carcinoma. The Journal of Pathology. 2010;**220**(3):392-400

[21] Pamula-Pilat J et al. Gene expression profiles in three histologic types, clear-cell, endometrioid and serous ovarian carcinomas. Journal of Biological Regulators and Homeostatic Agents. 2014;**28**(4):659-674

[22] Howlader N et al. SEER Cancer Statistics Review, 1975-2012. Bethesda, MD: National Cancer Institute; 2015

[23] Chang CM et al. Gene set-based functionome analysis of pathogenesis in epithelial ovarian serous carcinoma and the molecular features in different FIGO stages. International Journal of Molecular Sciences. 2016;**17**(6)

[24] Burks RT, Sherman ME, Kurman RJ. Micropapillary serous carcinoma of the ovary. A distinctive low-grade carcinoma related to serous borderline tumors. The American Journal of Surgical Pathology. 1996;**20**(11):1319-1330

[25] Seidman JD, Kurman RJ. Subclassification of serous borderline tumors of the ovary into benign and malignant types. A clinicopathologic study of 65 advanced stage cases. The American Journal of Surgical Pathology. 1996;**20**(11):1331-1345

[26] Malpica A et al. Interobserver and intraobserver variability of a two-tier system for grading ovarian serous carcinoma. The American Journal of Surgical Pathology. 2007;**31**(8):1168-1174

[27] O'Neill CJ et al. High-grade ovarian serous carcinoma exhibits significantly higher p16 expression than low-grade serous carcinoma and serous borderline tumour. Histopathology. 2007;**50**(6):773-779

[28] Lee SH et al. Genetic alteration and immunohistochemical staining patterns of ovarian high-grade serous adenocarcinoma with special emphasis on p53 immnnostaining pattern. Pathology International. 2013;**63**(5):252-259

[29] Vereczkey I et al. Molecular characterization of 103 ovarian serous and mucinous tumors. Pathology Oncology Research. 2011;**17**(3):551-559

[30] Al-Hussaini M et al. WT-1 assists in distinguishing ovarian from uterine serous carcinoma and in distinguishing between serous and endometrioid ovarian carcinoma. Histopathology. 2004;**44**(2):109-115

[31] O'Neill CJ et al. An immunohistochemical comparison between low-grade and high-grade ovarian serous carcinomas: Significantly higher expression of p53, MIB1, BCL2, HER-2/neu, and C-KIT in high-grade neoplasms. The American Journal of Surgical Pathology. 2005;**29**(8):1034-1041

[32] Dehari R et al. The development of high-grade serous carcinoma from atypical proliferative (borderline) serous tumors and low-grade micropapillary serous carcinoma: A morphologic and molecular genetic analysis. The American Journal of Surgical Pathology. 2007;**31**(7):1007-1012

[33] Boyd C, McCluggage WG. Low-grade ovarian serous neoplasms (low-grade serous carcinoma and serous borderline tumor) associated with high-grade serous carcinoma or undifferentiated carcinoma: Report of a series of cases of an unusual phenomenon. The American Journal of Surgical Pathology. 2012;**36**(3):368-375

[34] Gorringe KL et al. High-resolution single nucleotide polymorphism array analysis of epithelial ovarian cancer reveals numerous microdeletions and amplifications. Clinical Cancer Research. 2007;**13**(16):4731-4739

[35] Ahmed AA et al. Driver mutations in TP53 are ubiquitous in high grade serous carcinoma of the ovary. The Journal of Pathology. 2010;**221**(1):49-56

[36] Network TCGAR. Integrated genomic analyses of ovarian carcinoma. Nature. 2011;**474**(7353):609-615

[37] Turner N, Tutt A, Ashworth A. Hallmarks of 'BRCAness' in sporadic cancers. Nature Reviews Cancer. 2004;**4**(10):814-819

[38] Jazaeri AA et al. Gene expression profiles of BRCA1-linked, BRCA2-linked, and sporadic ovarian cancers. Journal of the National Cancer Institute. 2002;**94**(13):990-1000

[39] Network TCGA. Comprehensive molecular portraits of human breast tumours. Nature. 2012;**490**(7418):61-70

[40] Ciriello G et al. Emerging landscape of oncogenic signatures across human cancers. Nature Genetics. 2013;**45**(10):1127-1133

[41] Nakayama N et al. Gene amplification CCNE1 is related to poor survival and potential therapeutic target in ovarian cancer. Cancer. 2010;**116**(11):2621-2634

[42] Patch AM et al. Whole-genome characterization of chemoresistant ovarian cancer. Nature. 2015;**521**(7553):489-494

[43] Martins FC et al. Combined image and genomic analysis of high-grade serous ovarian cancer reveals PTEN loss as a common driver event and prognostic classifier. Genome Biology. 2014;**15**(12):526

[44] Integrated genomic analyses of ovarian carcinoma. Nature. 2011;**474**(7353):609-615

[45] Singer G et al. Diverse tumorigenic pathways in ovarian serous carcinoma. The American Journal of Pathology. 2002;**160**(4):1223-1228

[46] Salani R et al. Assessment of TP53 mutation using purified tissue samples of ovarian serous carcinomas reveals a higher mutation rate than previously reported and does not correlate with drug resistance. International Journal of Gynecological Cancer. 2008;**18**(3):487-491

[47] Fong PC et al. Inhibition of poly(ADP-ribose) polymerase in tumors from BRCA mutation carriers. The New England Journal of Medicine. 2009;**361**(2):123-134

[48] Audeh MW et al. Oral poly(ADP-ribose) polymerase inhibitor olaparib in patients with BRCA1 or BRCA2 mutations and recurrent ovarian cancer: A proof-of-concept trial. Lancet. 2010;**376**(9737):245-251

[49] Jenner ZB, Sood AK, Coleman RL. Evaluation of rucaparib and companion diagnostics in the PARP inhibitor landscape for recurrent ovarian cancer therapy. Future Oncology. 2016;**12**(12):1439-1456

[50] Drew Y et al. Phase 2 multicentre trial investigating intermittent and continuous dosing schedules of the poly(ADP-ribose) polymerase inhibitor rucaparib in germline BRCA mutation carriers with advanced ovarian and breast cancer. British Journal of Cancer. 2016;**114**(7):723-730

[51] Mirza MR et al. Niraparib maintenance therapy in platinum-sensitive, recurrent ovarian cancer. The New England Journal of Medicine. 2016

[52] Do TV et al. Aurora a kinase regulates non-homologous end-joining and poly(ADP-ribose) polymerase function in ovarian carcinoma cells. Oncotarget. 2017

[53] Sakai W et al. Secondary mutations as a mechanism of cisplatin resistance in BRCA2-mutated cancers. Nature. 2008;**451**(7182):1116-1120

[54] Bolton KL et al. Association between BRCA1 and BRCA2 mutations and survival in women with invasive epithelial ovarian cancer. JAMA. 2012;**307**(4):382-390

[55] Eyre R et al. Reversing paclitaxel resistance in ovarian cancer cells via inhibition of the ABCB1 expressing side population. Tumour Biology. 2014;**35**(10):9879-9892

[56] Sun KX et al. MicroRNA-186 induces sensitivity of ovarian cancer cells to paclitaxel and cisplatin by targeting ABCB1. Journal of Ovarian Research. 2015;**8**:80

[57] Wang SQ et al. Afatinib reverses multidrug resistance in ovarian cancer via dually inhibiting ATP binding cassette subfamily B member 1. Oncotarget. 2015;**6**(28):26142-26160

[58] Johnatty SE et al. ABCB1 (MDR 1) polymorphisms and progression-free survival among women with ovarian cancer following paclitaxel/carboplatin chemotherapy. Clinical Cancer Research. 2008;**14**(17):5594-5601

[59] Vaidyanathan A et al. ABCB1 (MDR1) induction defines a common resistance mechanism in paclitaxel- and olaparib-resistant ovarian cancer cells. British Journal of Cancer. 2016;**115**(4):431-441

[60] Surowiak P et al. ABCC2 (MRP2, cMOAT) can be localized in the nuclear membrane of ovarian carcinomas and correlates with resistance to Cisplatin and clinical outcome. Clinical Cancer Research. 2006;**12**(23):7149-7158

[61] Tian C et al. Common variants in ABCB1, ABCC2 and ABCG2 genes and clinical outcomes among women with advanced stage ovarian cancer treated with platinum and taxane-based chemotherapy: A Gynecologic oncology group study. Gynecologic Oncology. 2012;**124**(3):575-581

[62] Hamaguchi K et al. Cross-resistance to diverse drugs is associated with primary cisplatin resistance in ovarian cancer cell lines. Cancer Research. 1993;**53**(21):5225-5232

[63] Godwin AK et al. High resistance to cisplatin in human ovarian cancer cell lines is associated with marked increase of glutathione synthesis. Proceedings of the National Academy of Sciences of the United States of America. 1992;**89**(7):3070-3074

[64] Kajiyama H et al. Chemoresistance to paclitaxel induces epithelial-mesenchymal transition and enhances metastatic potential for epithelial ovarian carcinoma cells. International Journal of Oncology. 2007;**31**(2):277-283

[65] Haslehurst AM et al. EMT transcription factors snail and slug directly contribute to cisplatin resistance in ovarian cancer. BMC Cancer. 2012;**12**:91

[66] Crow J et al. Exosomes as mediators of platinum resistance in ovarian cancer. Oncotarget. 2017

[67] Au Yeung CL et al. Exosomal transfer of stroma-derived miR21 confers paclitaxel resistance in ovarian cancer cells through targeting APAF1. Nature Communications. 2016;**7**:11150

[68] Yew KH et al. Epimorphin-induced MET sensitizes ovarian cancer cells to platinum. PLoS One. 2013;**8**(9):e72637

[69] Vang R, Shih I-M, Kurman RJ. Ovarian low-grade and high-grade serous carcinoma: Pathogenesis, clinicopathologic and molecular biologic features, and diagnostic problems. Advances in Anatomic Pathology. 2009;**16**(5):267-282

[70] Bell KA, Smith Sehdev AE, Kurman RJ. Refined diagnostic criteria for implants associated with ovarian atypical proliferative serous tumors (borderline) and micropapillary serous carcinomas. The American Journal of Surgical Pathology. 2001;**25**(4):419-432

[71] Gershenson DM, Silva EG. Serous ovarian tumors of low malignant potential with peritoneal implants. Cancer. 1990;**65**(3):578-585

[72] Singer G et al. Mutations in BRAF and KRAS characterize the development of low-grade ovarian serous carcinoma. Journal of the National Cancer Institute. 2003;**95**(6):484-486

[73] Singer G et al. Patterns of p53 mutations separate ovarian serous borderline tumors and low- and high-grade carcinomas and provide support for a new model of ovarian

carcinogenesis: A mutational analysis with immunohistochemical correlation. The American Journal of Surgical Pathology. 2005;**29**(2):218-224

[74] Hunter SM et al. Molecular profiling of low grade serous ovarian tumours identifies novel candidate driver genes. Oncotarget. 2015;**6**(35):37663-37677

[75] Hsu CY et al. Characterization of active mitogen-activated protein kinase in ovarian serous carcinomas. Clinical Cancer Research. 2004;**10**(19):6432-6436

[76] Tone AA et al. Intratumoral heterogeneity in a minority of ovarian low-grade serous carcinomas. BMC Cancer. 2014;**14**:982

[77] Gershenson DM et al. Recurrent low-grade serous ovarian carcinoma is relatively chemoresistant. Gynecologic Oncology. 2009;**114**(1):48-52

[78] Crane EK et al. The role of secondary cytoreduction in low-grade serous ovarian cancer or peritoneal cancer. Gynecologic Oncology. 2015;**136**(1):25-29

[79] Della Pepa C et al. Low grade serous ovarian carcinoma: From the molecular characterization to the best therapeutic strategy. Cancer Treatment Reviews. 2015;**41**(2):136-143

[80] Farley J et al. Selumetinib in women with recurrent low-grade serous carcinoma of the ovary or peritoneum: An open-label, single-arm, phase 2 study. The Lancet Oncology. 2013;**14**(2):134-140

[81] Nikrui N. Survey of clinical behavior of patients with borderline epithelial tumors of the ovary. Gynecologic Oncology. 1981;**12**(1):107-119

[82] Hogg R et al. Microinvasion links ovarian serous borderline tumor and grade 1 invasive carcinoma. Gynecologic Oncology. 2007;**106**(1):44-51

[83] Okoye E, Euscher ED, Malpica A. Ovarian low-grade serous carcinoma: A clinicopathologic study of 33 cases with primary surgery performed at a single institution. The American Journal of Surgical Pathology. 2016;**40**(5):627-635

[84] Sherman ME et al. Survival among women with borderline ovarian tumors and ovarian carcinoma: A population-based analysis. Cancer. 2004;**100**(5):1045-1052

[85] Kaern J, Trope CG, Abeler VM. A retrospective study of 370 borderline tumors of the ovary treated at the Norwegian radium hospital from 1970 to 1982. A review of clinicopathologic features and treatment modalities. Cancer. 1993;**71**(5):1810-1820

[86] Malpica A, Wong KK. The molecular pathology of ovarian serous borderline tumors. Annals of Oncology. 2016;**27**(Suppl 1):i16-i19

[87] Zeppernick F et al. BRAF mutation is associated with a specific cell type with features suggestive of senescence in ovarian serous borderline (atypical proliferative) tumors. The American Journal of Surgical Pathology. 2014;**38**(12):1603-1611

[88] Ahn G et al. Low-grade serous carcinoma of the ovary: Clinicopathologic analysis of 52 invasive cases and identification of a possible noninvasive intermediate lesion. The American Journal of Surgical Pathology. 2016;**40**(9):1165-1176

[89] Brown J, Frumovitz M. Mucinous tumors of the ovary: Current thoughts on diagnosis and management. Current Oncology Reports. 2014;**16**(6):389

[90] Chiesa AG et al. Ovarian intestinal type mucinous borderline tumors: Are we ready for a nomenclature change? International Journal of Gynecological Pathology. 2010;**29**(2): 108-112

[91] Sampson JA. Endometrial carcinoma of the ovary, arising in endometrial tissue in that organ. Archives of Surgery. 1925;**10**(1):1-72

[92] Vercellini P et al. Site of origin of epithelial ovarian cancer: The endometriosis connection. BJOG. 2000;**107**(9):1155-1157

[93] Keita M et al. Endometrioid ovarian cancer and endometriotic cells exhibit the same alteration in the expression of interleukin-1 receptor II: To a link between endometriosis and endometrioid ovarian cancer. The Journal of Obstetrics and Gynaecology Research. 2011;**37**(2):99-107

[94] Wang Y et al. Tubal origin of ovarian endometriosis and clear cell and endometrioid carcinoma. American Journal of Cancer Research. 2015;**5**(3):869-879

[95] Prowse AH et al. Molecular genetic evidence that endometriosis is a precursor of ovarian cancer. International Journal of Cancer. 2006;**119**(3):556-562

[96] Zwart J, Geisler JP, Geisler HE. Five-year survival in patients with endometrioid carcinoma of the ovary versus those with serous carcinoma. European Journal of Gynaecological Oncology. 1998;**19**(3):225-228

[97] Bouchard-Fortier G et al. Endometrioid carcinoma of the ovary: Outcomes compared to serous carcinoma after 10 years of follow-up. Journal of Obstetrics and Gynaecology Canada. 2017;**39**(1):34-41

[98] Mangili G et al. Unraveling the two entities of endometrioid ovarian cancer: A single center clinical experience. Gynecologic Oncology. 2012;**126**(3):403-407

[99] Schwartz DR et al. Gene expression in ovarian cancer reflects both morphology and biological behavior, distinguishing clear cell from other poor-prognosis ovarian carcinomas. Cancer Research. 2002;**62**(16):4722-4729

[100] Schwartz DR et al. Novel candidate targets of beta-catenin/T-cell factor signaling identified by gene expression profiling of ovarian endometrioid adenocarcinomas. Cancer Research. 2003;**63**(11):2913-2922

[101] McConechy MK et al. Ovarian and endometrial endometrioid carcinomas have distinct CTNNB1 and PTEN mutation profiles. Modern Pathology. 2014;**27**(1):128-134

[102] Wiegand KC et al. ARID1A mutations in endometriosis-associated ovarian carcinomas. The New England Journal of Medicine. 2010;**363**(16):1532-1543

[103] Obata K et al. Frequent PTEN/MMAC mutations in endometrioid but not serous or mucinous epithelial ovarian tumors. Cancer Research. 1998;**58**(10):2095-2097

[104] Coward JI, Middleton K, Murphy F. New perspectives on targeted therapy in ovarian cancer. International Journal of Women's Health. 2015;**7**:189-203

[105] Mabuchi S et al. The PI3K/AKT/mTOR pathway as a therapeutic target in ovarian cancer. Gynecologic Oncology. 2015;**137**(1):173-179

[106] Riopel MA, Ronnett BM, Kurman RJ. Evaluation of diagnostic criteria and behavior of ovarian intestinal-type mucinous tumors: Atypical proliferative (borderline) tumors and intraepithelial, microinvasive, invasive, and metastatic carcinomas. The American Journal of Surgical Pathology. 1999;**23**(6):617-635

[107] Lee KR, Young RH. The distinction between primary and metastatic mucinous carcinomas of the ovary: Gross and histologic findings in 50 cases. The American Journal of Surgical Pathology. 2003;**27**(3):281-292

[108] Seidman JD, Kurman RJ, Ronnett BM. Primary and metastatic mucinous adenocarcinomas in the ovaries: Incidence in routine practice with a new approach to improve intraoperative diagnosis. The American Journal of Surgical Pathology. 2003;**27**(7):985-993

[109] Leitao MM Jr et al. Clinicopathologic analysis of early-stage sporadic ovarian carcinoma. The American Journal of Surgical Pathology. 2004;**28**(2):147-159

[110] Schiavone MB et al. Natural history and outcome of mucinous carcinoma of the ovary. American Journal of Obstetrics and Gynecology. 2011;**205**(5):480. e1-480. e8

[111] Kobel M et al. Differences in tumor type in low-stage versus high-stage ovarian carcinomas. International Journal of Gynecological Pathology. 2010;**29**(3):203-211

[112] Simons M et al. Relatively poor survival of mucinous ovarian carcinoma in advanced stage: A systematic review and meta-analysis. International Journal of Gynecological Cancer. 2017;**27**(4):651-658

[113] Vang R et al. Cytokeratins 7 and 20 in primary and secondary mucinous tumors of the ovary: Analysis of coordinate immunohistochemical expression profiles and staining distribution in 179 cases. The American Journal of Surgical Pathology. 2006;**30**(9):1130-1139

[114] Vang R et al. Ovarian mucinous tumors associated with mature cystic teratomas: Morphologic and immunohistochemical analysis identifies a subset of potential teratomatous origin that shares features of lower gastrointestinal tract mucinous tumors more commonly encountered as secondary tumors in the ovary. The American Journal of Surgical Pathology. 2007;**31**(6):854-869

[115] Vang R et al. Immunohistochemical expression of CDX2 in primary ovarian mucinous tumors and metastatic mucinous carcinomas involving the ovary: Comparison with CK20 and correlation with coordinate expression of CK7. Modern Pathology. 2006;**19**(11):1421-1428

[116] Moh M et al. SATB2 expression distinguishes ovarian metastases of colorectal and appendiceal origin from primary ovarian tumors of mucinous or endometrioid type. The American Journal of Surgical Pathology. 2016;**40**(3):419-432

[117] Ordonez NG. Value of PAX 8 immunostaining in tumor diagnosis: A review and update. Advances in Anatomic Pathology. 2012;**19**(3):140-151

[118] Hess V et al. Mucinous epithelial ovarian cancer: A separate entity requiring specific treatment. Journal of Clinical Oncology. 2004;**22**(6):1040-1044

[119] Wamunyokoli FW et al. Expression profiling of mucinous tumors of the ovary identifies genes of clinicopathologic importance. Clinical Cancer Research. 2006;**12**(3 Pt 1):690-700

[120] Zaino RJ et al. Advanced stage mucinous adenocarcinoma of the ovary is both rare and highly lethal: A Gynecologic oncology group study. Cancer. 2011;**117**(3):554-562

[121] Teer JK et al. Mutational heterogeneity in non-serous ovarian cancers. Scientific Reports. 2017;**7**(1):9728

[122] Cuatrecasas M et al. K-ras mutations in mucinous ovarian tumors: A clinicopathologic and molecular study of 95 cases. Cancer. 1997;**79**(8):1581-1586

[123] Lin WL et al. Identification of the coexisting HER2 gene amplification and novel mutations in the HER2 protein-overexpressed mucinous epithelial ovarian cancer. Annals of Surgical Oncology. 2011;**18**(8):2388-2394

[124] Ryland GL et al. Mutational landscape of mucinous ovarian carcinoma and its neoplastic precursors. Genome Medicine. 2015;**7**(1):87

[125] Gore ME et al. Multicentre trial of carboplatin/paclitaxel versus oxaliplatin/capecitabine, each with/without bevacizumab, as first line chemotherapy for patients with mucinous epithelial ovarian cancer (mEOC). American Society of Clinical Oncology. 2015;**33**:5528-5528

[126] McAlpine JN et al. HER2 overexpression and amplification is present in a subset of ovarian mucinous carcinomas and can be targeted with trastuzumab therapy. BMC Cancer. 2009;**9**:433

[127] McCaughan H et al. HER2 expression in ovarian carcinoma: Caution and complexity in biomarker analysis. Journal of Clinical Pathology. 2012;**65**(7):670-671; author reply 671-2

[128] Sugiyama T et al. Clinical characteristics of clear cell carcinoma of the ovary: A distinct histologic type with poor prognosis and resistance to platinum-based chemotherapy. Cancer. 2000;**88**(11):2584-2589

[129] Tung KH et al. Reproductive factors and epithelial ovarian cancer risk by histologic type: A multiethnic case-control study. American Journal of Epidemiology. 2003;**158**(7):629-638

[130] Kandalaft PL, Gown AM, Isacson C. The lung-restricted marker napsin a is highly expressed in clear cell carcinomas of the ovary. American Journal of Clinical Pathology. 2014;**142**(6):830-836

[131] Zorn KK et al. Gene expression profiles of serous, endometrioid, and clear cell subtypes of ovarian and endometrial cancer. Clinical Cancer Research. 2005;**11**(18):6422-6430

[132] Domcke S et al. Evaluating cell lines as tumour models by comparison of genomic profiles. Nature Communications. 2013;**4**:2126

[133] Tan DS et al. Genomic analysis reveals the molecular heterogeneity of ovarian clear cell carcinomas. Clinical Cancer Research. 2011;**17**(6):1521-1534

[134] Zannoni GF et al. Mutational status of KRAS, NRAS, and BRAF in primary clear cell ovarian carcinoma. Virchows Archiv. 2014;**465**(2):193-198

[135] Campbell IG et al. Mutation of the PIK3CA gene in ovarian and breast cancer. Cancer Research. 2004;**64**(21):7678-7681

[136] Alsop K et al. BRCA mutation frequency and patterns of treatment response in BRCA mutation-positive women with ovarian cancer: A report from the Australian ovarian cancer study group. Journal of Clinical Oncology. 2012;**30**(21):2654-2663

[137] Mabuchi S, Sugiyama T, Kimura T. Clear cell carcinoma of the ovary: Molecular insights and future therapeutic perspectives. Journal of Gynecologic Oncology. 2016;**27**(3):e31

[138] Oliver KE et al. An evaluation of progression free survival and overall survival of ovarian cancer patients with clear cell carcinoma versus serous carcinoma treated with platinum therapy: An NRG oncology/Gynecologic oncology group experience. Gynecologic Oncology. 2017

[139] Sancho-Torres I et al. Clear cell carcinoma of the ovary: Characterization of its CD44 isoform repertoire. Gynecologic Oncology. 2000;**79**(2):187-195

[140] Anglesio MS et al. IL6-STAT3-HIF signaling and therapeutic response to the angiogenesis inhibitor sunitinib in ovarian clear cell cancer. Clinical Cancer Research. 2011;**17**(8):2538-2548

[141] Fathalla MF. Incessant ovulation--a factor in ovarian neoplasia? Lancet. 1971;**2**(7716):163

[142] Fleming JS et al. Incessant ovulation, inflammation and epithelial ovarian carcinogenesis: Revisiting old hypotheses. Molecular and Cellular Endocrinology. 2006;**247**(1-2):4-21

[143] Fathalla MF. Incessant ovulation and ovarian cancer - a hypothesis re-visited. Facts, Views & Vision in ObGyn. 2013;**5**(4):292-297

[144] Banks RE et al. Circulating intercellular adhesion molecule-1 (ICAM-1), E-selectin and vascular cell adhesion molecule-1 (VCAM-1) in human malignancies. British Journal of Cancer. 1993;**68**(1):122-124

[145] Land JA. Ovulation, ovulation induction and ovarian carcinoma. Baillière's Clinical Obstetrics and Gynaecology. 1993;**7**(2):455-472

[146] Fredrickson TN. Ovarian tumors of the hen. Environmental Health Perspectives. 1987;**73**:35-51

[147] Lee J, Song G. The laying hen: An animal model for human ovarian cancer. Reproductive & Developmental Biology. 2013;**37**:41-49

[148] Godwin AK et al. Spontaneous transformation of rat ovarian surface epithelial cells: Association with cytogenetic changes and implications of repeated ovulation in the etiology of ovarian cancer. Journal of the National Cancer Institute. 1992;**84**(8):592-601

[149] Godwin AK, Testa JR, Hamilton TC. The biology of ovarian cancer development. Cancer. 1993;**71**(2 Suppl):530-536

[150] Perez RP et al. Transformation of rat ovarian epithelial and Rat-1 fibroblast cell lines by RAST24 does not influence cisplatin sensitivity. Cancer Research. 1993;**53**(16):3771-3775

[151] Testa JR et al. Spontaneous transformation of rat ovarian surface epithelial cells results in well to poorly differentiated tumors with a parallel range of cytogenetic complexity. Cancer Research. 1994;**54**(10):2778-2784

[152] Auersperg N et al. Expression of two mucin antigens in cultured human ovarian surface epithelium: Influence of a family history of ovarian cancer. American Journal of Obstetrics and Gynecology. 1995;**173**(2):558-565

[153] Godwin AK et al. Retroviral-like sequences specifically expressed in the rat ovary detect genetic differences between normal and transformed rat ovarian surface epithelial cells. Endocrinology. 1995;**136**(10):4640-4649

[154] Salazar H et al. Microscopic benign and invasive malignant neoplasms and a cancer-prone phenotype in prophylactic oophorectomies. Journal of the National Cancer Institute. 1996;**88**(24):1810-1820

[155] Dyck HG et al. Autonomy of the epithelial phenotype in human ovarian surface epithelium: Changes with neoplastic progression and with a family history of ovarian cancer. International Journal of Cancer. 1996;**69**(6):429-436

[156] Abdollahi A et al. Identification of a gene containing zinc-finger motifs based on lost expression in malignantly transformed rat ovarian surface epithelial cells. Cancer Research. 1997;**57**(10):2029-2034

[157] Abdollahi A et al. Genome scanning detects amplification of the cathepsin B gene (CtsB) in transformed rat ovarian surface epithelial cells. Journal of the Society for Gynecologic Investigation. 1999;**6**(1):32-40

[158] Kruk PA et al. Telomeric instability and reduced proliferative potential in ovarian surface epithelial cells from women with a family history of ovarian cancer. Gynecologic Oncology. 1999;**73**(2):229-236

[159] Roberts D et al. Decreased expression of retinol-binding proteins is associated with malignant transformation of the ovarian surface epithelium. DNA and Cell Biology. 2002;**21**(1):11-19

[160] Yang DH et al. Molecular events associated with dysplastic morphologic transformation and initiation of ovarian tumorigenicity. Cancer. 2002;**94**(9):2380-2392

[161] Roland IH et al. Loss of surface and cyst epithelial basement membranes and pre-neoplastic morphologic changes in prophylactic oophorectomies. Cancer. 2003;**98**(12): 2607-2623

[162] Flesken-Nikitin A et al. Induction of carcinogenesis by concurrent inactivation of p53 and Rb1 in the mouse ovarian surface epithelium. Cancer Research. 2003;**63**(13):3459-3463

[163] Kindelberger DW et al. Intraepithelial carcinoma of the fimbria and pelvic serous carcinoma: Evidence for a causal relationship. The American Journal of Surgical Pathology. 2007;**31**(2):161-169

[164] Lee Y et al. A candidate precursor to serous carcinoma that originates in the distal fallopian tube. The Journal of Pathology. 2007;**211**(1):26-35

[165] Rebbeck TR et al. Prophylactic oophorectomy in carriers of BRCA1 or BRCA2 mutations. The New England Journal of Medicine. 2002;**346**(21):1616-1622

[166] Olivier RI et al. Clinical outcome of prophylactic oophorectomy in BRCA1/BRCA2 mutation carriers and events during follow-up. British Journal of Cancer. 2004;**90**(8):1492-1497

[167] Cibula D et al. Tubal ligation and the risk of ovarian cancer: Review and meta-analysis. Human Reproduction Update. 2011;**17**(1):55-67

[168] Gross AL et al. Precursor lesions of high-grade serous ovarian carcinoma: Morphological and molecular characteristics. Journal of Oncology. 2010;**2010**:126295

[169] Crum CP et al. Lessons from BRCA: The tubal fimbria emerges as an origin for pelvic serous cancer. Clinical Medicine & Research. 2007;**5**(1):35-44

[170] Callahan MJ et al. Primary fallopian tube malignancies in BRCA-positive women undergoing surgery for ovarian cancer risk reduction. Journal of Clinical Oncology. 2007;**25**(25):3985-3990

[171] Piek JM et al. Dysplastic changes in prophylactically removed fallopian tubes of women predisposed to developing ovarian cancer. The Journal of Pathology. 2001;**195**(4):451-456

[172] Shaw PA et al. Candidate serous cancer precursors in fallopian tube epithelium of BRCA1/2 mutation carriers. Modern Pathology. 2009;**22**(9):1133-1138

[173] Medeiros F et al. The tubal fimbria is a preferred site for early adenocarcinoma in women with familial ovarian cancer syndrome. The American Journal of Surgical Pathology. 2006;**30**(2):230-236

[174] Folkins AK et al. A candidate precursor to pelvic serous cancer (p53 signature) and its prevalence in ovaries and fallopian tubes from women with BRCA mutations. Gynecologic Oncology. 2008;**109**(2):168-173

[175] Akbari MR et al. The spectrum of BRCA1 and BRCA2 mutations in breast cancer patients in the Bahamas. Clinical Genetics. 2014;**85**(1):64-67

[176] Tone AA et al. Gene expression profiles of luteal phase fallopian tube epithelium from BRCA mutation carriers resemble high-grade serous carcinoma. Clinical Cancer Research. 2008;**14**(13):4067-4078

[177] Karst AM, Levanon K, Drapkin R. Modeling high-grade serous ovarian carcinogenesis from the fallopian tube. Proceedings of the National Academy of Sciences of the United States of America. 2011;**108**(18):7547-7552

[178] Perets R et al. Transformation of the fallopian tube secretory epithelium leads to high-grade serous ovarian cancer in Brca;Tp53;Pten models. Cancer Cell. 2013;**24**(6):751-765

[179] Salvador S et al. Chromosomal instability in fallopian tube precursor lesions of serous carcinoma and frequent monoclonality of synchronous ovarian and fallopian tube mucosal serous carcinoma. Gynecologic Oncology. 2008;**110**(3):408-417

[180] Karst AM et al. Cyclin E1 deregulation occurs early in secretory cell transformation to promote formation of fallopian tube-derived high-grade serous ovarian cancers. Cancer Research. 2014;**74**(4):1141-1152

[181] Kuhn E et al. CCNE1 amplification and centrosome number abnormality in serous tubal intraepithelial carcinoma: Further evidence supporting its role as a precursor of ovarian high-grade serous carcinoma. Modern Pathology. 2016;**29**(10):1254-1261

[182] McDaniel AS et al. Next-generation sequencing of tubal intraepithelial carcinomas. JAMA Oncology. 2015;**1**(8):1128-1132

[183] Wicha MS, Liu S, Dontu G. Cancer stem cells: An old idea–a paradigm shift. Cancer Research. 2006;**66**(4):1883-1890; discussion 1895-6

[184] Marsden CG et al. Breast tumor-initiating cells isolated from patient core biopsies for study of hormone action. Methods in Molecular Biology. 2009;**590**:363-375

[185] Singh SK et al. Identification of a cancer stem cell in human brain tumors. Cancer Research. 2003;**63**(18):5821-5828

[186] Collins AT et al. Prospective identification of tumorigenic prostate cancer stem cells. Cancer Research. 2005;**65**(23):10946-10951

[187] Ricci-Vitiani L et al. Identification and expansion of human colon-cancer-initiating cells. Nature. 2007;**445**(7123):111-115

[188] Kreso A, Dick JE. Evolution of the cancer stem cell model. Cell Stem Cell. 2014;**14**(3):275-291

[189] Capel B. Ovarian epithelium regeneration by Lgr5(+) cells. Nature Cell Biology. 2014;**16**(8):743-744

[190] Ng A et al. Lgr5 marks stem/progenitor cells in ovary and tubal epithelia. Nature Cell Biology. 2014;**16**(8):745-757

[191] Bowen NJ et al. Gene expression profiling supports the hypothesis that human ovarian surface epithelia are multipotent and capable of serving as ovarian cancer initiating cells. BMC Medical Genomics. 2009;**2**:71

[192] Flesken-Nikitin A et al. Ovarian surface epithelium at the junction area contains a cancer-prone stem cell niche. Nature. 2013;**495**(7440):241-245

[193] Kessler M et al. The notch and Wnt pathways regulate stemness and differentiation in human fallopian tube organoids. Nature Communications. 2015;**6**:8989

[194] Paik DY et al. Stem-like epithelial cells are concentrated in the distal end of the fallopian tube: A site for injury and serous cancer initiation. Stem Cells. 2012;**30**(11):2487-2497

[195] Wang Y et al. Identification of quiescent, stem-like cells in the distal female reproductive tract. PLoS One. 2012;**7**(7):e40691

[196] Hellner K et al. Premalignant SOX2 overexpression in the fallopian tubes of ovarian cancer patients: Discovery and validation studies. eBioMedicine. 2016;**10**:137-149

[197] Ziogas A et al. Cancer risk estimates for family members of a population-based family registry for breast and ovarian cancer. Cancer Epidemiology, Biomarkers & Prevention. 2000;**9**(1):103-111

[198] Bewtra C et al. Hereditary ovarian cancer: A clinicopathological study. International Journal of Gynecological Pathology. 1992;**11**(3):180-187

[199] Lynch HT, Krush AJ. Carcinoma of the breast and ovary in three families. Surgery, Gynecology & Obstetrics. 1971;**133**(4):644-648

[200] Lynch HT et al. Familial association of carcinoma of the breast and ovary. Surgery, Gynecology & Obstetrics. 1974;**138**(5):717-724

[201] Miki Y et al. A strong candidate for the breast and ovarian cancer susceptibility gene BRCA1. Science. 1994;**266**(5182):66-71

[202] Wooster R et al. Localization of a breast cancer susceptibility gene, BRCA2, to chromosome 13q12-13. Science. 1994;**265**(5181):2088-2090

[203] Wooster R et al. Identification of the breast cancer susceptibility gene BRCA2. Nature. 1995;**378**(6559):789-792

[204] Peto J et al. Prevalence of BRCA1 and BRCA2 gene mutations in patients with early-onset breast cancer. Journal of the National Cancer Institute. 1999;**91**(11):943-949

[205] Whittemore AS et al. Prevalence of BRCA1 mutation carriers among U.S. non-Hispanic whites. Cancer Epidemiology, Biomarkers & Prevention. 2004;**13**(12):2078-2083

[206] Struewing JP et al. The risk of cancer associated with specific mutations of BRCA1 and BRCA2 among Ashkenazi Jews. The New England Journal of Medicine. 1997;**336**(20):1401-1408

[207] Rubin SC et al. BRCA1, BRCA2, and hereditary nonpolyposis colorectal cancer gene mutations in an unselected ovarian cancer population: Relationship to family history and implications for genetic testing. American Journal of Obstetrics and Gynecology. 1998;**178**(4):670-677

[208] Ford D et al. Risks of cancer in BRCA1-mutation carriers. Breast cancer linkage consortium. Lancet. 1994;**343**(8899):692-695

[209] Easton DF, Ford D, Bishop DT. Breast and ovarian cancer incidence in BRCA1-mutation carriers. Breast cancer linkage consortium. American Journal of Human Genetics. 1995;**56**(1):265-271

[210] Chen S, Parmigiani G. Meta-analysis of BRCA1 and BRCA2 penetrance. Journal of Clinical Oncology. 2007;**25**(11):1329-1333

[211] Kuchenbaecker KB et al. Risks of breast, ovarian, and contralateral breast cancer for BRCA1 and BRCA2 mutation carriers. JAMA. 2017;**317**(23):2402-2416

[212] Antoniou A et al. Average risks of breast and ovarian cancer associated with BRCA1 or BRCA2 mutations detected in case series unselected for family history: A combined analysis of 22 studies. American Journal of Human Genetics. 2003;**72**(5):1117-1130

[213] King MC, Marks JH, Mandell JB. Breast and ovarian cancer risks due to inherited mutations in BRCA1 and BRCA2. Science. 2003;**302**(5645):643-646

[214] Sogaard M, Kjaer SK, Gayther S. Ovarian cancer and genetic susceptibility in relation to the BRCA1 and BRCA2 genes. Occurrence, clinical importance and intervention. Acta Obstetricia et Gynecologica Scandinavica. 2006;**85**(1):93-105

[215] Rebbeck TR et al. Association of type and location of BRCA1 and BRCA2 mutations with risk of breast and ovarian cancer. JAMA. 2015;**313**(13):1347-1361

[216] Mavaddat N et al. Pathology of breast and ovarian cancers among BRCA1 and BRCA2 mutation carriers: Results from the consortium of investigators of modifiers of BRCA1/2 (CIMBA). Cancer Epidemiology, Biomarkers & Prevention. 2012;**21**(1):134-147

[217] Ramus SJ et al. Ovarian cancer susceptibility alleles and risk of ovarian cancer in BRCA1 and BRCA2 mutation carriers. Human Mutation. 2012;**33**(4):690-702

[218] Antoniou AC et al. RAD51 135G-->C modifies breast cancer risk among BRCA2 mutation carriers: Results from a combined analysis of 19 studies. American Journal of Human Genetics. 2007;**81**(6):1186-1200

[219] Osorio A et al. DNA glycosylases involved in base excision repair may be associated with cancer risk in BRCA1 and BRCA2 mutation carriers. PLoS Genetics. 2014;**10**(4):e1004256

[220] Couch FJ et al. Genome-wide association study in BRCA1 mutation carriers identifies novel loci associated with breast and ovarian cancer risk. PLoS Genetics. 2013;**9**(3):e1003212

[221] Ding YC et al. A nonsynonymous polymorphism in IRS1 modifies risk of developing breast and ovarian cancers in BRCA1 and ovarian cancer in BRCA2 mutation carriers. Cancer Epidemiology, Biomarkers & Prevention. 2012;**21**(8):1362-1370

[222] Jakubowska A et al. Association of PHB 1630 C>T and MTHFR 677 C>T polymorphisms with breast and ovarian cancer risk in BRCA1/2 mutation carriers: Results from a multicenter study. British Journal of Cancer. 2012;**106**(12):2016-2024

[223] Castilla LH et al. Mutations in the BRCA1 gene in families with early-onset breast and ovarian cancer. Nature Genetics. 1994;**8**(4):387-391

[224] Tonin P et al. Frequency of recurrent BRCA1 and BRCA2 mutations in Ashkenazi Jewish breast cancer families. Nature Medicine. 1996;**2**(11):1179-1183

[225] Berman DB et al. A common mutation in BRCA2 that predisposes to a variety of cancers is found in both Jewish Ashkenazi and non-Jewish individuals. Cancer Research. 1996;**56**(15):3409-3414

[226] Bergthorsson JT et al. Identification of a novel splice-site mutation of the BRCA1 gene in two breast cancer families: Screening reveals low frequency in Icelandic breast cancer patients. Human Mutation. 1998;(Suppl 1):S195-S197

[227] Liu G et al. Differing clinical impact of BRCA1 and BRCA2 mutations in serous ovarian cancer. Pharmacogenomics. 2012;**13**(13):1523-1535

[228] Candido-dos-Reis FJ et al. Germline mutation in BRCA1 or BRCA2 and ten-year survival for women diagnosed with epithelial ovarian cancer. Clinical Cancer Research. 2015;**21**(3):652-657

[229] Gorodnova TV et al. High response rates to neoadjuvant platinum-based therapy in ovarian cancer patients carrying germ-line BRCA mutation. Cancer Letters. 2015;**369**(2):363-367

[230] Goode EL et al. A genome-wide association study identifies susceptibility loci for ovarian cancer at 2q31 and 8q24. Nature Genetics. 2010;**42**(10):874-879

[231] Kuchenbaecker KB et al. Identification of six new susceptibility loci for invasive epithelial ovarian cancer. Nature Genetics. 2015;**47**(2):164-171

[232] Engel C et al. Association of the variants CASP8 D302H and CASP10 V410I with breast and ovarian cancer risk in BRCA1 and BRCA2 mutation carriers. Cancer Epidemiology, Biomarkers & Prevention. 2010;**19**(11):2859-2868

[233] Ratner E et al. A KRAS-variant in ovarian cancer acts as a genetic marker of cancer risk. Cancer Research. 2010;**70**(16):6509-6515

[234] Potapova A et al. Promoter hypermethylation of the PALB2 susceptibility gene in inherited and sporadic breast and ovarian cancer. Cancer Research. 2008;**68**(4):998-1002

[235] Walker LC et al. Evaluation of copy-number variants as modifiers of breast and ovarian cancer risk for BRCA1 pathogenic variant carriers. European Journal of Human Genetics. 2017;**25**(4):432-438

[236] Bojesen SE et al. Multiple independent variants at the TERT locus are associated with telomere length and risks of breast and ovarian cancer. Nature Genetics. 2013;**45**(4):371-384 384e1-2

[237] Walsh T et al. Mutations in 12 genes for inherited ovarian, fallopian tube, and peritoneal carcinoma identified by massively parallel sequencing. Proceedings of the National Academy of Sciences of the United States of America. 2011;**108**(44):18032-18037

[238] Pennington KP, Swisher EM. Hereditary ovarian cancer: Beyond the usual suspects. Gynecologic Oncology. 2012;**124**(2):347-353

[239] Song H et al. Contribution of germline mutations in the RAD51B, RAD51C, and RAD51D genes to ovarian cancer in the population. Journal of Clinical Oncology. 2015;**33**(26):2901-2907

[240] Ketabi Z et al. Ovarian cancer linked to lynch syndrome typically presents as early-onset, non-serous epithelial tumors. Gynecologic Oncology. 2011;**121**(3):462-465

[241] Crispens MA. Endometrial and ovarian cancer in lynch syndrome. Clinics in Colon and Rectal Surgery. 2012;**25**(2):97-102

[242] Malander S et al. The contribution of the hereditary nonpolyposis colorectal cancer syndrome to the development of ovarian cancer. Gynecologic Oncology. 2006;**101**(2): 238-243

[243] Gwinn ML et al. Pregnancy, breast feeding, and oral contraceptives and the risk of epithelial ovarian cancer. Journal of Clinical Epidemiology. 1990;**43**(6):559-568

[244] Rice MS, Hankinson SE, Tworoger SS. Tubal ligation, hysterectomy, unilateral oophorectomy, and risk of ovarian cancer in the Nurses' health studies. Fertility and Sterility. 2014;**102**(1):192-198 e3

[245] Gaitskell K et al. Tubal ligation and ovarian cancer risk in a large cohort: Substantial variation by histological type. International Journal of Cancer. 2016;**138**(5):1076-1084

[246] Kauff ND et al. Risk-reducing salpingo-oophorectomy for the prevention of BRCA1- and BRCA2-associated breast and gynecologic cancer: A multicenter, prospective study. Journal of Clinical Oncology. 2008;**26**(8):1331-1337

[247] Beral V et al. Ovarian cancer and oral contraceptives: Collaborative reanalysis of data from 45 epidemiological studies including 23,257 women with ovarian cancer and 87,303 controls. Lancet. 2008;**371**(9609):303-314

[248] Havrilesky LJ et al. Oral contraceptive pills as primary prevention for ovarian cancer: A systematic review and meta-analysis. Obstetrics and Gynecology. 2013;**122**(1):139-147

[249] Moorman PG et al. Oral contraceptives and risk of ovarian cancer and breast cancer among high-risk women: A systematic review and meta-analysis. Journal of Clinical Oncology. 2013;**31**(33):4188-4198

[250] Bassuk SS, Manson JE. Oral contraceptives and menopausal hormone therapy: Relative and attributable risks of cardiovascular disease, cancer, and other health outcomes. Annals of Epidemiology. 2015;**25**(3):193-200

[251] Wentzensen N et al. Ovarian cancer risk factors by histologic subtype: An analysis from the ovarian cancer cohort consortium. Journal of Clinical Oncology. 2016;**34**(24):2888-2898

[252] Havrilesky LJ et al. Oral contraceptive use for the primary prevention of ovarian cancer. Evidence report/technology assessment (Full Report). 2013;**212**:1-514

[253] Hankinson SE et al. A prospective study of reproductive factors and risk of epithelial ovarian cancer. Cancer. 1995;**76**(2):284-290

[254] Adami HO et al. Parity, age at first childbirth, and risk of ovarian cancer. Lancet. 1994;**344**(8932):1250-1254

[255] Tsilidis KK et al. Oral contraceptive use and reproductive factors and risk of ovarian cancer in the European prospective investigation into cancer and nutrition. British Journal of Cancer. 2011;**105**(9):1436-1442

[256] Schildkraut JM et al. Age at natural menopause and the risk of epithelial ovarian cancer. Obstetrics and Gynecology. 2001;**98**(1):85-90

[257] Pearce CL et al. Increased ovarian cancer risk associated with menopausal estrogen therapy is reduced by adding a progestin. Cancer. 2009;**115**(3):531-539

[258] Morch LS et al. Hormone therapy and ovarian cancer. JAMA. 2009;**302**(3):298-305

[259] Hildebrand JS et al. Postmenopausal hormone use and incident ovarian cancer: Associations differ by regimen. International Journal of Cancer. 2010;**127**(12):2928-2935

[260] Beral V et al. Menopausal hormone use and ovarian cancer risk: Individual participant meta-analysis of 52 epidemiological studies. Lancet. 2015;**385**(9980):1835-1842

[261] Eeles RA et al. Adjuvant hormone therapy may improve survival in epithelial ovarian cancer: Results of the AHT randomized trial. Journal of Clinical Oncology. 2015;**33**(35):4138-4144

[262] Luan NN et al. Breastfeeding and ovarian cancer risk: A meta-analysis of epidemiologic studies. The American Journal of Clinical Nutrition. 2013;**98**(4):1020-1031

[263] Beral V et al. Ovarian cancer and smoking: Individual participant meta-analysis including 28,114 women with ovarian cancer from 51 epidemiological studies. The Lancet Oncology. 2012;**13**(9):946-956

[264] Jordan SJ et al. Does smoking increase risk of ovarian cancer? A systematic review. Gynecologic Oncology. 2006;**103**(3):1122-1129

[265] Gram IT et al. Cigarette smoking and risk of histological subtypes of epithelial ovarian cancer in the EPIC cohort study. International Journal of Cancer. 2012;**130**(9):2204-2210

[266] Gwinn ML et al. Alcohol consumption and ovarian cancer risk. American Journal of Epidemiology. 1986;**123**(5):759-766

[267] Genkinger JM et al. Alcohol intake and ovarian cancer risk: A pooled analysis of 10 cohort studies. British Journal of Cancer. 2006;**94**(5):757-762

[268] Rota M et al. Alcohol drinking and epithelial ovarian cancer risk. A systematic review and meta-analysis. Gynecologic Oncology. 2012;**125**(3):758-763

[269] Olsen CM et al. Obesity and risk of ovarian cancer subtypes: Evidence from the ovarian cancer association consortium. Endocrine-Related Cancer. 2013;**20**(2):251-262

[270] Cannioto RA, Moysich KB. Epithelial ovarian cancer and recreational physical activity: A review of the epidemiological literature and implications for exercise prescription. Gynecologic Oncology. 2015;**137**(3):559-573

[271] Ness RB, Cottreau C. Possible role of ovarian epithelial inflammation in ovarian cancer. Journal of the National Cancer Institute. 1999;**91**(17):1459-1467

[272] Trabert B et al. Aspirin, nonaspirin nonsteroidal anti-inflammatory drug, and acetaminophen use and risk of invasive epithelial ovarian cancer: A pooled analysis in the ovarian cancer association consortium. Journal of the National Cancer Institute. 2014;**106**(2):djt431

4

Locally Advanced Cervical Carcinoma Management

Achille Manirakiza, Sumi Sinha and
Fidel Rubagumya

Abstract

Cervical cancer is a public health burden to Low and Middle Income countries. Whereas strides are being made in the management of malignancies worldwide, resources limited settings are confronted with the paucity of basic awareness, health professionals, diagnosis and management modalities, all contributing to cervical cancer disease late presentation. Among available treatment modalities, the mainstay of treatment for locally advanced cervical cancer remains radiation therapy combined with chemotherapy. Radiation is delivered through external radiation and brachytherapy. The evidence leading to the decision making, the modern management modalities and the general side effects, will be reviewed here.

Keywords: cervical cancer, radiation, brachytherapy

1. Introduction

Cervical cancer represents the second most common malignancy and the third overall cause of cancer mortality in Low and Middle Income Countries (LMICs) [1]. Such countries contribute the majority of the cervical cancer burden worldwide.

The FIGO classification system, endorsed by the American Joint Commission on Cancer 2017, defines locally advanced cervical cancer, as a disease found between stages IB2 to IVA [2]. This subset of diseases is visible on clinical examination and usually predict worse outcome in terms of recurrence and survival rates when compared to early stage disease.

Several studies focusing on the different stages at initial presentation have shown consistently high rates of advanced disease in LMICs (**Table 1**).

Studies	Type	Country	Patients (N)	Stage (rate percentage) at presentation
Chirenje et al. [5]	CS[2]	Zimbabwe	196	Stages IIB - IVA: (80.3%)
Musa et al. [4]	R[1]	Nigeria	65	IA (1.5%) -
				IB (6.1%);
				IIA (20%);
				IIB (35.4%);
				IIIA (9.2%),
				IIIB (24.6%);
				IVA (3.1%)
Mlange et al. [6]	CS[2]	Tanzania	212	IA (1.4%),
				IB (28.2%),
				IIA (6.4%),
				IIB (20.4%),
				IIIA (15.8%),
				IIIB (17.3%),
				IVA (7.4%)
Sharma et al. [3]	R[1]	India	227	IA (3.9%),
				IB (8.7%),
				IIA (6.8%),
				IIB (32.5%),
				IIIA (6.8%),
				IIIB (30.7%),
				IVA (8.7%); IVB (1.9%)

[1]R = retrospective review.
[2]CS = cross-sectional study.

Table 1. Summary of rates of cervical carcinoma disease stage at presentation in LMICs.

Advanced stages present a considerable challenge to achieving adequate treatment. This is compounded by the absence of modern treatment modalities and technologies that are available in high-income countries (HIC).

LMICs face a double burden where patients for different reasons including health system factors presents at hospital with advanced diseases and at the same time there is a pronounced lack of infrastructure to take care of these patients. This leads to an overall poor survival rates.

2. Disease evaluation

Staging with full nodal evaluation remains a crucial aspect of the management of locally advanced cervical carcinoma.

The pattern of spread of cervical cancer follows principles seen in numerous other solid malignancies namely, local extension, lymphatic spread and distant metastasis.

The disease usually spreads directly distally to the vagina, with extension along the parametria, the uterine ligaments (commonly utero-sacral) and the peri-rectal area.

Lymphatic spread occurs by echelon from the pelvic nodes, usually proximally toward the para-aortic nodes, and could substantially lead to left supraclavicular lymph node involvement in rare cases.

There is a high correlation between nodal status and disease outcomes. Contemporary studies have estimated close to 40% of survival at 5-years follow-up if evidence of para-aortic node involvement is established. Risk of nodal metastasis increases approximately by 15% for each stage, from FIGO stage I to III.

A Computed-Tomography (CT) guided biopsy is needed for nodal disease confirmation. For expert centers, an F-18 fluorodeoxyglucose-based positron emission tomography (PET) scan is necessary to establish nodal disease.

The patient needs also to be screened for competing risk factors. Importantly, patients should be evaluated for present or acquired (by local extension, Stage IIIB) kidney disease as the management of locally advanced cervical carcinoma incorporates the use of platinum-based chemotherapy as a radio-sensitizer. Corrections to the management protocols related to the renal disease stage have been suggested and carry promising grounds for further prospective studies.

Disease staging provides ground for prognosis, local control and survival prediction in the presence of adequate management modalities. Survival rates vary across studies and are inversely related to stage, with disease control and 5-year overall survival both ranging from 90% for stage IB to only close to 30% for stage IVA, in recent studies.

For aggregate analyses of locally advanced cervical carcinoma management outcome-based studies, newer treatment techniques are providing encouraging survival data.

3. Locally advanced cervical carcinoma management

The standard of care for advanced cervical carcinoma is Radiation Therapy alone (in case of palliation), or in combination with cisplatin-based chemotherapy.

Overall survival is usually a function of disease-free interval rates, highlighting the scarcity of salvage therapy options in case of recurrence.

With limited options for salvage in cases of recurrences, disease-free interval rates directly correlate to Overall Survival and comorbidities of the patients.

Generally, management of cervical carcinoma includes definitive surgery for selected cases, upfront radiation therapy and chemo-radiation. Surgery and radiation therapy amount to the same effect yet with drastic differences in terms of debilitating toxicities, hence surgery alone is the treatment of choice for initial smaller lesions (<4 cm) with other treatment modalities offered as a salvage in case of recurrence.

4. Primary chemoradiation vs. surgery

As cited above, the widely used treatment scheme for locally advanced cervical carcinoma consists of upfront radiotherapy concurrently with a platinum-based chemotherapy.

Surgery has been proven to not be superior to chemo-radiation, but carries twice a risk of increased toxicity rates.

Adverse features arising post-surgery could be similar to other advanced diseases, including high grade disease, lympho-vascular space invasion (LVSI), positive lymph nodes, prompting the use of multiple modalities of treatment with subsequent considerable toxicities.

The largest comparison study to date by Landoni, compared 343 patients with early disease, contemporarily included in the locally advanced stage (IB - IIA) disease, to undergo an extensive surgery with pelvic lymph node dissection, with a possibility of Radiation Therapy boost in the presence residual disease. This arm was compared with upfront Radiation Therapy. The comparison yielded no differences in survival, but showed considerable difference in toxicity rates [7].

Chemo-radiation has been proven to offer a high survival benefit which is greatly influenced by disease stage. Additionally, concurrent chemo-radiation decreases the recurrence risk.

Radiation consists of external beam radiotherapy session and a stage-variable boosting dose achieved by brachytherapy. Details on patient simulation, field size and dose specification are found below.

5. Combined radiation and chemotherapy regimen

5.1. Chemotherapy regimens

Concurrent radiation with chemotherapy has come to age relatively recently, with cisplatin-based chemotherapy rising at the dawn of the twenty-first century.

Before this era, numerous institutional trials had been published with various chemotherapy regimens selections.

Among previously suggested regimens, hydroxyurea was used in the 1960s, perceived as being a radiosensitizer. Hydroxyurea induces a block on the G1-S phase of the cell cycle, hence enhancing cell kill by radiation; prevention of sub-lethal damage repair has also been proven.

A Gynecological Oncology Group (GOG 56) study confirmed the benefit of added hydroxyurea to radiation therapy, with a higher Progression Free interval, though no significant survival benefit was found [8]. This study was controversial in its setting and the recommendations were not applied widely. Hydroxyurea involves a high risk of myelosuppression, and prospects of considering it as a viable combination therapy to radiation were abandoned overtime.

5-Fluorouracil has also been considered as an alternative chemotherapy regimen for combination therapy. However, the few published studies failed to prove local disease control and survival benefit with an added 5-Fluorouracil regimen [9].

Based on a five-study analysis, cisplatin added to radiation therapy was confirmed to have a superior survival when compared to radiation alone.

A large systematic review of 18 trials combining radiation and chemotherapy for locally advanced cervical carcinoma proved the survival benefit of adding chemotherapy. Platinum based chemotherapy was not seen to be significantly different from non-platinum based chemotherapy (HR: 0.84 vs. 0.76, $p = 0.48$). Platinum-based regimens were also found to have a non-significant increased toxicity trend. However, single agent platinum offered an important alternative with regards to local disease control, adherence to treatment and ease of administration.

Historically, the GOG 120 compared different chemo-radiation regimens, combined with a brachytherapy boost. The arms had a cisplatin alone, a hydroxyurea alone and a cisplatin/5-Fluorouracil/Hydroxyurea components. The arms containing cisplatin had improved survival and disease down-staging was achieved. Subsequent studies removed hydroxyurea and compared upfront radiation therapy with concurrent cisplatin (with or without 5-Fluorouracil) with radiation therapy, which established the standard of care of adding chemotherapy to radiation therapy, as it was shown to increase survival and decrease recurrence risks.

The rationale behind adding cisplatin to radiation is that it acts as a radiosensitizer, by preventing the Non-Homologous End Joining pathway, which is paramount in the Double Strand Breaks repair. Double Strand Breaks in DNA are induced by high energy radiation therapy.

Cisplatin is given on a weekly basis, a few hours before radiation therapy, and care needs to be taken for its administration. As a nephrotoxic agent, adequate hydration is to be ensured, before and after cisplatin infusion. Together with knowing prior the renal status of the patient, dosing can be altered to prevent toxicity. Carboplatin has been shown to provide a suitable alternative to cisplatin for patients who are not candidates to cisplatin infusion (**Table 2**).

Gemcitabine could also be a choice when cisplatin is contraindicated. However, in the absence of level I evidence, and with the increased toxicity risk associated with Gemcitabine, carboplatin remains the preferred choice in case of intolerance to cisplatin, and deranged renal function tests.

5.2. Radiation therapy

Radiation Therapy is provided by both External Beam Radiation (EBRT) and brachytherapy (BT) to increase local control.

Cisplatin - dosage and premedications	Details
Prior to Treatment Work-up	Complete Blood Count - with a low Absolute Neutrophil Count, consider adding Filgrastim (if available) prior to chemotherapy infusion
	Renal Function Tests - use the Glomerular Filtration Rate to determine fitness of the patient to receive cisplatin
	Serum Electrolytes (K^+, Na^+)
Dosage	40 mg/m^2 IV weekly
Pre-medications	Hydration – 2 l Normal Saline (0.9%) over 2 hours prior and after a cisplatin infusion
	Ondansetron 16 mg IV and Dexamethasone 16 mg IV, both mixed with 100 ml of Normal Saline (0.9%)

Table 2. Summary—cisplatin treatment planning and dosage.

Total doses above 45 Gy are preferred as they are proven to offer a survival advantage.

Radiation therapy is offered to post-operative patients confirmed to have adverse features (mainly Lympho-Vascular Space Invasion, positive pelvic nodes, involved parametria and positive surgical margins), with stages IA2, IB. It is also the definitive treatment, with concurrent chemotherapy for stage IIB- IVA.

The typical dose given by EBRT varies between 45 and 50 Gy depending on the stage and prior treatment. For patients treated with a prior hysterectomy, lower doses (typically below 45 Gy) are preferred to avoid radiation induced bowel toxicity; higher doses are safe to be delivered on an intact uterus and cervix.

Current RTOG and GOG protocols suggest total doses for cervical carcinoma treated with definitive radiation therapy to be around 80–90 Gy to a point defined within the paracervical triangle, namely the point A.

The point A has been varied over the years, and is defined as being at 2 cm above the external cervical os and 2 cm lateral to uterus midline. This corresponds to the paracervical triangle, where the uterine vessels cross the ureter, medial to the broad ligament.

Given the proximity of the cervix to the major pelvic organs and the femoral heads, the external beam radiation doses are limited to an overall dose of 50 Gy. Institutional practices vary, some preferring doses below 45 Gy before proceeding to brachytherapy, with options of lowering the field size to boost to gross residual and nodal disease to doses up to 50 Gy.

Addition of brachytherapy has shown high rates of cancer-specific and overall survival benefits when compared to external beam radiation therapy alone. The objective of brachytherapy addition is to reach the desired total dose of 80–90 Gy to the disease site while minimizing toxicity to organs at risk.

5.3. External beam radiation techniques

The distal most part of the disease needs to be marked with radiopaque gold seeds for disease localization prior to treatment imaging. In the absence of gold seeds, radiopaque materials such as lead or steel-made wires can be used for disease localization. The same needs to be applied to the vagina and anus areas.

For a 4-field (antero-posterior, postero-anterior and lateral fields) treatment, the simulation is done in the supine position and CT or Fluoroscopic images taken. Patients are positioned with arms on the chest, knees and lower legs immobilized. Anterior and lateral tattoos are marked and aligned with lasers for lateral rotation prevention. Obese patients may benefit from prone belly boards, to avoid small bowel inclusion in the radiation volume.

Intra-venous contrast CT scans are taken to help highlight the pelvic vessels used as reference to delineate the pelvic nodes.

For centers using two-dimensional planning and fluoroscopic imaging, the same marking has to be done, with fluorescent markers, and tattoos where applicable.

The borders are:

- Superior: Lumbar spine level 4/5

- Lateral: 1.5–2 cm away from the pelvic brim

- Anterior: 1 cm anterior to pubic symphysis

- Posterior: Entire Sacrum to be included

- Inferior: Below the ischial tuberosity or the inferior obturator foramen if bony landmarks are used

For advanced disease involving the lower vagina (stage IIIA), include at least a margin of 3 cm away from the distal most part of the disease.

Extensive Radiation Therapy has been suggested in the presence of para-aortic lymph nodes, with the superior-most border being T12/L1, with kidney blocks [10].

Stage IIIA is associated with inguinal nodes, and the field needs to include the vaginal introitus as the inferior border; with a common iliac nodes disease presence, the superior border is to be raised up to L3/4.

Dosing should be up to 50 Gy delivered in 25 equal fractions, daily. This is usually given within 5 days a week for 5 weeks, allowing a 2-day rest between weeks of treatment.

Dose limiting organs are mainly the bladder, rectum, femoral heads, and with a lower instance, the small bowel and ovaries.

5.4. Brachytherapy

As per the American Brachytherapy Society guidelines, brachytherapy for cervical cancer needs to be applied for a disease not exceeding a size of 5 cm.

The preferred brachytherapy technique is the High Dose Rate Brachytherapy, delivering above 12 Gy/hour.

The point of interest for brachytherapy delivery is defined in the contemporary method as per the Manchester point A - 2 cm superior to the external cervical os and 2 cm lateral to the central uterine canal. The objective is to deliver a cumulative dose of 80–90 Gy.

Due to nodal disease associated with locally advanced cervical cancer, a Manchester point B is defined at 3 cm lateral to point A. With this system, bladder, vaginal and rectal points are also defined. Care needs to be taken to minimize the radiation dose to the bladder and rectum by anteriorly and posteriorly packing through the vagina and around the brachytherapy applicators.

Brachytherapy delivery is provided once weekly over a time interval of 3–6 weeks. Total radiotherapy treatment (EBRT and BT) should be completed within a time period of 7–8 weeks.

6. Complications

Acute complications commonly include local features, consisting with dry and moist skin desquamation, vaginitis, cystitis, and proctitis. Management of these complications varies between anti-inflammatory medications and anti-microbial drugs given for prophylaxis.

Brachytherapy side effects are mainly due to neighboring organ toxicity and include vaginitis, cystitis and uterine perforation.

Late complications include vaginal stenosis, recto-vaginal and vesico-vaginal fistula and intestinal perforation.

7. Conclusions

With increasing rates of advanced cervical cancer disease in Low and Middle Income countries, adherence to evidence-based literature for treatment is key. Radiation therapy combined with chemotherapy are the mainstay of management for locally advanced cervical carcinoma. The treatment should ideally not exceed eight (8) weeks after the baseline work-up and disease evaluation to maximize disease control.

Author details

Achille Manirakiza[1]*, Sumi Sinha[2] and Fidel Rubagumya[1]

*Address all correspondence to: achille.manirakiza@gmail.com

1 Department of Clinical Oncology, School of Medicine, Muhimbili University of Health and Allied Sciences, Dar es Salaam, Tanzania

2 Department of Radiation Oncology, University of California, San Francisco, USA

References

[1] Torre LA, Bray F, Siegel RL, Ferlay J, Lortet-Tieulent J, Jemal A. Global cancer statistics, 2012. CA: A Cancer Journal for Clinicians. 2015;65(2):87

[2] Pecorelli S, Zigliani L, Odicino F. Revised FIGO staging for carcinoma of the cervix. International Journal of Gynaecology and Obstetrics. 2009;105(2):107. Epub 2009 Apr 1

[3] Sharma A, Kulkarni V, Bhaskaran U, Singha M, Mujtahedi S, Chatrath A, Sridhar M, Thapar R, Mithra PP, Kumar N, Holla R, Darshan BB, Kumar A. Profile of cervical cancer patients attending Tertiary Care Hospitals of Mangalore, Karnataka: A 4 year retrospective study. Journal of Natural Science, Biology, and Medicine. 2017 Jan-Jun;8(1):125-112

[4] Musa J, Nankat J, Achenbach CJ, Shambe IH, Taiwo BO, Mandong B, Daru PH, Murphy RL, Sagay AS. Cervical cancer survival in a resource-limited setting-North Central Nigeria. Infectious Agents and Cancer. 2016 Mar 24;11:15

[5] Chirenje ZM, Rusakaniko S, Akino V, Mlingo M. A review of cervical cancer patients presenting in Harare and Parirenyatwa Hospitals in 1998. The Central African Journal of Medicine. 2000 Oct;46(10):264-267

[6] Mlange R, Matovelo D, Rambau P, Kidenya B. Patient and disease characteristics associated with late tumour stage at presentation of cervical cancer in northwestern Tanzania. BMC Women's Health. 2016 Jan 25;16:5

[7] Landoni F, Maneo A, Colombo A, Placa F, Milani R, Perego P, Favini G, Ferri L, Mangioni C. Randomised study of radical surgery versus radiotherapy for stage Ib-IIa cervical cancer. Lancet. 1997;9077(350):535-540

[8] Hreshchyshyn MM, Aron BS, Boronow RC, Franklin EW, Shingleton HM, Blessing JA. Hydroxyurea or placebo combined with radiation to treat stages iiib and iv cervical cancer confined to the pelvis. International Journal of Radiation Oncology, Biology, Physics. 1979;5(3):317-322

[9] Whitney CW, Sause W, Bundy BN, et al. Randomized comparison of fluorouracil plus cisplatin versus hydroxyurea as an adjunct to radiation therapy in stage IIB–IVA carcinoma of the cervix with negative para-aortic lymph nodes: A Gynecologic Oncology Group and Southwest Oncology Group study. Journal of Clinical Oncology. 1999;17:1339-1348

[10] Eifel PJ, Winter K, Morris M, et al. Pelvic irradiation with concurrent chemotherapy versus pelvic and para-aortic irradiation for high-risk cervical cancer an update of Radiation Therapy Oncology Group trial (RTOG) 90-01. Journal of Clinical Oncology. 2004;22:972-880

5

Ascites in Advanced Ovarian Cancer

Katarina Cerne and Borut Kobal

Abstract

The presence of ascites is one of the general ovarian cancer (OC) symptoms detected at initial diagnosis and can be present at an early stage but is most often seen in advanced disease. In newly diagnosed OC patients, ascites is treated by the standard treatment for the underlying disease. However, once the chemoresistant and recurrent features of the disease develop, management of a large volume of ascites can be a major problem. By increasing abdominal pressure, ascites can cause severe symptoms; thus, palliation of symptomatic patients is the main goal. The elimination of fluid accumulation in OC patients with these symptoms will certainly improve their quality of life and may even prolong survival. Unfortunately, no standard treatment for OC-associated ascites exists. There are several traditional therapies for ascites, with limited effectiveness and significant adverse effects. Catumaxomab is the only medicine approved for intraperitoneal treatment of malignant ascites in patients with EpCAM-positive carcinomas. Advances in our understanding of malignant ascites aetiology and more effective treatment strategies for ascites and OC will help reduce the symptoms associated with ascites.

Keywords: advanced ovarian cancer, malignant ascites, aetiology, treatment, diagnosis

1. Introduction

Ascites is an abnormal accumulation of serous fluid (>50 mL) in the peritoneal cavity between the membrane lining the abdominal wall and the membrane covering the abdominal organs. Although ascites is most commonly observed in patients with cirrhosis, 7–10% of patients with ascites develop it secondary to malignancy. The commonest primary tumour associated with the development of ascites is ovarian cancer (OC) [1]. Large amounts of ascites in a patient with OC usually indicate the presence of peritoneal metastasis; therefore, ascites is found in the majority of patients (89%) with advanced disease (FIGO stages III and IV). However, the absence of ascites may not exclude malignant disease, since ascites is rarely

(17%) observed in the early disease (FIGO stages I and II) and is absent in nearly half of borderline tumours. Unlike in primary OC, recurrent disease is not strongly associated with ascites, which was found in 38% of patients with recurrent OC [2].

Throughout history, ascites has always been regarded as a poor prognostic sign. In the 1700s, Sir Thomas Spencer Wells wrote "surgeons stood and trembled on the brink of ovarian waters" [3]. Studies addressing the prognostic significance of ascites in patients with stage III or IV have shown a significantly poorer survival [4]. Ascites is also associated with pharmacoresistance [4]. Patch et al. showed that matched primary ascites (tumour cells isolated from ascites) share most genomic changes of acquired resistance with primary tumour samples across the whole genome [5].

In newly diagnosed ovarian cancer patients, ascites is treated by using the standard treatment for the underlying disease. However, once the chemoresistant and recurrent features of the disease develop, management of a large volume of ascites can be a major problem. Palliation of symptomatic patients is therefore the foremost goal, and elimination of fluid accumulation in patients with these symptoms will certainly improve their quality of life and may even prolong survival [6, 7]. An understanding of malignant ascites aetiology is of utmost importance if more effective treatment strategies for ascites and OC are to emerge in the future.

This chapter considers the aetiology and pathophysiology of malignant ascites in OC as well as current diagnostic modalities and explores the best form of management.

2. Mechanisms of malignant ascites formation

The word ascites originates from the ancient Greek askos, meaning a sac or bag. Celsus (c.30 BC–c.50 AD) postulated a link between ascites and renal disease, and he coined the term [8]. The peritoneal cavity, located between the parietal and visceral peritoneum, contains approximately 100 mL of serous fluids. Free fluid in the peritoneal cavity acts as a lubricant of the serosal surfaces and originates from the transduction of plasma through capillary membranes of the peritoneal serosa. Healthy women may normally have as much as 20 mL of free peritoneal fluid, depending on the phase of the menstrual cycle [9]. Under physiological conditions, transudation is balanced by efflux of the peritoneal fluid via lymphatic vessels. Tumour growth eventually disrupts the normal regulation of intraperitoneal fluid flow and the maintenance of a steady state in the peritoneal cavity by simultaneously causing a greater fluid inflow and a reduced outflow. Four major factors that contribute to the formation of ascites: two cause increased influx due to tumour-related factors and two cause decreased efflux due to lymphatic obstruction and mechanical obstruction by accumulation of tumour cells at the peritoneal surface (**Figure 1**) [1, 10]. The percentage of cases with a greater ascites volume increased as the stage of ovarian malignancy progressed [1].

2.1. Efflux from the peritoneal cavity into the blood

The peritoneal lymphatic system collects excess fluid, proteins, other macromolecules (>16 kDa) and cells and returns them to systemic circulation [11]. Decreased efflux from the peritoneal cavity due to lymphatic obstruction by tumour cells was first proposed as a hypothesis for ascites

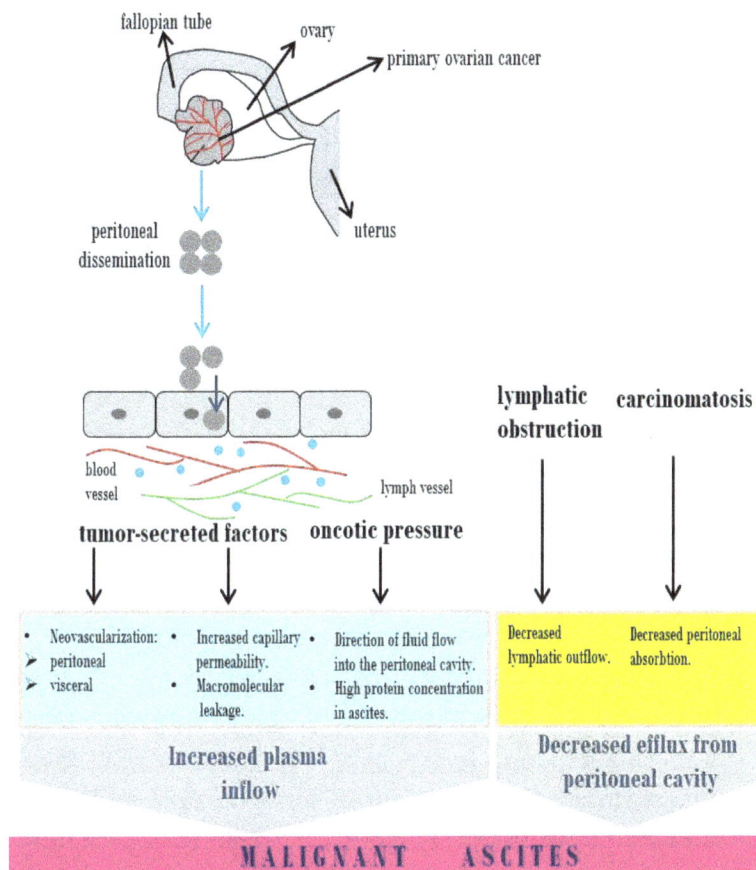

Figure 1. Aetiology of malignant ascites in ovarian cancer.

formation by Holm-Nielsen more than 60 years ago [12]. Published data using lymphoscintig-raphy showed that patients with malignant ascites had no activity above the diaphragm after intraperitoneal injection of the isotope, in contrast to control patients with no ascites or cirrhotic ascites. Bronskill et al. [13] showed that OC patients with persistent, intractable ascites, who were approaching their terminal illness, had low peritoneal drainage rates (below 50 ml/h). This result generally indicates obstruction of the diaphragmatic plexus [13]. Initial events that lead to fluid accumulation were studied by Nagy et al. [14] who showed that in mice efflux the perito-neal cavity of ^{125}I-labelled human serum albumin and ^{51}Cr-labelled red blood cells is markedly reduced (fivefold) within 1 day of *i.p.* ovarian tumour cell line injection. A significant reduction preceding a detectable increase in tumour cell number was not attributable to the blockage of peritoneal lymphatics by tumour cells and by itself did not provoke peritoneal fluid accumula-tion. These results suggest a prominent role for nonobstructive mechanisms, including con-traction of lymph vessels induced by secretion of tumour cell product(s). At later periods, the absorption of fluid from the peritoneal cavity might also be affected due to carcinomatosis [14].

2.2. Influx into the peritoneal cavity

Nagy et al. studied the influx of fluid into the peritoneal cavity of mice [14]. They found that after *i.p.* ovarian tumour cell line injection, influx of ^{125}I-labelled human serum albumin rose between days 5 and 7 to values 13- to 25-fold higher than control values, when the tumour cell number had increased >500-fold. By day 10, influx had increased sufficiently to exceed efflux, resulting in net accumulation of fluid [14]. An increase in influx is a result of various factors: (1) increased capillary permeability, (2) angiogenesis, (3) increased area for filtration and (4) decreased oncotic pressure difference. In malignant ascites, various factors secreted by tumour cells are present, which increase vascular permeability and induce angiogenesis. An early step leading to angiogenesis is partial proteolysis of vascular basal lamina, resulting in hyperpermeability. Vascular endothelial growth factor (VEGF) is the most potent and specific angiogenic factor, secreted by a large variety of tumours, peritoneal mesothelial cells, monocyte/macrophages in malignant ascites and even tumour-infiltrating T cells [7]. Additionally, VEGF increases the permeability of vessels to plasma proteins, including albumin and fibrinogen, with a potency 10,000 times higher than histamine [15, 16]. Other factors that may also induce angiogenesis have been identified in malignant ascites and include basic fibroblast growth factor (bFGF), angiogenin, transforming growth factor alpha and beta (TGF-alpha, TGF-beta), interleukin-8, placental growth factor (PlGF) and platelet-derived endothelial cell growth factor (PD-EGF) [11]. Influx into the peritoneal cavity after *i.p.* ovarian tumour cell line injection rose significantly when the surface area for filtration also increased; the size and number of vessels lining the peritoneal cavity increased as much as 15-fold [16]. The protein content of malignant ascites is greater than in peritoneal fluid of healthy women [11]. The oncotic pressure difference between plasma and ascites therefore decreases, and as a consequence, reabsorption decreases and interstitial fluid accumulation results [11]. Liver metastasis causing hepatic vein obstruction may be an important aetiology factor in some cases of malignant ascites [1].

3. Diagnosis

The absence of symptoms or the presence of symptoms that mimic other conditions often results in diagnostic delay with OC, and this worsens prognosis. Evaluation consists of physical examination, imaging [ultrasonography, computerized tomography (CT), magnetic resonance image (MRI)], serum tumour markers analysis and ascitic fluid analysis (visual inspection, biochemical analysis, cytology and tumour markers). Diagnostic laparoscopy is an additional investigation and may be useful in patients with whom simple investigations have failed to determine the cause of ascites (**Figure 2**) [6, 17–21].

3.1. Symptoms

The most common complaint in the presentation of OC is abdominal swelling or bloating [17]. These symptoms are commonly associated with the physical and surgical finding of ascites. As the amount of fluid increases, ascites can cause significant symptoms referable to the gastrointestinal and genitourinary tracts. Malignant ascites is associated with abdominal and pelvic pain, while liver disease tends to be relatively painless [6, 17].

3.2. Imaging

Transabdominal and transvaginal ultrasonographies are the most sensitive techniques for the detection of ascitic fluid (**Figure 3**) [19]. Uncomplicated ascites appears as ahomogeneous, freely mobile, anechoic collection in the peritoneal cavity that demonstrates deep acoustic enhancement. Generally, free ascites do not displace organs situated between them

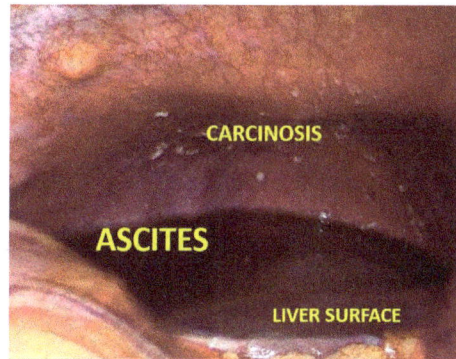

Figure 2. Diagnostic laparoscopy showing ascites and peritoneal carcinosis.

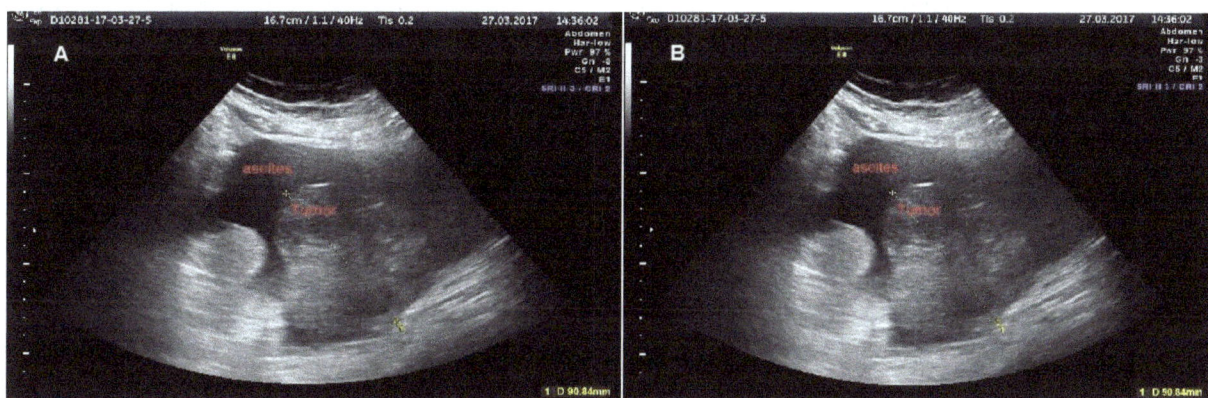

Figure 3. Ultrasound images of ascites. (A) Transabdominal ultrasound image demonstrates ascites and ovarian tumour. (B) Transvaginal ultrasound image demonstrates ascites and intestinal carcinosis.

(**Figure 3A**) [20]. Sometimes, bowel loops do not float freely but may be tethered along the posterior abdominal wall, plastered to organs or surrounded by loculated fluid collections (**Figure 3B**) [21]. When small amounts of ascitic fluid localise in the Morison pouch and the pouch of Douglas, CT scan demonstrated the best sensitivity [21, 22].

3.3. Ascitic fluid analysis

In patients with new-onset ascites of unknown origin, peritoneal fluid analysis may provide some information regarding the origin of the disease. However, it remains difficult to differentiate malignant ascites from other types [23].

On inspection, most ascitic fluids are transparent and tinged yellow. In the case of malignancy, it could also appear pink or red (when at least 10,000 red blood cells/µL are present). Any inflammatory condition can cause an elevated white blood cell count. In case of malignant ascites, lymphocytes usually predominate [24].

Conventional cytological examination shows high specificity, but its sensitivity is low (58–75%) [23]. The cellular components of malignant ascites contain a complex mixture of cell populations, including tumour cells and stromal cells [25]. Immunohistochemistry (ICH) staining and cytological diagnosis by using cell block (CB) sections prepared with the ascites cytological specimen are useful in delineation of the primary origin of the tumour cells. Since multiple sections can be obtained by the CB method, this technique is particularly valuable when the ICH staining is required for a battery of markers. Typically, primary ovarian epithelial cancers are positive for ER/PR, PAX8, CK7 and negative for CK20 and CDX2. The reverse is true for gastrointestinal cancers. By using a combination of cytological conventional smears and CB methods, the primary site could be detected with 81% accuracy [26, 27].

A number of soluble factors are present in abundance in malignant ascites, but few have been validated for their biomarker potential [28].

4. Treatment

Many factors influence the optimal therapeutic interventions. The aim is palliation in a significant number of patients; only in a selected subgroup is it to improve survival [29].

4.1. Non-pharmacological treatment of ascites

Surgical treatment of malignant ascites involves a variety of different options, each with a certain degree of efficacy but not without risks [30]. Very few studies concern the benefits and harm of differing surgical interventions for intra-peritoneal fluid drainage. Numerous questions, such as how long should the drain stay in place, whether the volume of fluid drained should be replaced intravenously, whether the drain should be clamped to regulate the drainage of fluid and whether any particular vital observations should be regularly recorded, remain partially unanswered [31]. The most common surgical option for ascites drainage is abdominal paracentesis followed, in recent years, by the insertion of permanent tunnelled catheters (PleurX®) and peritoneal-venous shunts.

4.1.1. Paracentesis

Paracentesis (needle drainage of fluid) is an effective and widely used procedure for the management of treatment-resistant, recurrent malignant ascites [32]. It can provide good short-term symptomatic relief in up to 90% of hospital cases, although it may also be offered as a day-case procedure [33].

The procedure involves the placement of a fine tube into the peritoneal cavity to drain ascitic fluid. The procedure can be done all at once but, especially for large volume paracentesis, the catheter can remain in place for several hours and sometimes for days [31]. The volume of drained fluid can vary according to the patient's general conditions, from a few litres up to a maximum of 20 l [30]. Complications of the procedure may include peritonitis, sepsis, visceral injuries, bleeding and fluid leak. Moreover, especially for large volume drainage or repeated procedures, paracentesis may be associated with significantly higher incidence of hypotension and renal impairment [32, 34].

In general, intravenous fluid replacement is not routinely required for paracentesis with less than 5 l removed, but it depends on the patient's clinical condition [32]. However, some reports suggest the use of 5% dextrose infusion during the procedure to avoid severe hypotensive episodes [30, 34]. There is no evidence albumin infusion is of benefit during paracentesis for malignant ascites, even though many studies focusing on cirrhosis related ascites have demonstrated great benefits of albumin infusion (6–8 g per litre of ascites removed) to maintain intravascular volume [30].

4.1.2. Peritoneal-venous shunting

Common peritoneal-venous shunts drain ascites from the peritoneal cavity into the superior vena cava and have a one-way valve that prevents reflux of blood [32, 34]. They are rarely used due to the high rate of complications such as occlusion, infection, coagulopathy and the widespread dissemination of malignant cells [35]. The only advantage compared to other techniques is related to saving electrolytes and proteins, preserving the body fluid balance [30, 32]. Two shunts are commonly used: the older LeVeen and the most recent Denver shunt, which require different pressures to open the valves [32, 36].

Contraindications of shunt positioning are as follows: congestive heart disease or renal failure due to the significant hemodilution and blood volume overload produced by the shunt, portal hypertension, and severe pleural effusion and clotting disorders [35].

A novel type of technique, automated low-flow ascites pump, drains ascites from the peritoneal cavity to the bladder. This novel device seems effective (even though tested only on liver disease patients) for symptom relief, although data about safety (especially linked to catheter dislodgement and infections) are only preliminary [37].

4.1.3. Catheter drainage

In cases of recurrent or refractory malignant ascites, when frequent paracentesis is required, patients may benefit from an indwelling catheter [32]. This device allows easy and self-drainage, eliminating the need for hospitalisation and frequent paracentesis. The most common permanent catheters are the tunnelled PleurX®, Tenckhoff, Port-a-Cath and cope-type loop catheters [30, 38]. Most authors prefer tunnelled catheters due to greater stability (higher long-term patency rate and success rate) and lower infection rate [30, 39]. Recent trials have suggested that untunnelled catheters have a 21–34% risk of developing peritonitis compared to 4.4% with tunnelled Tenckhoff and 2.5% for tunnelled PleurX® [30].

Catheter placement can be performed with ultrasound guidance or with CT guidance in cases of particular anatomical conditions or widespread carcinomatosis [30]. Antibiotic prophylaxis is recommended for catheter placement [39]. Patients should be instructed to drain the fluid frequently enough to avoid the development of tense ascites, usually once or twice per week. Intravenous fluid replacement and/or albumin supplementation is indicated according to clinical conditions and ascites volume [30, 39].

The safety and cost-effective profiles of tunnelled catheters for the management of recurrent malignant ascites have been demonstrated by several observational studies [38, 40].

4.2. Pharmacological treatment of ascites

If the patient's malignant disease is sensitive to chemotherapy, reduction of ascites production and relief of symptoms may be achieved. However, most patients with ascites have already been treated with several lines of treatment, and their disease has become refractory to chemotherapy, and carcinomatosis may not be amenable to surgery. For such patients, no pharmacological therapy has been approved except catumaxomab in the EU. The effectiveness of other drugs to treat ascites has been explored in a few studies, with the majority of treatments having been studied in a small series.

4.2.1. Catumaxomab

Catumaxomab (Removab®; Fresenius Biotech) was approved in 2009 by the European Medicine Agency (EMA) for the intraperitoneal treatment of malignant ascites in adults with EpCAM-positive carcinomas, where standard therapy is not available or no longer feasible [41]. Catumoxomab is a trifunctional rat-mouse hybrid monoclonal antibody that is specifically directed against the epithelial cell adhesion molecule (EpCAM) and CD3 antigen (**Figure 4**). EpCAM (CD326) antigen is overexpressed in epithelial ovarian cancer of serous (68%), endometrioid (82%), clear cell (92%) and mucinous (49%) histological subtypes. EpCAM correlates with lower overall survival [42]. Over 80% of ovarian cancer patients have EpCAM over-expressed in tumour cells present in ascites [43]. EpCAM has been reported to initiate cell proliferation by upregulating the oncogene c-myc and to dampen antitumour immunity by blocking antigen presentation in dendritic cells [44, 45]. Mesothelial cells do not express EpCAM on their surface, so catumaxomab applied to the peritoneal cavity specifically targets epithelial tumour cells but not the normal tissue. CD3, as a second antigen, is expressed in mature T-cells as a component of the T-cell receptor. A third functional binding site in the Fc-region of catumaxomab enables the interaction with accessory immune cells (macrophages, dendritic cells and NK cells) via Fcγ receptors. Due to catumaxomab's binding properties, tumour cells and immune effector cells come in close proximity, and complex "crosstalk"

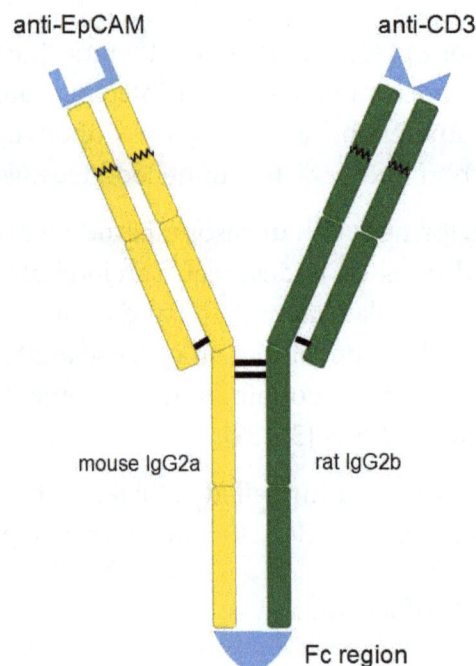

Figure 4. Schematic structure of catumaxomab.

between the T cell and accessory cell can occur, which includes cytokines and co-stimulatory signalling necessary for T-cell activation cascade, resulting in the killing of tumour cells [41].

The clinical efficacy of catumaxomab in the treatment of malignant ascites has been demonstrated in two clinical studies: a phase I/II study (STP-REM-01) and a pivotal phase II/III study (IP-REM-AC-01) [41]. In the first study treatment resulted in a significant reduction of the ascites flow rate from a median of 105 mL/h at baseline to 23 mL/h 1 day after the fourth infusion. Twenty-two of 23 patients did not require paracentesis between the last infusion and the end of the study. Tumour cell-count monitoring revealed a mean reduction up to 99.9% of EpCAM-positive malignant cells in ascites. In a pivotal study, 129 ovarian cancer patients with recurrent symptomatic malignant ascites were randomised to treatment with catumaxomab (as four 6-h *i.p.* infusions on days 0, 3, 7, and 10 at doses 10, 20, 50, and 150 µg, respectively) plus paracentesis or paracentesis alone (the control group). The median time to the next paracentesis was significantly longer for catumaxomab plus paracentesis than paracentesis alone: 77 versus 13 days (P < 0.0001) [41].

The safety profile of catumaxomab was established from five completed studies (STP-REM-01, IP-REM-AC-01, IP-REM-PC-01-DE, AGO-Ovar-2.10 and IP-REM-PK-01-EU) [41]. A total of 258 patients were treated with *i.p.* administration of catumaxomab and 207 (80%) patients completed treatment, underlining the good tolerability for the drug. Catumaxomab may cause symptoms related to local and systemic cytokine release: pyrexia, nausea and vomiting. In 48% of patients, abdominal pain was reported, which is considered in part a consequence of the *i.p.* route of administration. All mentioned adverse drug reactions (ADRs) are fully reversible. One hundred and twenty-seven (49%) patients had at least one ADR of grade 3/4, according to the Terminology Criteria for Adverse Events (CTCAE). Abdominal pain, pyrexia and vomiting were the most common symptomatic grade 3 ADRs. Grade 4 ADRs were isolated cases (1%), mostly related to the progression of the underlying malignant disease, such as ileus. In 1% of patients, symptoms of systemic inflammatory response syndrome (SIRS) were observed within 24 h after catumaxomab infusion, such as tachycardia, fever and dyspnea. These reactions resolve under symptomatic treatment. Conditions such as hypovolemia, hypoproteinaemia, hypotension, circulatory decompensation and acute renal impairment must be resolved before each infusion. Since patients with severe hepatic or renal impairment have not been investigated, treatment of these patients should only be considered after a thorough evaluation of benefit/risk. Catumaxomab is potentially immunogenic when administered to humans. In clinical studies, almost all patients (94%) developed human anti-mouse antibodies (HAMAs) or human anti-rat antibodies (HARAs) 1 month after the last infusion; however, patients who developed HAMAs 8 days after the fourth infusion showed a better clinical outcome as measured by puncture-free survival, compared with HAMA-negative patients, suggesting that HAMA development may be a biomarker for catumaxomab response. No hypersensitivity reactions were observed [41].

4.2.2. Other immunological approaches

Evidence to suggest that an immunological approach to the treatment of malignant ascites in OC may be effective and has been observed in small studies of intraperitoneal administration of triamcinolone (long acting corticosteroid), interferons and TNFα [10, 46].

Interferon alpha-2b (IFNα-2b), administered *i.p.* inserted with a 9-French catheter, was evaluated in a study by Sartory et al. Twelve of 41 patients had OC. A complete response (no fluid recurrence) within 30 days of treatment (six courses with an interval of 4 days with six or nine million units depending on a body weight) occurred in 65% of OC patients. The fluid reaccumulated after 11.4 days before and 70.5 days after the treatment. Adverse effects were flu-like symptoms, vomiting and infection with staphylococcus (two patients). If there is no response after the first three courses, the treatment should be stopped [47].

TNFα, installed inside the abdomen of advanced OC patients for 24–48 h (the procedure was repeated on day 8 at a dose of 0.08–0.014 mg/m^2), was evaluated in a study by Kaufmann et al. Production of ascites was supressed or reduced to a minimum for at least 4 weeks in 87% of patients. The treatment was not effective in patients with malignant ascites due to mucinous OC. Patients often suffer from flu-like symptoms, which can be reduced by taking indomethacin or paracetamol before the infusion [47].

4.2.3. Bevacizumab

Bevacizumab (Avastin®, Genentech, Inc., a member of the Roche Group) was approved as an *i.v.* infusion in 2014 by the Food and Drug Administration (FDA) and by EMA in combination with paclitaxel, topotecan, or pegylated liposomal doxorubicin, for the treatment of adult patients with recurrent epithelial ovarian cancer that is resistant to platinum-containing chemotherapy. Bevacizumab is a humanised monoclonal antibody directed against vascular endothelial growth factor (VEGF). Bevacizumab binds to VEGF and thereby prevents the binding of VEGF to its receptors, Flt-1 (VEGFR-1) and KDR (VEGFR-2), on the surface of endothelial cells. Neutralising the biological activity of VEGF regresses the vascularisation of tumours and inhibits the formation of a new tumour vasculature and thereby inhibits tumour growth. Interestingly, the delay of tumour growth induced by anti-VEGF antibody was mainly attributed to the blockage of ascites development and vascular permeability and to a lesser degree to the inhibition of VEGF-induced angiogenesis [7].

Approval of bevacizumab in the USA and EU was based on results of a phase III AURELIA study that involved 361 women with recurrent, platinum-resistant OC, who received either chemotherapy or bevacizumab in combination with chemotherapy. In the subgroup of patients with ascites at baseline, the absence of paracentesis after the first bevacizumab dose suggests that adding bevacizumab to chemotherapy improved the control of ascites [48]. Bevacizumab has been associated with serious (but rare) side effects, and the use of bevacizumab remains significantly more expensive than cytotoxic therapies. The identification of predictive clinical and biological factors that could be utilised to select patients with a greater likelihood of clinical benefit therefore remains a high priority. Using data from Phase III trial GOG218 (Gynaecologic Oncology Group), ascites as a prognostic factor and as a predictor of efficacy for bevacizumab in advanced OC was investigated. In multivariate survival analysis, ascites was prognostic of poor overall survival (OS) but not progression-free survival (PFS). In predictive analysis, patients without ascites treated with bevacizumab had no significant improvement in either PFS or OS, whereas patients with ascites treated with bevacizumab had significantly improved PFS (p < 0.001) and OS (p = 0.014). These findings support the plausible biologic rational that patients with malignant ascites have cancer with a phenotype representative of the initiation phase of angiogenesis and are therefore more likely to respond to anti-VEGF therapy. If these findings could be validated through a similar analysis of data from one or more independent randomised phase III trials, the clinical determination of malignant ascites could be a simple and cost-effective way of selecting patients with the greatest probability of benefit from bevacizumab. However, it is possible that volume of ascites could be a more robust predictor of the degree of benefit from VEGF-targeted therapy [49].

Intraperitoneal administration of bevacizumab has also been explored, although only very few OC patients with malignant ascites have received this route of administration. In all patients, ascites resolved after a single *i.p.* dose (5 mg/kg) without re-accumulation or repeat paracentesis over a median observation period >2 months. Moreover, no grade 2–5 adverse events were observed [50]. To evaluate the great potential that preclinical data and clinical case reports have suggested for *i.p.* administration of bevacizumab, clinical trials should be undertaken regarding the safety of treatment, specifically for the palliation of ascites. Bevacizumab may have the potential advantage so that it could be used in patients with reduced performance [47].

4.2.4. Aflibercept (VEGF-TRAP)

Aflibercept (Zaltrap®, Sanofi-Aventis group) was approved for the treatment of adult metastatic colorectal cancer that is resistant or has progressed after an oxalipatin-containing regimen. Aflibercept, also known as VEGF trap (it binds to VEGF trapping it and inhibiting it) in the scientific literature, is a fusion protein, comprising a portion of human VEGF receptor Fit-1 (VEGFR-1) + KDR (VEGFR-2) extracellular domains fused to the Fc-portion of human IgG. Aflibercept binds to VEGF-A, VEGF-B and placental growth factor (PlGF). By acting as a ligand trap, aflibercept prevents binding of endogenous ligands to their cognate receptors and thereby blocks receptor-mediated signalling. VEGF-A acts via VEGFR-1 and VEGFR-2 present on the surface of endothelial cells. PlGF and VEGF-B bind only to VEGFR-1, which is also present on the surface of leucocytes. Excessive activation of receptors by VEGF-A can result in pathological neovascularisation and excessive vascular permeability. PlGF is also linked to pathological neovascularisation and recruitment of inflammatory cells into tumours [51]. In addition to the approved indication, aflibercept has demonstrated the ability to reduce the formation of ascites in patients with advanced epithelial OC [10, 52, 53]. In pre-clinical xenograft models, aflibercept inhibited tumour growth, angiogenesis, reduced blood vessel density and inhibited metastases [10]. The safety and efficacy of aflibercept, administrated *i.v.* at a dosage of 4 mg/kg every 2 weeks, was tested in two-phase II clinical trials in chemoresistant advanced OC patients with recurrent symptomatic ascites [52, 53]. In a randomised, double blind, placebo-controlled, parallel trial, 29 patients were treated. The mean time to paracentesis was significantly (*p* = 0.0019) longer in the aflibercept arm (55.1 days) than in the placebo arm (23.3 days). Two patients receiving aflibercept did not need paracentesis for a period of 6 months. The most common grade 3 or 4 adverse effects were dyspnea, fatigue or asthenia, and dehydration. The frequency of fatal gastrointestinal perforation was higher with aflibercept (three-bowel perforation) than with the placebo. In spite of the effectiveness of aflibercept in the reduction of malignantascites, the authors acknowledge that the limitation of this treatment is the risk of significant morbidity associated with bowel perforation in patients with very advanced OC. Thus, the advantages of aflibercept over bevacizumab are unclear [53].

4.2.5. Matrix metalloproteinase inhibitors (MMPIs)

MMPs, mainly MMP9, play a role in the release of biologically active VEGF and, consequently, play a role in the formation of ascites. Batistamat, a potent reversible inhibitor of a broad spectrum of MMP, has been developed and has been shown to resolve ascites when given *i.p.* to mice ascites secondary to an ovarian carcinoma xenograft; treatment was accompanied by a 6.5-fold increase in survival [54]. Sixteen patients with OC (out of 23 patients) were included in a Phase I study of *i.p.* administration of batistamat after drainage of ascites. Patients acquired a predicted survival of 1 month or more. Of the 23 patients in the study, 16 did not require redrainage within 28 days of the initial treatment. Five of the 23 patients neither reaccumulated ascites nor died up to 112 days after dosing. Seven patients died without reaccumulating ascites. Adverse effects considered at least possibly related to the treatment occurred in 16 patients, the most common of which were fatigue, fever, vomiting and abdominal pain [46]. MMP inhibitors may warrant further study.

4.2.6. Intraperitoneal chemotherapy

Intraperitoneal chemotherapy is an effective way to palliate malignant ascites. By destroying the surface cancer, it induces a progressive fibrotic process, which will prevent the formation of fluid. If the sclerotic process is not complete, it may produce fluid loculation, which will interfere with uniform drug distribution, may cause obstructions and makes subsequent paracentesis difficult and risky [29]. Intraperitoneal therapy with cisplatin has been evaluated for the first-line treatment of optimal debulked OC patients with FIGO stage III. Despite a 16-month survival advantage, the catheter-related complications rate was 34%, and only 42% of women in the trial completed six cycles of chemotherapy [46].

The procedure called intraperitoneal hyperthermic chemotherapy (HIPEC) is an attempt to increase the cytotoxicity of selected cytotoxic drugs by a hyperthermic medium (40.5–43°C), thereby improving tissue penetration and reducing drug resistance. The primary objective is an increase of PFS and OS, not the control of ascites itself [47]. Finally, aggressive cytoreductive surgery combined with laparoscopic installation of HIPEC is reserved for selected patients with malignant ascites. In well-selected patients, results are encouraging, and this procedure not only controls ascites, but prolongation of OS is possible [29].

Laparoscopic installation of HIPEC has been recently reported as an option to treat resistant malignant ascites not suitable for surgery. The biggest series published, which also included patients with OC, was by Valle et al. [55], who achieved complete remission of ascites in 94% of 52 patients after 1 month of follow-up. There were no complications of the procedure, demonstrating the feasibility and safety of this technique [55].

4.2.7. Diuretics

Some patients with liver metastasis and malignant ascites have raised plasma renin concentrations, and these patients showed a good response to aldosterone competitive antagonist spironolactone, which decreases reabsorption of water and sodium in the renal collecting duct. Packros et al. [56] found that 13 of 15 patients treated with increasing doses of spirono-lactone had a good response, with eight remaining free of ascites until death. Renin levels were raised in all of these patients [56].

5. Role of ascites in translational science

Ascites is often therapeutically removed from patients and is therefore an available source of valuable tumour material. Representing the local tumour environment, ascites is composed of cellular and acellular components. In addition to tumour cells present, either as single cells or as spheroids, the cellular component of ascites is composed of stromal cells, including fibroblasts, mesothelial cells, endothelial cells, adipocytes and inflammatory cells. Cells in ascites communicate with each other through acellular components, including cytokines, proteins, metabolites and exosomes. All these components work in coordination to create a tumour-friendly micro-environment. Better knowledge of the tumour microenvironment represented by ascites would thus certainly help to overcome the limitations of current anticancer treatments [23].

Targeting ascites components that cause immunosuppression of T-cells is an interesting future therapeutic option. T-cells present in ovarian tumour ascites do not respond properly to stimulation via the T-cell receptor. Since these T-cells were assayed in the absence of ascites, they gained their normal function, but when ascites was added to T-cells, this effect was rapidly reversed. This might explain why human tumours grow despite the presence of T-cells and other cells of immunological response [10].

In the study by Latifi et al. [57], it was demonstrated that cells in malignant ascites belong to two types of tumour cells, adherent cells (expressed mesenchymal features) and non-adherent cells with an epithelial phenotype, as expressed by EpCAM and cytokeratin 7. Patients with chemo-resistant tumours had more tumorogenic, non-adherent cells in the ascites than non-tumoro-genic adherent cells. Non-adherent cells featured increased mRNA expression of cancer stem cell-associated genes [10]. Since catumaxomab selectively kills epithelial tumour cells belonging to the non-adherent cell type, this might explain why it is beneficial for patients with OC.

Ascites is highly attractive as a source for biomarker discovery study. The concentrations of cancer-associated soluble factors are usually much higher in ascites than in serum [47, 58]. Moreover, investigation of the relationship between biomarker concentrations in ascites and serum in OC patients may help elucidate whether concentration changes in the local environment can be detected with a blood test [58].

6. Conclusions

The development of malignant ascites is probably dependent on a combination of factors, which disrupts the normal regulation of intraperitoneal fluid flow and the maintenance of a steady state in the peritoneal cavity. Each factor plays a greater or lesser role in each individual patient, so the results of available treatment alternatives are inconsistent. In advanced OC, palliation of symptomatic patients is the foremost goal, and elimination of fluid accumulation in a patient with these symptoms will certainly improve the patient's quality of life and may even prolong survival. However, effective palliation of malignant ascites remains a difficult management issue. Present treatments have been developed, particularly for malignant ascites, with the primary aim of prolonging the time until a need for subsequent paracentesis. Further clinical trials are therefore necessary in order to investigate the influence on ascites-triggered intervention not only for symptomatic relief but also for the prolongation of both PFS and OS. For the use of targeted therapeutics in malignant ascites (catumaxomab, bevacizumab, aflibercept), it is mandatory to select patients carefully and to identify their risk factors so that the incidence of adverse effects can be minimised. The identification of predictive clinical and biological factors that could be utilised to select patients with a greater likelihood of clinical benefit remains a high priority. With advances in our understanding of malignant ascites pathophysiology, more effective treatment strategies for malignant ascites and ovarian cancer will emerge in the future.

Acknowledgements

This work was supported by the Slovenian Research Agency through the research programs P3-067 and by the University Medical Centre Ljubljana (Project No.: 20160084). The authors thank Nevenka Dolžan for technical assistance and Martin Cregeen for language editing.

Author details

Katarina Cerne[1]* and Borut Kobal[2,3]

*Address all correspondence to: katarina.cerne@mf.uni-lj.si

1 Department of Pharmacology and Experimental Toxicology, Faculty of Medicine, University Ljubljana, Ljubljana, Slovenia

2 Department of Gynaecology, Division of Gynaecology and Obstetrics, University Medical Centre Ljubljana, Ljubljana, Slovenia

3 Department of Gynaecology and Obstetrics, Faculty of Medicine, University Ljubljana, Ljubljana, Slovenia

References

[1] Parsons SL, Watson SA, Steele RJC. Malignant ascites. British Journal of Surgery. 1996; **83**:6-14

[2] Forstner R. CT and MRI in ovarian carcinoma. In: Hamm B, Forstner R, editors. MRI and CT of the Female Pelvis. New York: Springer; 2007. pp. 233-265

[3] Speert H. Gynecology. In: Speert H, editor. Obstetrics and Gynecology: A History and Iconography, 2nd ed. San Francisco: Norman Publishing; 1994. p. 455

[4] Puls LE, Duniho T, Hunter JE, Kryscio R, Blackhurst D, Gallion H. The prognostic implication of ascites in advanced-stage ovarian cancer. Gynecologic Oncology. 1996; **61**(1):109-112

[5] Patch AM, Christie EL, Etemadmoghadam D, Garsed DW, George J, Fereday S, et al. Whole-genome characterization of chemoresistant ovarian cancer. Nature. 2015; **521**(7553):489-494. DOI: 10.1038/nature14410

[6] Ahmed N, Stenvers KL. Getting to know ovarian cancer ascites: Opportunities for targeted therapy-based translational research. Frontiers in Oncology. 2013;**3**:256. DOI: 10.3389/fonc.2013.00256

[7] Kobold S, Hegewisch-Becker S, Oechsle K, Jordan K, Bokemeyer C, Atanackovic D. Intraperitoneal VEGF inhibition using bevacizumab: A potential approach for the symptomatic treatment of malignant ascites? The Oncologist. 2009;**14**(12):1242-1251. DOI: 10.1634/theoncologist.2009-0109

[8] BioEtymology. Origin of biomedical terms [Internet]. 2011. Available from: http://bioetymology.blogspot.si/ [Accessed: March 18, 2017]

[9] Maathuis JB, Van Look PF, Michie EA. Changes in volume, total protein and ovarian steroid concentrations of peritoneal fluid throughout the human menstrual cycle. The Journal of Endocrinology. 1978;**76**(1):123-133

[10] Smolle E, Taucher V, Haybaeck J. Malignant ascites in ovarian cancer and the role of targeted therapeutics. Anticancer Research. 2014;**34**(4):1553-1561

[11] Stanojević Z, Rančić G, Radić S, Potić-Zečević N, Đorđević B, Marković M, et al. Pathogenesis of malignant ascites in ovarian cancer patients. Archive of Oncology. 2004; **12**(2):115-118

[12] Holm-Nielsen P. Pathogenesis of ascites in peritoneal carcinomatosis. Acta Pathologica et Microbiologica Scandinavica. 1953;**33**:10-21

[13] Bronskill MJ, Bush RS, Ege GN. A quantitative measurement of peritoneal drainage in malignant ascites. Cancer. 1977;**40**:2375-2380

[14] Nagy JA, Herzberg KT, Dvorak JM, Dvorak HF. Pathogenesis of malignant ascites formation: Initiating events that lead to fluid accumulation. Cancer Research. 1993;**53**:2631-2643

[15] Senger DR, Galli SJ, Dvorak AM, et al. Tumor cells secrete a vascular permeability factor that promotes accumulation of ascites fluid. Science. 1983;**219**:983-985

[16] Nagy JA, Morgan ES, Herzberg KT, Manseau EJ, Dvorak AM, Dvorak HF. Pathogenesis of ascites tumor growth: Angiogenesis, vascular remodeling, and stroma formation in the peritoneal lining. Cancer Research. 1995;**55**(2):376-385

[17] Flam F, Einhorn N, Sjövall K. Symptomatology of ovarian cancer. European Journal of Obstetrics, Gynecology, and Reproductive Biology. 1988;**27**(1):53-57

[18] Tarn AC, Lapworth R. Biochemical analysis of ascitic (peritoneal) fluid: What should we measure? Annals of Clinical Biochemistry. 2010;**47**(5):397-407. DOI: 10.1258/acb.2010.010048

[19] Zhang T, Li F, Liu J, Zhang S. Diagnostic performance of the gynecology imaging reporting and data system for malignant adnexal masses. International Journal of Gynaecology and Obstetrics. 2017;**137**(3):227-349. DOI: 10.1002/ijgo.12153

[20] Timmerman D, Testa AC, Bourne T, Ameye L, Jurkovic D, Van Holsbeke C, et al. Simple ultrasound-based rules for the diagnosis of ovarian cancer. Ultrasound in Obstetrics & Gynecology. 2008;**31**(6):681-690. DOI: 10.1002/uog.5365

[21] Thoeni RF. The role of imaging in patients with ascites. AJR. American Journal of Roentgenology. 1995;**165**(1):16-18. DOI: 10.2214/ajr.165.1.7785576

[22] Ferrandina G, Sallustio G, Fagotti A, Vizzielli G, Paglia A, Cucci E, et al. Role of CT scan-based and clinical evaluation in the preoperative prediction of optimal cytoreduction in advanced ovarian cancer: A prospective trial. British Journal of Cancer. 2009;**101**(7):1066-1073. DOI: 10.1038/sj.bjc.6605292

[23] Kim S, Kim B, Song YS. Ascites modulates cancer cell behavior, contributing to tumor heterogeneity in ovarian cancer. Cancer Science. 2016;**107**(9):1173-1178. DOI: 10.1111/cas.12987

[24] Jang M, Yew PY, Hasegawa K, Ikeda Y, Fujiwara K, Fleming GF, et al. Characterization of T cell repertoire of blood, tumor, and ascites in ovarian cancer patients using next generation sequencing. Oncoimmunology. 2015;**4**(11):e1030561

[25] Worzfeld T, Pogge von Strandmann E, Huber M, Adhikary T, Wagner U, Reinartz S, et al. The unique molecular and cellular microenvironment of ovarian cancer. Frontiers in Oncology. 2017;**7**:24. DOI: 10.3389/fonc.2017.00024

[26] Shivakumarswamy U, Arakeril SU, Karigowdar MH, Yelikar BR. The role of the cell block method in the diagnosis of malignant ascetic fluid effusions. Journal of Clinical and Diagnostic Research. 2012;**6**(7):1280-1283

[27] Wang Y, Zheng W. Cytologic changes of ovarian epithelial cancer induced by neaadjuvant chemotherapy. International Journal of Clinical and Experimental Pathology. 2013;**6**(10):2121-2128

[28] Zhu FL, Ling AS, Wei Q, Ma J, Lu G. Tumor markers in serum and ascites in the diagnosis of benign and malignant ascites. Asian Pacific Journal of Cancer Prevention. 2015;**16**(2):719-722

[29] Adam RA, Adam YG. Malignant ascites: past, present, and future. Journal of the American College of Surgeons. 2004;**198**(6):999-1011

[30] Cavazzoni E, Bugiantella W, Graziosi L, Franceschini MS, Donini A. Malignant ascites: Pathophysiology and treatment. International Journal of Clinical Oncology. 2013;**18**(1):1-9. DOI: 10.1007/s10147-012-0396-6

[31] Keen A, Fitzgerald D, Bryant A, Dickinson HO. Management of drainage for malignant ascites in gynaecological cancer. Cochrane Database of Systematic Reviews. 2010;**1**:CD007794. DOI: 10.1002/14651858.CD007794.pub2

[32] Management of ascites in Ovarian Cancer patients [internet]. 2014. Available from: https://www.rcog.org.uk/globalassets/documents/guidelines/scientific-impact-papers/sip45ascites.pdf [Accessed: April 18, 2017]

[33] Harding V, Fenu E, Medani H, Shaboodien R, Ngan S, Li HK, et al. Safety, cost-effectiveness and feasibility of daycase paracentesis in the management of malignant ascites with a focus on ovarian cancer. British Journal of Cancer. 2012;**107**(6):925-930. DOI: 10.1038/bjc.2012.343

[34] Becker G, Galandi D, Blum HE. Malignant ascites: Systematic review and guideline for treatment. European Journal of Cancer. 2006;**42**(5):589-597

[35] Stange A. Malignant ascites – Current treatment and novel therapeutic options. Magazine of European Medical Oncology. 2012;**5**:43-46. DOI: 10.1007/s12254-012-0338-z

[36] Martin LG. Percutaneous placement and management of the Denver shunt for portal hypertensive ascites. AJR. American Journal of Roentgenology. 2012;**199**(4):W449-W453

[37] Bellot P, Welker MW, Soriano G, von Schaewen M, Appenrodt B, Wiest R, et al. Automated low flow pump system for the treatment of refractory ascites: A multi-center safety and efficacy study. Journal of Hepatology 2013;**58**(5):922-927. DOI:10.1016/j.jhep.2012.12.020

[38] Narayanan G, Pezeshkmehr A, Venkat S, Guerrero G, Barbery K. Safety and efficacy of the PleurX catheter for the treatment of malignant ascites. Journal of Palliative Medicine. 2014;**17**(8):906-912. DOI: 10.1089/jpm.2013.0427

[39] Fleming ND, Alvarez-Secord A, Von Gruenigen V, Miller MJ, Abernethy AP. Indwelling catheters for the management of refractory malignant ascites: A systematic literature overview and retrospective chart review. Journal of Pain and Symptom Management. 2009;**38**(3):341-349. DOI: 10.1016/j.jpainsymman.2008.09.008

[40] Qu C, Xing M, Ghodadra A, McCluskey KM, Santos E, Kim HS. The impact of tunneled catheters for ascites and peritoneal Carcinomatosis on patient Rehospitalizations. Cardiovascular and Interventional Radiology. 2016;**39**(5):711-716. DOI: 10.1007/s00270-015-1258-1

[41] EMEA Assessment Report for REMOVAB. Doc. Ref.: EMEA/CHMP/100434/2009 [internet]. 2009. Available from: http://www.ema.europa.eu/docs/en_GB/document_library/EPAR_-_Public_assessment_report/human/000972/WC50 0051808.pdf [Accessed: April 11, 2017]

[42] Went P, Lugli A, Meier S, Bundi M, Mirlacher M, Sauter G, et al. Frequent EpCAM protein expression in human carcinomas. Human Pathology. 2004;**35**:122-128

[43] Maguire B, Whitaker D, Carrello S, Spagnolo D, et al. Monoclonal antibody Ber-EP4:Its use in the differential diagnosis of malignant mesothelioma and carcinoma in cell blocks of malignant effusions and FNA specimens. Diagnostic Cytopathology. 1994;**10**:130-134

[44] Munz M, Kieu C, Mack B, Schmitt B, Zeidler R, Gires O, et al. The carcinoma-associated antigen EpCAM upregulates c-myc and induces cell proliferation. Oncogene. 2004;**23**:5748-5758

[45] Gutzmer R, Li W, Sutterwala S, Elizalde JI, Urtishak SL, Behrens EM, et al. A tumor-associated glycoprotein that blocks MHC class II-dependent antigen presentation by dendritic cells. Journal of Immunology. 2004;**173**:1023-1032

[46] Kipps E, Tan DS, Kaye SB. Meeting the challenge of ascites in ovarian cancer: New avenues for therapy and research. Nature Reviews. Cancer. 2013;**13**(4):273-282. DOI: 10.1038/nrc3432

[47] Woopen H, Sehouli J. Current and future options in the treatment of malignant ascites in ovarian cancer. Anticancer Research. 2009;**29**(8):3353-3359

[48] Pujade-Lauraine E, Hilpert F, Weber B, Reuss A, Poveda A, Kristensen G, et al. Bevacizumab combined with chemotherapy for platinum-resistant recurrent ovarian cancer: The AURELIA open-label randomized phase III trial. Journal of Clinical Oncology. 2014; **32**(13):1302-1308. DOI: 10.1200/JCO.2013.51.4489

[49] Ferriss JS, Java JJ, Bookman MA, Fleming GF, Monk BJ, Walker JL, et al. Ascites predicts treatment benefit of bevacizumab in front-line therapy of advanced epithelial ovarian, fallopian tube and peritoneal cancers: An NRG oncology/GOG study. Gynecologic Oncology. 2015;**139**(1):17-22. DOI: 10.1016/j.ygyno.2015.07.103

[50] El-Shami K, Elsaid A, El-Kerm Y. Open-label safety and efficacy pilot trial of intraperitoneal bevacizumab as palliative treatment in refractory malignant ascites. Journal of Clinical Oncology. 2007;**25**(18):9043

[51] Zaltrap, Annex I Summary of product characteristics[internet]. Available from: http:// www.ema.europa.eu/docs/en_GB/document_library/EPAR_-_Product_Information/ human/002532/WC500139484.pdf [Accessed: April 12, 2017]

[52] Colombo N, Mangili G, Mammoliti S, Kalling M, Tholander B, Sternas L, et al. A phase II study of aflibercept in patients with advanced epithelial ovarian cancer and symptomatic malignant ascites. Gynecologic Oncology. 2012;**125**(1):42-47

[53] Gotlieb WH, Amant F, Advani S, Goswami C, Hirte H, Provencher D, et al. Intravenous aflibercept for treatment of recurrent symptomatic malignant ascites in patients with advanced ovarian cancer: A phase 2, randomised, double-blind, placebo-controlled study. The Lancet Oncology. 2012;**13**(2):154-162

[54] Davies B, Brown PD, East N, Crimmin MJ, Balkwill FR. A synthetic matrix metalloproteinase inhibitor decreases tumor burden and prolongs survival of mice bearing human ovarian carcinoma xenografts. Cancer Research. 1993;**53**(9):2087-2091

[55] Valle M, Federici O, Garofalo A. Patient selection for cytoreductive surgery and hyperthermic intraperitoneal chemotherapy, and role of laparoscopy in diagnosis, staging, and treatment. Surgical Oncology Clinics of North America. 2012;**21**(4):515-531. DOI: 10.1016/j.soc.2012.07.005

[56] Pockros PJ, Esrason KT, Nguyen C, Duque J, Woods S. Mobilization of malignant ascites with diuretics is dependent on ascitic fluid characteristics. Gastroenterology. 1992; **103**:1302-1306

[57] Latifi A, Luwor RB, Bilandzic M, Nazaretian S, Stenvers K, Pyman J, et al. Isolation and characterization of tumor cells from the ascites of ovarian cancer patients: Molecular phenotype of chemoresistant ovarian tumors. PLoS One. 2012;**7**(10):e46858

[58] Kobal B, Jerman KG, Karo J, Verdenik I, Cerne K. (forthcoming 2016). Relationship of ovarian cancer tumour markers concentration between local fluid and serum: Comparison of malignant to benign condition. European Journal of Gynaecological Oncology. 2017

6

Uterine Cervical Cancer Screening

Doris Barboza and Esther Arbona

Abstract

Cervical cancer is the fourth most common cancer and the third cause of death among women worldwide. More than 85% of the cases occur in developing countries. In Latin America, cervical cancer is the most common cause of cancer deaths among women, primarily in young women with devastating social impact. It is mostly the consequence of lack of a health care infrastructure that allows cervical cancer screening suitable for detecting pre-malignant lesions. With the knowledge that human papillomavirus (HPV) infection is the main cause of cervical cancer, two major preventive interventions have emerged: HPV vaccination and screening, which involve the detection and treatment of cervical dysplasia and early-stage cervical cancer. HPV 16 and 18 cause up to 70% of all cervical cancer cases in Latin America and are covered in all available vaccines. Since tests for high-risk HPV types and HPV vaccines are expensive and they have not been included in immunization programs and given free of charge to eligible women in Venezuela and most less developed regions, screening campaigns with cytology and direct visualization of the cervix with VIN continue to be the major interventions that can prevent cervical cancer in these countries; they need to be implemented in a large scale.

Keywords: cervical cancer screening, human papillomavirus, HPV vaccine, PAP test, Papanicolaou, cytology, acetic acid, oncogenic HPV

1. Introduction

Cervical cancer is a public health problem in adult women in developing countries of South America, Central and Sub-Saharan Africa, meridional and Sub-oriental Asia [1]. It is the fourth most common cancer and the third cause of death among women worldwide [2]. Nine percent (529,800) of new cancer and 8% (275,100) of all cancer deaths in 2008 were caused by cervical cancer. More than 85% of the cases occur in developing countries. Twenty-seven percent (77,100) of all cervical cancer deaths occurred in India, the second most populous country in the world (**Figure 1**).

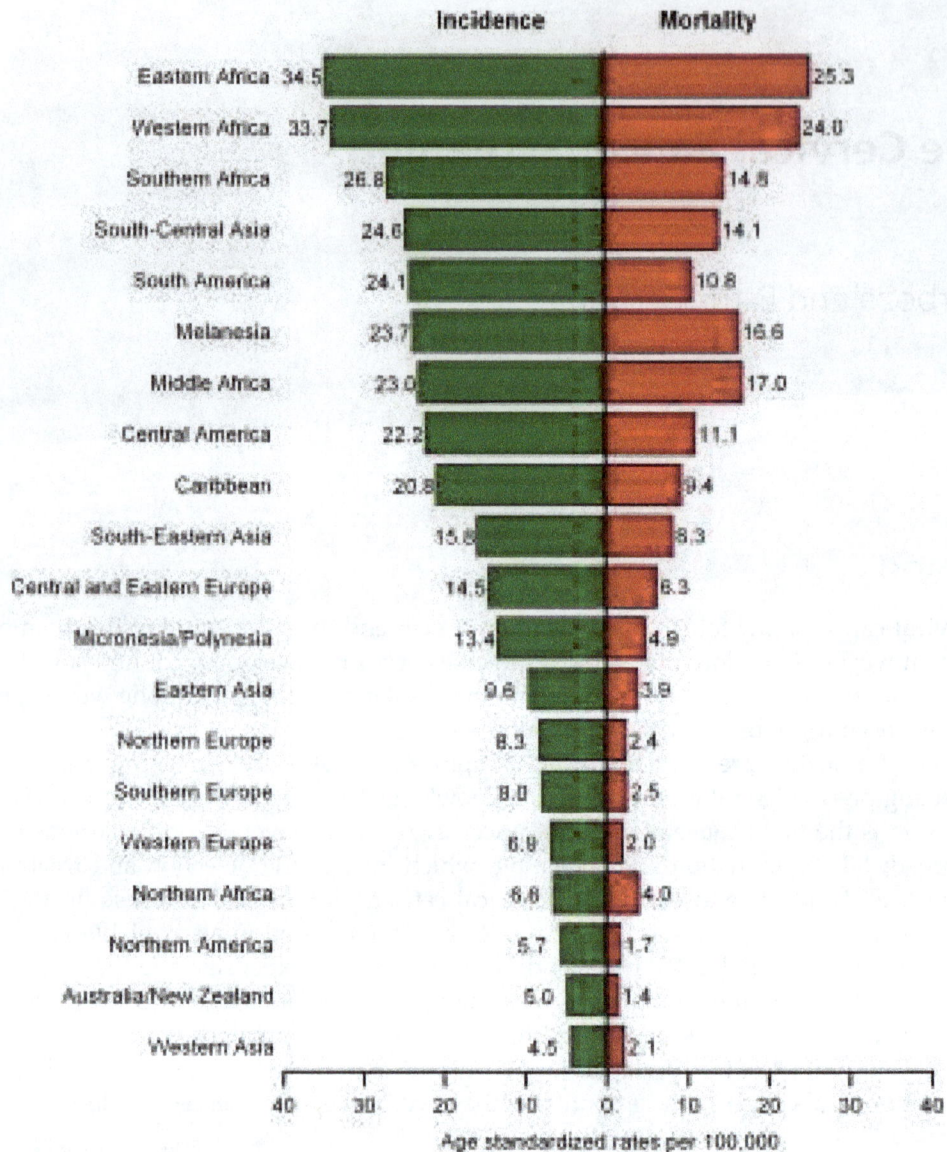

Figure 1. Age-standardized cervical cancer: Incidence and mortality. Rates by world area. GLOBOCAN 2008.

In 2017, the American Cancer Society (Cancer Statistic Center) estimated that there will be 12,820 new cervical cancer patients and 4210 deaths. The incidence rate for cervical cancer from 2009 through 2017 is 7.6 per 100,000 women; the rate of death from 2010 through 2014 is 2.3 per 100,000 women. The incidence and death rates for cervical cancer in Latin America are still high; for example, in Venezuela, the annual average of new cervical cancer cases from 2010 through 2014 was 4019, with a standardized rate on 2014 of 24.88.

In developed countries, most patients are diagnosed in the early stage of the disease or with pre-malignant lesions susceptible to effective treatment. Nevertheless, with the current migratory movement of women, there is an upturn of advanced stage cervical cancer, especially among women who miss their routine gynecologic evaluation or belong to immigrant's groups without suitable medical assistance.

In Latin America, cervical cancer occupies the second position after breast cancer and is the most common cause of cancer deaths among women, primarily in young women. For public health, the principal importance is that cervical cancer mainly affects young women from low income households, with a devastating impact on them and their families with lot of orphans. Despite it being an easily preventable disease, prevention and screening of cervical cancer are not up to the mark in these regions. If prevention and screening programs do not improve, it is estimated that the annual cases will increase with estimation for 2025 of 126,000 new cases [3].

The highest incidence and mortality of cervical cancer in developing countries and other medically unattended areas is mostly the consequence of lack of a health care infrastructure that allows screening suitable for detecting pre-malignant lesions [4]. The most efficient and profitable screening techniques [5] are cytology-based screening (the Pap test) and HPV DNA screening. A clinical trial in one of India's rural areas with low income households found than 1 round of HPV DNA screening was related with a 50% reduction in probability of developing cervical cancer [6].

Screening programs fail because of substandard quality of pap-smear sampling techniques, methodology errors, limited geographical and population coverage with emphasis on high-risk women, and sub-optimal follow-up.

With the knowledge that HPV infection is the main cause of cervical cancer, two major interventions that can prevent cervical cancer have emerged: HPV vaccination and screening, which involves the detection and treatment of cervical dysplasia and early-stage cervical cancer.

All HPV vaccines currently available cover HPV 16 and 18 that cause up to 70% of all cervical cancer cases in Latin America [7]. Cervarix from GlaxoSmithKline is a bivalent vaccine that covers only HPV 16/18; Gardasil from Merck & Co is a quadrivalent vaccine that covers HPV 16/18 and HPV 6/11, which cause genital warts. Both vaccines prevent primary VPH infection, CNI2 and CNI3 related to HPV 16 and HPV 18, when 3 doses are completed. The 9-valent vaccine (Gardasil 9 from Merck & Co.) covers seven HPV types related to cervical cancer, including HPV 16/18 and HPV 6/11 [8, 9].

HPV vaccine is recommended for girls aged 9–26 years of age to prevent cancers of the cervix, vagina, and vulva related with HPV 16 or 18, or genital warts (HPV 6 or HPV 11), and lesions related with other HPV types, cervical adenocarcinoma in situ, vulvar or vaginal intraepithelial neoplasia [10]. In addition, women must be vaccinated before their first sexual activity, prior to exposure to HPV. HPV vaccination is also recommended for women with weakened immune systems (including people with HIV infection), given their higher risk of having HPV infection.

By mid-2016, 65 countries had introduced HPV vaccines, mostly developing countries, but including an increasing number of middle and low-income countries. Unfortunately, HPV vaccines are expensive and they have not been included in immunization programs and given free of charge to eligible women in Venezuela and most less-developed regions. Thus, screening continues to be the major intervention that can prevent cervical cancer in these countries.

2. Risk factors

Most of the risk factors for developing cervical cancer are associated with a compromised immune response that allows HPV infection, the etiologic agent of nearly all cases of cervical cancer. These factors include the following.

- Early first sexual intercourse; the risk increases if the first sexual activity is before 21 years of age [11, 12], being approximately 1.5% when first sexual activity is at 18–20 years of age and younger.

- Multiple sexual partners.

- High-risk sexual partner, for example, a partner with multiple sexual partners or with HPV infection.

- Squamous vulvar intraepithelial neoplasia or vaginal neoplasia (highly associated with HPV infection) in the past.

- History of sexually transmitted disease (chlamydia, genital herpes) [13, 14].

- Immunosuppression: VIH-positive women have consistently shown to be at an increased risk for high-grade cervical dysplasia. [14]

- Young age at first full-term pregnancy (less than 20 years of age) and high parity are exogenous cofactors associated with an increased risk of cervical carcinoma; these factors are thought to increase the risk through the maintenance of the transformation zone on the exocervix for a prolonged time, which facilitates exposure to HPV [15].

- Low income/socio-economic status is associated with cervical cancer; incidence and mortality are higher in high-poverty communities [16].

- Oral contraceptives: The data analysis of 24 epidemiologic studies [17] found that the risk of cervical cancer increases with increasing duration of oral contraceptive use (5 years or more of using oral contraceptives vs. non-users); the relative risk was 95% and it decreased after use of oral contraceptives has ceased; the same analysis estimated that 10-year use of oral contraceptives that started at 20–30 years of age increases incidence of cervical cancer in middle-age women

- In current smokers, a doubling in risk of developing cervical cancer has been observed, with a positive correlation with the habit intensity; nicotine and smoke derivates from tobacco discovered on cervical mucus suggest a possible biologic mechanism through immunosuppression that favor infectious agent such as HPV; tobacco smoking is associated with squamous cervical cancer [18]

- Some daughters of women, especially young women, who took diethylstilbestrol during pregnancy have developed clear cell adenocarcinoma of the cervix and vagina [19, 20]

- High incidence of cervical cancer is observed in Afro-Americans, Latins, and ethnic groups with low incomes and socio-economic conditions with limited access to effective screening and health system [18]

3. Genetic factors

There is no established model for a genetic base, although population studies have found increased risk in familiar groups. In the past, it was attributed to ambient environmental exposure and shared risk factors; however, subsequent data comparing sisters and half-sisters far exceed shared environments.

Research has been done to identify genetic alterations that can make women more susceptible to cervical cancer because of less resistance to HPV infection and persistent infection.

To date, results show a large polymorphism diversity in a wide variety of genes, including those regulating immunity and susceptibility [19–21] and generating a large amount of immune mechanism (cytokines production, angiogenesis, tumor suppression pathways, transcription activation) [22–24].

4. Human papillomavirus

The causal role of HPV in all common and non-common histologic types has been firmly established biologically and epidemiologically and has led to a new carcinogenic model for cervical cancer: HPV acquisition, HPV persistence, progression of pre-malignant lesion to invasive cancer [25, 26]. Human papillomavirus is acquired through sexual contact; most population prevalence reaches its peak few years after the median age of initiation of sexual intercourse.

Most HVP infections are transient, lasting no more than 1 or 2 years [27]. Persistent HPV infection for 1–2 years, especially by HPV 16 predicts development of CIN 3 (cervical intraepithelial neoplasia) or malignant changes. The probability of untreated CIN 3 transforming into an invasive cancer is 30%, although 1% of treated CIN 3 transforms into an invasive cancer [28].

There are more than 100 HPV types; high-risk types 16, 18, 31, 35, and 39 are linked to malignant transformation [29]. Type 18 infection progresses with bad prognosis based on recorded survival rates.

High-risk HPV infection may generate some of the following cell biologic alterations leading to malignant transformation. Two of the eight proteins encoded by the HPV genome, E6 and E7, accounts for most carcinogenic effects of high-risk HPV types. They promote carcinogenesis in several ways:

- They interfere with important tumor suppressor pathways; E6 inhibits the p53 tumor suppressor by promoting its proteasomal degradation, while E7 disrupts the retinoblastoma (Rb) pathway [30, 31], or activates oncogenes via EGFR (epidermal growth factor receptor) [32, 33].

- They induce telomerase enzyme activation related with the unlimited potential of neoplastic cells replication [34].

- E6 and E7 abrogate cell cycle checkpoints and induce genomic instability. Both can induce abnormal centrosome numbers and centrosome abnormalities. They also have synergistic effects on centrosome abnormalities and chromosomal instability [35, 36].

Progression of HPV infection to uterine cervical cancer is associated with progressive histologic changes. Cervical intraepithelial neoplasia (CIN) is a histologic change corresponding to dysplasia of cervical squamous epithelium associated with HPV infection and is considered a potential precursor of uterine cervical cancer. They are classified into three grades: CIN grade I, mild dysplasia, or abnormal cell growth confined to the basal 1/3 of the cervical epithelium; CIN grade II, moderate dysplasia confined to the basal 2/3 of the epithelium; and CIN grade 3, severe dysplasia that spans more than 2/3 of the epithelium, and may involve the full thickness.

Historical data demonstrated that the majority (71–90%) of CIN 1 lesions *regress spontaneously* in contrast with persistence and progression rates for CIN 2 and CIN 3, estimated in 57 and 70% respectively [37].

There are mainly four steps implicated in the development of uterine cervical cancer:

1. Oncogenic HPV infection of squamous cells in the transformation zone of the cervix, which is in the union area of the squamous epithelium of the exocervix and the endocervical glandular epithelium.

2. Persistent HPV infection.

3. Progression of persistent HPV epithelial cells infected to a pre-malignant lesion.

4. Development of invasive carcinoma: Tumor cells in the epithelium cross the basement membrane and invade the stroma.

Formal epidemiological evidence of the association between HPV and cervical cancer did not exist until the early 1990s, although molecular characterization of one of the first types of HPV in the 1980s made it possible to develop tests of hybridization to obtain fragments of HPV genes in human tissue. Using hybridization studies based on polymerase chain reaction (PCR), studies have been conducted for the identification of HPV DNA. One of the pioneer studies in Latin America was carried out by the Agency for Research of Cancer, between Colombia and Spain. The results of this study have been considered as the first evidence of the causal association between HPV and cervical cancer. Subsequently, similar studies were carried out in 9 countries (Algeria, Brazil, India, Mali, Morocco, Peru, Paraguay, Thailand, and Philippines) between 1985 and 1988 to evaluate the role of the virus of HPV in the etiology of CIN 3. The DNA was obtained by cytology and was evaluated by Virapap and PCR. In Spain, HPV prevalence based on PCR was detected in 63.2% of the cases and for controls was observed in 47%. In Colombia, HPV DNA was detected in 63.2% of the cases and in 10.5% of the controls. VPH 16 was the most predominant type of virus and showed stronger association with the development of CIN 3. HPV of unknown origin was common in positive cases (18.3% in Spain and 38.0% in Colombia [28]. In 2006, a study was carried out at the gynecologic department of the Padre Machado Hospital, in Venezuela; it included 58 patients with uterine cervical cancer. Typification of human papillomavirus by PCR for types 6, 11, 16, 18, 31,33, and 35 were performed; other variables such as age, stage, and histological type were also analyzed. The purpose of this study was typification of HPV in women with invasive uterine cervical cancer in Venezuela, identification of the country's most frequent HPV type, and comparison with worldwide incidence of VPH. HPV DNA sequences were associated in 52.3% of the patients, VPH 16 in 24.52%, and HPV 18 in 7.4% of their population. These results suggest the imperative need of large-scale epidemiological studies as these results do not reflect the results reported in other countries [38].

5. Uterine cervical cancer screening

Screening of uterine cervix decreases the incidence and mortality of cervical cancer. Cervical cancer has two main histological types: squamous and adenocarcinoma. Screening can detect precursors and early stage for both types, and treatment of precursors can prevent the development of invasive cancer. Currently, in addition to screening, test for high-risk human papillomavirus types, which form the foundation of uterine cervical cancer pathogenesis, has been included. In view of the high incidence and mortality of cervical cancer, its significance as a global public health problem, and the difficulties involved in establishing effective screening in different regions of the world, the American Society of Oncology (ASCO), in the year 2013 [39], released a world guide for cervical screening and follow-up of positive cases, as well as guidelines for treatment for pre-malignant lesions. The main recommendation was screening for cervical pre-cancers for all women in appropriate age groups and establishing consistent minimum standards for screening considering and based on resource levels and health systems infrastructure.

Based on the results of a large clinical trial in India that demonstrated that cervical cancer screening with acetic acid (vinegar) could prevent thousands of deaths each year in developing countries [39], initial visual inspection with acetic acid (vinegar) was incorporated in the global screening guideline.

Cancer of the cervix is a highly preventable disease; low-income countries lack large-scale screening and vaccination programs against HPV. As a result, more than 85% of the world's cervical cancer diagnoses and deaths occur in less developed regions. Access to programs of detection and treatment of cervical cancer varies not only between countries but also within them. Standards were established in four different areas of health: basic, enhanced, and maximum limited. These levels correspond not only to the financial resources of a country or region, but also the strengths of the health care including personnel, infrastructure, and access to health systems.

ASCO's guideline builds upon WHO's recommendations by providing a minimum set of standards across all countries based on their existing resources, and by accounting for the 2013 VIA study and other recent data. HPV DNA testing is recommended in all resource settings and VIA may be used while HPV testing becomes available. If VIA, as a primary screening, gives abnormal results, women should receive treatment. After a positive HPV DNA testing result, VIA is recommended for follow-up in basic and limited settings. For other settings, HPV genotyping and/or cytology may be used for triage. Women with abnormal triage results should receive immediate treatment in basic and limited settings, or colposcopy in all other settings. Screening is recommended for women of ages 25–65 years every 5 years and for ages 30–65 years, and if two consecutive tests are negative at 5-year intervals, then every 10 years. In the context of limited setting, screening is recommended for ages 30–49 years, every 10 years and for basic settings, for ages 30–49 years, one or more screens in a lifetime. When a precursor lesion is diagnosed, the recommended treatment includes LEEP, or ablative treatments (cryotherapy, cold coagulation) with a 12-month post-treatment follow-up for all settings. For women who are HIV positive, those who had recently given birth, and those who have undergone a hysterectomy, separate screening recommendations have been provided.

Screening methods include Papanicolaou (PAP) test (cytology) and tests for high-risk human papillomavirus types. Cervical cancer screening detects precancerous lesions in the early stages and their treatment decreases uterine cervical cancer incidence and mortality. In the United States, PAP was adopted in 1950 and in the mid-1980s [40], the incidence of cervical cancer had decreased to 70% [41]. The benefit of screening is that it decreases mortality and the incidence of cancer of the cervix, but information provided by the PAP must be evaluated since infection can be transient and dysplasia can regress spontaneously, especially in young women [42]. Major adverse outcomes of screening are derived for furthers consequence to methods used for treatment of injuries. The effects on the reproductive system include stenosis, loss of pregnancy in the second trimester, premature births, and rupture of the membrane [43].

Most episodes of HPV infection and many cases of CIN 1 and CNI2 are transient and fail to develop into CIN 3 or cancer. Potential problems associated with positive screening tests are stigmatization of a sexually transmitted disease and inconvenience associated with additional diagnostic and treatment procedures [44]. Getting a positive test at any time of life may contribute to the perception that one is at an increased risk of cancer and a desire for more tests with the consequent possibility of another positive test, the monetary costs involving the control procedures after a positive result, and the higher cost, from the health perspective, of developing cancer [45]. Although any false-positive test has the potential to induce anxiety, quality of life test is usually not included in screening trials. As a result, the number of colposcopies related to CIN 3 and cancer has been regulated. Cervical cancer is rare in young women and adolescents and may not be prevented by cytological screening. The incidence has not changed in developed countries, but in low-income countries, it presents in earlier ages [46].

Screening in adolescents leads to an unnecessary evaluation and treatment of lesions with high potential of spontaneous regression with reproductive long-term problems. Cancer prevention programs in adolescent should focus on massive vaccination for HPV [47].

Among the 21 to 29 year-olds, screening is recommended with PAP every 3 years. For women aged 21 to 29, with two or more consecutive negative cytologic findings [48, 49], there is no evidence that supports a greater interval for detection (3 or more years). For women less than 30 years of age, HPV screening is not recommended, given high chance of transient HPV infections. Positive predictive value of these tests limits the usefulness of them as screening methods. Randomized studies have shown that HPV testing for women less than 30 years of age [48–50] results in high detection of transient infections by HPV and the women undergo unnecessary colposcopies [51].

For women older than 30 years, PAP is recommended every 3 years with co-tests (PAP and HPV) every 5 years if both initial tests were negative. For women older than 30 years, HPV infection has a greater chance of being persistent; it also has uncertain clinical significance. Any other determination of HPV test increases the probability of positive results, with largest number of colposcopies with uncertain results [52].

In women older than 65 years, tests are not recommended if they meet the following criteria:

- No risk factors: No history of abnormal test; not a habitual smoker, or currently smoking; no disease related to HPV; not new couples; not immunocompromised; no exposure to diethylstilbestrol in utero

- Optimal screening: Two consecutive negative tests, co-tests, or three PAP tests in the last 20 years, latest during five previous years [53, 54]

- No history of high grade dysplasia or more

There are some clinical conditions where increased risk of developing CIN and cervical cancer are observed, as in human immunodeficiency virus (HIV)-infected women. This conclusion is based on several trials including the study of Wright et al. [55] where the definition of cervical intraepithelial neoplasia (CIN) prevalence, validity of PAP tests, and the association of risk factors in women infected with HPV virus, demonstrated that these patients are more likely to have a persistent infection with the virus, increased rate of high grade cervical dysplasia, and higher risk of developing cervical cancer.

Immunosuppressed women: Patients with immunosuppressive therapy (organ /bone marrow transplants, prolonged treatment with steroids, systemic disease), infected with HIV present greater persistence of infection with minor ability to regress spontaneously and therefore, they have higher rates of cervical dysplasia and cancer. Information about immunosuppressed women are based on the results of screening women with systemic lupus erythematosus (SLE). High grade dysplasia and subtype of high-risk HPV persistence rates are significantly higher in women with SLE who receive immunosuppressive therapy, than immunosuppressed patients treated for other conditions, or patients with minor SLE receiving treatment [56, 57].

At present, for this group of patients, who are immunocompromised or HIV-infected, it is recommended to start screening at age 21, or PAP and HPV tests should be done at the age when participating in the first sexual relationship.

Women with total hysterectomy, no history of CIN or cervical cancer, operated for benign pathologies have a very low risk of developing cervical cancer and need not undergo screening for cancer of the cervix [58, 59]. Women with sub-total hysterectomy probably share the same risks as patients with preserved cervix and must follow the general guidelines. For those women with hysterectomy and a history of CIN 2/3 or adenocarcinoma in situ, if the diagnosis was made prior to surgery or hysterectomy, the ACOG recommends screening at least 20 years after treatment [60]. The most recent summary of recommendations [61] includes the following:

- Start screening no sooner than age 21, regardless of the age of onset of sexual activity or other risk factors. Between 21 and 29 years of age, PAP smear must be done every 3 years. Between 30 and 65 years, co-testing (cytology more than an HPV test) every 5 years is preferable; if not possible, single cytology every 3 years is acceptable. After the age of 65 years, screening can be discontinued if previous screening has been done and found negative and not CIN 2 (+) during the previous 20 years.

- Screening can be discontinued if there is total hysterectomy (with removal of cervix) and a history of CIN 2 (+).

These suggestions are valid for developed countries that allow the implementation of adequate screening campaigns with all the resources available. However, for developing countries with limited resources, cytology and direct visualization of the cervix with VIN are valid methods.

Author details

Doris Barboza[1]* and Esther Arbona[2]

*Address all correspondence to: dorisbarbozad@gmail.com

1 Medical Institute La Floresta, Oncological Radiotherapy Service, Group GURVE, Caracas, Venezuela

2 Internal Medicine Infectious Disease Department, Dana–Farber Cancer Institute, Boston, USA

References

[1] Wrigt TC Jr, Blumenthal P, Bradley J, Denny L, Esmuy PD, Jayant K, Jayant K, Nene BM, Rajkumar R, Sankaranrayaanan R, Sellor JLD, Shastri SS, Serris J. Diagnostic Cytopathology. 2007 Dec;**35**(12):845

[2] Jemal A, Bray F, Center MM, et al. Global cáncer statistics CA. Cáncer Journal of Clinicians. 2011;**61**:69

[3] Kahn JA. HPV vaccination for the prevention of cervical intraepithelial neoplasia. New England Journal of Medicien. 2009;**361**:271

[4] Mathew A, George PS. Trends in incidence and mortality rate of squamous cell carcinoma and Adenocarcinoma of cérvix-Worlwide Asia Pac. Journal of Cancer Prevention. 2009;**10**:645-650

[5] Vizcaino AP, Moreno V, Bosch FX, et al. International trends in incidence of cervical cancer II. Squamous cell Carcinoma. International Journal of Cancer. 2000;**86**:429-435ia

[6] Sankaranarayanam R, Nene BM, Shastri SS. HPV screening for cervical cancer in rural Indian. England Journal of Medicine. 2009;**360**(14):385-1394

[7] Parking DM, Almonte M, Bruni L, Clifford G, Curado MP. Pineus burden and trends of type-specific human papillomavirus and related disease in Latin America an Caribbean Region. Vaccine. 2008;**26**(sup I:II):L1-L5

[8] Villa LL, Costa RL, Petta CA, et al. Prophylactic quadrivalent human papillovirus (types 6, 11, 16 and 18) L1 virus-like particle vaccine in young women: A randomised doublé blind placebo-controlled multicenter phase II efficacy trial. Lancet Oncology. 2005;**6**:271-278

[9] Sankaranarayanan R. HPV vaccination: The promise & problems. India Journal of Research. 2009;**130**:322-326

[10] Saslow Castle PE, Cox JT, et al. American Cancer Society Guideline for human papillovirus(and its precursors. HPV) vaccine use to prevent cervical cancer. CA Cancer Journal of Clinicians. 2007;**57**:7

[11] Wallim KL, Wiklund F, Angstrôm T, et al. Type-specific persistence of human papillomavirus DNA before the development of invasive cervical cancer. New England Journal of Medicine. 1999;**341**:572

[12] Ho GY, Bierman R, Beardsley L, et al. Natural history of cervicovaginal papillomavirus infection in young women. England Journal of Medicine. 1998;**338**:423

[13] Committee on practice Bulletins Gynecology. Practice Bulletin No. 168: Cervical Cancer Screening and Prevention. Obstetrics and Gynecology. 2016;**128**:e111

[14] Klumb EM, Araujo ML Jr, Jesus GR, et al. Is higher prevalence of cervical intraepithelial neoplasia in women with lupus due to immunosuppession? Journal of Clinical Rheumatology. 2010;**16**:153

[15] Muñoz N, Francheschi S, Bosetti C, et al. Role of parity and human papillovirus in cervical cancer. The IARC multricentic case-control study. Lancet. 2002;**359**:1093

[16] Jemal A, Simmard EP, Dorell C, et al. Annual Report to Nation on Status of Cancer, 1975-2009. Feature the burden and trends in human papillomavirus (HPV)-associated cancers and HPV vaccination coverage levels. Journal of National Cancer Institute. 2013;**105**:17

[17] Cervical cancer screening programs I. Epidemiology and natural history of carcinoma of the cervix. Canadian Medical Association Journal. 1976;**114**:1003

[18] International Collaboration of epidemiology studies of cervical cancer; Appleby P, Beral V, et al. Carcinoma of the cervix and tobacco smoking. Collaborative reanalysis of individual data on 13.541 women without carcinoma of the cervix from 23 epidemiological studies. International Journal of Cancer. 2006;**1181**:1481. http://Cancertopics/cause/des/persons-exposed-to-des [Accessed: June 14, 2012]

[19] National Cancer Institute. Clinical information: Identification and management of persons to DES (Diethylstilbestrol)

[20] Siegel R, Ward E, Brawley O, Jemal A. Cancer statistics, 2011: Impact of eliminating socioeconomic and racial disparities on premature cancer deaths. CA Cancer Journal of Clinicians. 2011;**61**:212

[21] Liu L, Yang X, Chen X, et al. Association between TNF polymorphisms and cervical cancer risk: a meta- analysis. Molecular Biology Reports. 2012;**39**:2683

[22] Wang Q, Zhang C, Walay S, et al. Association between cytokine gene polymorphisms and cervical cancer in a Chinese population. European Journal of Obstetrics and Gynecology and Reproductive Biology. 2011;**158**:330

[23] Craveiro R, Bravo I, Catarino R, et al. The role of p73 G4C 14 polymorphism in the susceptibility to cervical cancer. DNA and Cell Biology. 2012;**31**:224

[24] Whang K, Zhou B, Zhang J, et al. Association signal of signal transducer and activator of transcription 3 gene polymorphisms with cervical cancer in Chinese women. DNA and Cell Biology. 2011;**30**(11):931

[25] Jemal A, Simard EP, Dorell C, et al. Annual Report to the Nation on the Status of Cancer, 1975-2009, featuring the burden and trends in hu infman papillovirus (HPV)-associated cancers and HPV vaccination coverage levels. Journal of National Cancer Institute. 2013;**105**:175

[26] Koutsky LA, Holmes KK, Critchlow CW, Stevens CE, Paavone J, Beckmann AM, et al. A cohort study of the risk of cervical intraephitelial grade 2 or 3 in relation to papillomavirus infection. England Journal of Medicine. 1992;**327**:1272-1278

[27] Kjaer SK, Van der Brule AJ, Paul IG, Svare EI, Sherman ME, Thomsem BL, et al. Type specific persistent of high risk human papillovirus (HPV) as indicator of high grade cervical squamous intraepithelial lesions in young women: Population based prospective follow up study. BMJ. 2002;**325**(7364)

[28] Bosch FX, Muñoz N, De Sanjose, Navarro C, Moreo P, Ascunce N, Gonzalez LC, Tafur L, Gili M, Larrañaga I, et al. Human pavillomavirus and cervical intraepithelial neoplastic grado III/carcinoma in situ: A case control study in Spain and Colombia. Cancer Epidemiology Biomarkers Prevention. 1993 Sep-Oct;**2**(5):415-422

[29] Muñoz N, Bravo LE. Colombia Medica. 2012 Oct-Dec;**43**:296-304

[30] Werness Ba, Levine AJ, Howley PM. Association of human papillomavirus types 16 and 18 E6 proteins with p53. Science. 1990;**248**:76-79

[31] Vogelstein B, Kinzler K. The multistep nature of cancer. Trends in Genetics. 1993;**9**:138-141

[32] Hu G, Lui Mendelsohn J, Ellis LM, Radinsky R, Andreeff M, et al. Expression of epidermal growth factor receptor and papillomavirus E6/E7 proteins in cervical carcinoma cells. Journal of National Cancer Institute. 1997;**89**:1271-1276

[33] Sizemore N, Rorke E. Human papillomavirus16 immortalization of normal human ectocervical epithelial cells alters retinoic acid regulation of cell growth and epidermal growth factor receptor expression. Cancer Research. 1993;**53**:4511-4517

[34] Lee D, Kin HZ, Jeong KW, Shim YS, Horikawa L, Barret JC, et al. Human papillomavirus E2 down-regulates the human telomerase reverse transcriptase promoter. Biological Chemistry. 2002:27748-27745

[35] Duensing S,Duensing A, Crum CP, Mûnger K. Human papillomavirus type 16 E7 oncoprotein- induced abnormal centrosome synthesis is an early event in the evolving malignant phenotype. Cancer Research. 2001;**61**:2356-2360

[36] Zhang A, Mâner S, Betz R, Angstrôm T, Stendhal U, et al. Genetic alterations in cervical carcinomas: frequent low-level amplifications of oncogenes are associated with human papillomavirus infection. International Journal of Cancer. 2002;**101**:427-433

[37] Schiffman Castle PE, Jeronimo J, et al. Human papillomavirus and cervical cancer. Lancet. 2007;**370**(390)

[38] Suarez CM, Briñez A, Castillo L, Briceño JM, et al. Identify and typify Human papilloma virus in patients with Cancer Uterine Cervix in Venezuela. Revista Venezolana de Oncologia. 2006;**18**:221-225

[39] Shastri SS, Mittra I, Misha G, Dikshit SGR, Badwer R. Journal of Clincal Oncology. 2013 31.18 supple.2. Plenary session ASCO JUN 2,2013

[40] Nanda K, McCrroy DC, Myers ER, et al. Accuracy of the Papanicolau test screening for and up cervical cytology abnormalities: A systematic review. Annals of Internal Medicine. 2000;**132**:810

[41] Vesco KK, Whitlock EP, Eder M, et al. Risk factors and other epidemiologic considerations for cervical cancer screening: a narrative review for the U.S. Preventive Services Task Force. Annals of Internal Medicine. 2011;**155**:698

[42] Gibb RK, Martens MG. The impact of liquid-based cytology in decreasing the incidence of cervical cancer. Reviews in Obstetrics and Gynecology. 2011;**4**:S2

[43] Jama L, Saftlas A, Wang W, Exerter M, Whittaker J. Mccowam Treatment for cervical intraepithelial neoplasia and risk of preterm delivery. Jama. 2004 May 5;**291**(17):2100-2106

[44] Bell S, Porter M, Kitchener H, et al. Psychological response to cervical screening. Preventive Medicine. 1995;**24**:610

[45] Gray NM, Sharp L, Cotton SC, et al. Psychological effects of a low-grade abnormal cervical smear test result: Anxiety and associated factors. British Journal of General Practice. 1999;**49**:348

[46] American College of Obstetricians and Gynecologists. ACOG. Committee Opinion No 463: Cervical cancer in adolescents: screening, evaluation, and management. Obstetrics Gynecology. 2010;**116**:469

[47] Mount SL, Papillo JL. A study of 10.296 pediatric and adolescent Papanicolaou smear diagnoses in northern New England. Pediatrics. 1999;**103**:539

[48] Moyer VA, U.S. Preventive Services Task Force. Screening for cervical cancer; U.S Preventive Service Task Force recommendation statement. Annals of Internal Medicine. 2012;**156**:880

[49] Huh WK, Ault KA, Chelmow D, et al. Use of primary high-risk human papillomavirus testing for cervical cancer screening: Interim clinical guidance. Obstetrics Gynecology. 2015;**125**:330

[50] Committee on Practice Bulletins-Gynecology. Practice Bulletin No 168: Cervical Cancer Screening and Prevention Obstetrics Gynecology. 2016;**128**:e111

[51] Saslow D, Solomon D, Lawson HW, et al. American Cancer Society for Colposcopy and Cervical Pathology, and American Society for Clinical Pathology screening guidelines for the prevention and early detection of cervical cancer. CA Cancer Journal of Clinicians. 2012;**62**:147

[52] Sawaya GF, Kerlikowske K, Lee NC, et al. Frequency of cervical smear abnormalities within 3 years of normal cytology. Obstetrics Gynecology. 2000;**96**:219-223

[53] Sawaya GF, Grady D, Kerlikowske K, et al. The positive predictive value of cervical smears in previously screened postmenopausal women: The Heart and Estrogen/progestin Replacement Study (HERS). Annals of Internal Medicine. 2000;**133**:942

[54] Saad RS, Dabbs DJ, Kordunsky L, et al. Clinical significance of cytology diagnosis of atypical squamous cells, cannot exclude high grade, in perimenopausal and postmenopausal women. American Journal of Clinical Pathology. 2006;**126**:381

[55] Wright TC Jr, Ellerbrock TV, Chiasson MA, et al. Cervical intraepithelial neoplasia in women infected with human immudeficienciency virus: Prevalence, risk factors, and validity of Papanicolau smears. New York Cervical Disease Study. Obstetrics Gynecology. 1994;**84**:591

[56] Nath R, Mant C, Luxton J, et al. High risk of human papillomavirus type 16 infections and of development of cervical squamous intraepithelial lesions in systemic lupus erythematosus patients. Arthritis and Rheumatology. 2007;**57**:619

[57] Klumb EM, Pinto AC, Jesus GR, et al. Are women with lupus at higher risk of Hpv infection? Lupus. 2010;**19**:1485

[58] Rositch AF, Nowak RG, Gravitt PE. Increased age and race- specific incidence of cervical cancer after correction for hysterectomy prevalence in the United States from 2000 to 2009. Cancer. 2014;**120**:2032

[59] Fetters MD, Fischer G, Reed BD. Effectiveness of vaginal Papanicolaou smear screening after total hysterectomy for benign disease. JAMA. 1996;**275**:940

[60] Committee on Practice Bulletins Gynecology. ACOG Practice Bulletin Number 131: Screening for cervical cancer. Obstetrics Gynecology. 2012;**120**:1222

[61] ACOG. Clinical. Guidelines. 2012

7

New Insights into the Pathogenesis of Ovarian Cancer: Oxidative Stress

Ghassan M. Saed, Robert T. Morris and
Nicole M. Fletcher

Abstract

Ovarian cancer is the leading cause of death from gynecologic malignancies yet the underlying pathophysiology is not clearly established. Epithelial ovarian cancer (EOC) has long been considered a heterogeneous disease with respect to histopathology, molecular biology, and clinical outcome. Treatment of ovarian cancer includes a combination of cytoreductive surgery and combination chemotherapy, with platinums and taxanes. Despite initial success, over 75% of patients with advanced disease will relapse around 18 months and the overall 5-year survival is approximately 50%. Cancer cells are known to be under intrinsic oxidative stress, which alters their metabolic activity and reduces apoptosis. Epithelial ovarian cancer has been shown to manifest a persistent pro-oxidant state as evident by the upregulation of several key oxidant enzymes in EOC tissues and cells. In the light of our scientific research and the most recent experimental and clinical observations, this chapter provides the reader with up to date most relevant findings on the role of oxidative stress in the pathogenesis and prognosis of ovarian cancer, as well as a novel mechanism of apoptosis/survival in EOC cells.

Keywords: ovarian cancer, oxidative stress, chemoresistance, apoptosis, nitrosylation, caspase-3

1. Introduction

Ovarian cancer is the fifth leading cause of cancer death; the leading cause of death from gynecologic malignancies, and the second most commonly diagnosed gynecologic malignancy; yet the underlying pathophysiology continues to be delineated [1, 2]. Epithelial ovarian cancer has long been considered a heterogeneous disease with respect to histopathology, molecular biology, and clinical outcome. It comprises at least five distinct histological subtypes, the most common and well-studied being high-grade serous ovarian cancer (HGSOC) [3]. The majority of advanced-stage tumors are of epithelial cell origin and can arise from serous, mucinous, or endometrioid cells on the surface epithelium of the ovary or the fallopian tube [2]. The most obvious clinical implication of tumor heterogeneity is that molecular-targeted therapy, while being effective at one tumor site, may not be as effective at all of them [3].

Because early-stage ovarian cancer presents with nonspecific symptoms, most often diagnosis is not made until after the malignancy has spread beyond the ovaries [4]. Mortality rates for this type of malignancy are high because of a lack of a sensitive and specific early-stage screening method [4]. Surgical cytoreduction followed by platinum/taxane chemotherapy results in complete clinical response in 50–80% of patients with stage III and IV disease, but most will relapse within 18 months and ultimately develop chemoresistant disease [2]. Resistance to chemotherapy can either be intrinsic, occurring at the onset of treatment, or acquired, when the disease recurs despite an initially successful response [5–7]. Attempts to overcome drug resistance are central to both clinical and basic molecular research in cancer chemotherapy [5, 8]. Cancer cells are known to be under intrinsic oxidative stress, resulting in increased DNA mutations or damage, genome instability, and cellular proliferation [9–13]. The persistent generation of cellular reactive oxygen species (ROS) is a consequence of many factors including exposure to carcinogens, infection, inflammation, environmental toxicants, nutrients, and mitochondrial respiration [14–17].

The origin and causes of ovarian tumors remains under debate. Injury to surface epithelial ovarian cells due to repeated ovulation is thought to induce tumorigenesis in these cells and is known as the "incessant ovulation hypothesis." Additionally, hormonal stimulation of the surface epithelium of the ovary has been described to initiate tumorigenesis in surface epithelial cells and is known as the "gonadotropin hypothesis." Moreover, the fallopian tube, and not the ovary, has been suggested to be the origin for most epithelial ovarian cancer [2, 18, 19]. Nevertheless, many cases of ovarian cancer continue to be described as *de novo*.

Histopathologic, clinical and molecular genetic profiles were successfully utilized to clearly discriminate between type I and type II ovarian tumors [19]. Accordingly, type I ovarian tumors develop from benign precursor lesions that implant on the ovary and include clear cell, endometrioid, low-grade serous carcinomas, mucinous carcinomas and malignant Brenner tumors [19]. Type II ovarian tumors develop from intraepithelial carcinomas of the fallopian tube and can then spread to involve both the ovary as well as other sites, such as high-grade serous carcinomas which comprise morphologic and molecular subtypes [19]. Additionally, high-grade endometrioid, poorly differentiated ovarian cancers, and carcinosarcomas are also classified as type II tumors.

Attempts to identify specific genes in ovarian tumors to help in early detection of the disease and serve as targets for improved therapy had failed to identify reproducible prognostic indicators [2, 20–22]. Several oncogenic mutations and pathways have been identified in ovarian cancer. Specific inherited mutations in the BRCA1 and BRCA2 genes that produce tumor suppressor proteins, are known to be associated with a 15% increased risk of ovarian cancer overall [2]. Ovarian cancers associated with BRCA1 and BRCA2 mutations are much more common in younger age patients as compared with their nonhereditary counterparts. Additionally, somatic gene mutations in RAD51C and D, HNPCC, NF1, RB1, CDK12, P53, BRAF, KRAS, PIK3CA, and PTEN have been identified in epithelial ovarian cancer. Somatic mutations in BRAF and KRAS genes are relatively common in type I tumors, while p53 mutations, RAS signaling and PIK3CA are common in type II. Additional genetic variations have been hypothesized to act as low to moderate alleles, which contribute to ovarian cancer risk, as well as other diseases [23].

Ovarian tumors are distinct from many other type of cancers as they rarely metastasize outside of the peritoneal cavity [24]. Ovarian tumors are spread into the peritoneal cavity when cells from the primary tumor detach and travel into the peritoneum where they implant into the mesothelial lining [25]. Metastases beyond the peritoneum are usually restricted to recurrent or advanced disease; however, pleural metastases were reported to be present at initial diagnosis. Moreover, the recent discovery of ovarian cancer stem cells, which manifest properties of typical cancer stem cells, in ascites is a new additional contributing factor to not only to metastasis but also to chemoresistance [25, 26].

2. Oxidative stress

Homeostasis, the balance between the production and elimination of oxidants, is maintained by mechanisms involving oxidants and antioxidant enzymes and molecules. If this balance is altered, it leads to an enhanced state of oxidative stress that alters key biomolecules and cells of living organism [13]. Oxidant molecules are divided into two main groups; oxygen-derived or nitrogen-containing molecules. Oxygen-derived molecules, also known as reactive oxygen species (ROS), includes free radicals such as hydroxyl ($HO^{\bullet}$), superoxide ($O_2^{\bullet-}$), peroxyl ($RO_2^{\bullet}$), and alkoxyl ($RO^{\bullet}$), as well as oxidizing agents such as hydrogen peroxide (H_2O_2), hypochlorous acid (HOCl), ozone (O_3), and singlet oxygen ($^1O_2$) that can be converted to radicals [13, 27]. Nitrogen containing oxidants, also known as reactive nitrogen species (RNS), are derived from nitric oxide (NO) that is produced in the mitochondria in response to hypoxia [13]. Exposure to inflammation, infection, carcinogens, and toxicants are major sources of ROS and RNS, *in vivo* [13, 16, 27, 28]. Additionally, RNS and ROS can be produced by various enzymes including cytochrome P450, lipoxygenase, cyclooxygenase, nicotinamide adenine dinucleotide phosphate (NAD(P)H) oxidase complex, xanthine oxidase (XO), and peroxisomes (**Figure 1**) [13, 28, 29].

To maintain the redox balance, ROS and RNS are neutralized by various important enzyme systems including superoxide dismutase (SOD), catalase (CAT), glutathione S-transferase (GST), glutathione (GSH), thioredoxin coupled with thioredoxin reductase, glutaredoxin, glutathione peroxidase (GPX), and glutathione reductase (GSR) (**Figure 1**) [27]. Superoxide dismutase is known to convert $O_2^{\bullet-}$ to H_2O_2, which is then converted to water by CAT. Glutathione S-transferase is involved in detoxification of carcinogens and xenobiotics by catalyzing their conjugation to GSH that will aid in expulsion from the cell (**Figure 1**) [27]. Indeed, the GSH-to-oxidized-GSH (GSH/GSSG) ratio is a good indicator of cellular redox buffering capacity [30, 31]. Under enhanced oxidative stress, the GSH/GSSG complex is known to stimulate the activity of the GS-X-MRP1 efflux pump, which removes toxins from cells. This mechanism has been investigated in the development of resistance to chemotherapeutic drugs [30, 31].

iNOS   Hypoxia   Toxins/Drugs   Export out of the cell

NAD(P)H Oxidase
Xanthine Oxidase
Cytochrome P450 Reductase
Mitochondria e− transport chain

GST

GSR

+ H_4B
+ L-Arg

−H_4B
−L-Arg

Citrulline

$H_2O + \frac{1}{2} O_2$ 2 GSH   GSSG

CAT

H_2O_2 NO $O_2^{\bullet-}$ SOD H_2O_2 GPX   2 $H_2O + O_2$

Fenton & Haber-Weiss
Reaction

Cl^- MPO

Fe^{2+}

H^+

Fe^{3+}

HOCl $NO^{\bullet+}$ NO_2^- $ONOO^-$ $O_2 + H_2O + HO$

H_2O_2

NO_3^-

H_2O

$^1O_2 + Cl^-$

Oxidative Damage

-DNA
-Proteins
-Lipids

Peroxidation
Protein Chlorination

Protein Nitration
Protein nitrosylation
Nitrotyrosine

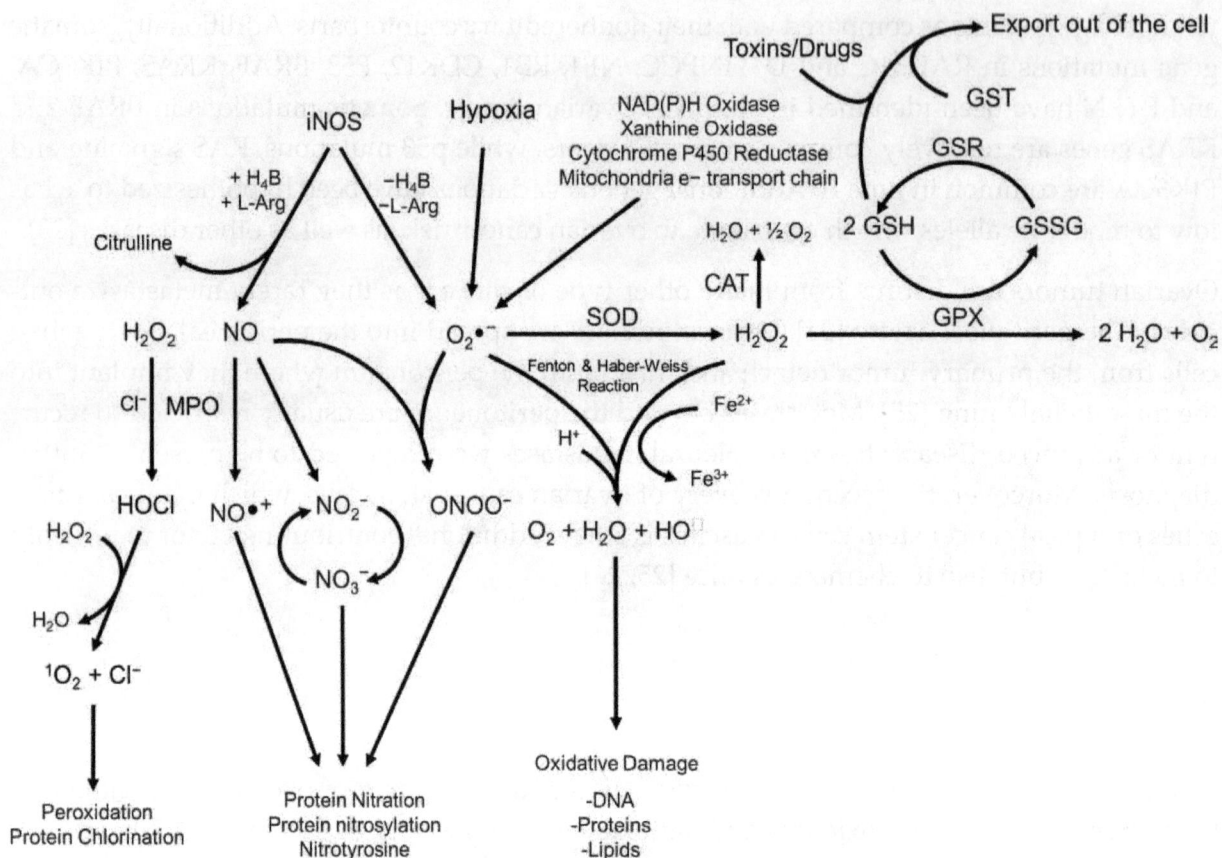

Figure 1. Summary of key oxidant and antioxidants in cancer [1]. Abbreviations are CAT, catalase; Cl^-, chloride ion; Fe_2^+, iron (II); Fe_3^+, iron (III); GPX, glutathione peroxidase; GSH, glutathione; GSR, glutathione reductase; GSSG, reduced glutathione; GST, glutathione S-transferase; H_2O_2, hydrogen peroxide; H_4B, tetrohydrobiopterin; $HO^{\bullet}$, hydroxyl radical; HOCl, hypochlorous acid; iNOS, inducible nitric oxide synthase; L-Arg, L-arginine; MPO, myeloperoxidase; NAD(P)H, nicotinamide adenine dinucleotide phosphate; $NO^{\bullet+}$, nitrosonium cation; NO_2^-, nitrite; NO_3^-, nitrate; $O_2^{\bullet-}$, superoxide; $ONOO^-$, peroxynitrite; SOD, superoxide dismutase.

3. Oxidative stress and cancer

Oxidative stress has been implicated in the etiology of several diseases, including cancer. Alteration of the cellular redox balance modulates the initiation, promotion, and progression of tumor cells [13, 27]. The continuous generation of oxidants and free radicals affects key cellular mechanisms that control the balance of cell proliferation and apoptosis, which play a major role in the initiation and development of several cancers. Depending on the concentration of ROS and RNS in the cellular environment, oxidants can initiate and promote the oncogenic phenotype or induce apoptosis, and thus act as antitumor agents [32]. Several transcription factors that modulate the expression of genes critical to the development and metastasis of cancer cells are known to be controlled by oxidative stress. This includes hypoxia inducible factor (HIF)-1α, nuclear factor (NF)-κB, peroxisome proliferator-activated receptor (PPAR)-γ, activator protein (AP)-1, β-catenin/Wnt, and Nuclear factor erythroid 2-related factor 2 (Nrf2) [13]. The transcription factor regulator Nrf2 is known to control the expression of some key antioxidant enzymes that are needed to scavenge oxidants and free radicals [13, 33]. The activation of Nrf2 involves the suppressor protein, Kelch-like ECH-associated protein 1

(Keap1), that binds Nrf2 in the cytoplasm and prevents its translocation into the nucleus, where it binds to promoters of antioxidant enzymes [13, 33]. Additionally, oxidative stress is known to activate certain signaling pathways, specifically, the MAPK/AP-1 and NF-κB pathways, which are critical for the initiation and maintenance of the oncogenic phenotype [34].

More importantly, ROS and RNS are known to induce genetic mutations that alter gene expression as well as induce DNA damage, and thus have been implicated in the etiology of several diseases, including cancer [2, 13, 35]. Damage to DNA by ROS and RNS is now accepted as a major cause of cancer, and has been demonstrated in the initiation and progression of several cancers including breast, hepatocellular carcinoma, and prostate cancer [34]. Oxidative stress is known to modify all the four DNA bases by base pair substitutions rather than base deletions and insertions. Modification of GC base pairs usually results in mutations, whereas, modification of AT base pairs does not [36]. Modification of guanine in cellular DNA, causing G to T transversions, is commonly induced by ROS and RNS [34]. If not repaired, the transversion of G to T in the DNA of oncogenes or tumor suppressor genes can lead to initiation and progression of cancer. Oxidation of DNA bases, such as thymidine glycol, 5-hydroxymethyl-2′-deoxyuridine, and 8-OHdG are now accepted markers of cellular DNA damage by free radicals [35].

Oxidants and free radicals are known to enhance cell migration contributing to the enhancement of tumor invasion and metastasis, main causes of death in cancer patients [2, 13]. Reactive oxygen species, through the activation of NF-κB, regulate the expression of intercellular adhesion protein-1 (ICAM-1), a cell surface protein in various cell types [13]. In response to oxidative stress, the interleukin 8 (IL-8)-induced enhanced expression of ICAM-1 on neutrophils enhances the migration of neutrophils across the endothelium, which is key in tumor metastasis [13]. Another important player that controls cell migration and consequently, tumor invasion, is the upregulation of specific matrix metalloproteinases (MMPs), essential enzymes in the degradation of most components of the basement membrane and extracellular matrix, such as type IV collagen [13, 37]. The expression of MMPs, such as MMP-2, MMP-3, MMP-9, MMP-10, and MMP-13 is enhanced by free radicals, specifically H_2O_2 and NO, through the activation of Ras, ERK1/2, p38, and JNK, or the inactivation of phosphatases [13, 37]. Indeed, the major source of cellular ROS, the NAD(P)H oxidase family of enzymes, has been linked to the promotion of survival and growth of tumor cells in pancreatic and lung cancers [2, 13].

Oxidants and free radicals are also known to enhance angiogenesis, a key process for the survival of solid tumors [13]. Angiogenesis involves the upregulation of vascular endothelial growth factor (VEGF) or the downregulation of thrombospondin-1 (TSP-1), an angiogenesis suppressor in response to oxidative stress [13]. This process is controlled by several oncogenes and tumor-suppressor genes such as Ras, c-Myc, c-Jun, mutated p53, human epidermal growth factor receptor-2, and steroid receptor coactivators [38, 39]. Additionally, oxidants and free radicals are known to stabilize HIF-1α protein and induce the production of angiogenic factors by tumor cells.

4. Cancer cells are under intrinsic oxidative stress

Cancer cells are continuously exposed to high levels of intrinsic oxidative stress due to increased aerobic glycolysis (Warburg effect), a known process in cancer cell metabolism [10, 40].

Thus, cancer cells trigger several critical adaptations that are essential for their survival such as suppression of apoptosis, alteration of glucose metabolism, and stimulation of angiogenesis [10, 29]. Oxygen depletion, due to a hypoxic microenvironment, significantly stimulates mitochondria to produce high levels of ROS and RNS which is known to activate HIF-1α and consequently promote cell survival in such an environment [29]. The half-life of HIF-1α is extremely short as it is rapidly inactivated through hydroxylation reactions mediated by dioxygen, oxaloglutarate, and iron-dependent prolyl 4-hydroxylases, located in the nucleus and cytoplasm [40, 41]. Nitric oxide and other ROS, as well as H_2O_2 efflux into the cytosol due to dismutation of $O_2^{\bullet-}$, can inhibit prolyl 4-hydroxylases activity, leading to the stabilization of HIF-1α [29, 42]. More importantly, stabilization of HIF-1α, under hypoxic conditions, can be blocked when inhibiting ROS production in mitochondria that lack cytochrome c [29, 43].

Pro-oxidant enzymes such as myeloperoxidase (MPO), inducible nitric oxide synthase (iNOS) and NAD(P)H oxidase have been associated with initiation, progression, survival, and increased risk in cancers such as breast, ovarian, lung, prostate, bladder, colorectal and malignant melanoma [21, 44]. Moreover, the expression of those key pro-oxidant enzymes was found to change based on the histological type and grade of the tumor [21, 45, 46]. Likewise, antioxidants have also been associated with initiation, progression, survival, and increased risk in cancers such as lung, head and neck, and prostate cancer [47–50]. The expression of GSR and GPX, key antioxidant enzymes, has also been reported to be altered in various types of cancer [21]. The activity and expression of SOD, a powerful antioxidant enzyme, has been reported to be decreased in colorectal carcinomas, pancreatic, lung, gastric, ovarian, and breast cancers [21, 45, 46]. Likewise, the expression and activity of CAT, a key antioxidant enzyme, was reported to be decreased in breast, bladder, and lung cancers but increased in brain cancer [21, 45, 46]. Antioxidant enzymes play a critical role in maintaining the redox balance in the presence of microenvironment stress, and thus, alteration of this balance may provide a unique and complex microenvironment for cancer cell survival.

5. Ovarian cancer cells manifest a persistent pro-oxidant state

Recent evidence suggests that oxidative stress is a critical factor in the initiation and development of several cancers, including ovarian cancer [40, 51]. Consistently, it has been reported that ovarian cancer patients manifested significantly decreased levels of antioxidants and higher levels of oxidants [10, 22, 40, 51–53]. An enhanced redox state, resulting from increased expression of key pro-oxidant enzymes and decreased expression of antioxidant enzymes, has been extensively described in epithelial ovarian cancer (EOC) [52–54]. We have previously reported that MPO, a hemoprotein present solely in myloid cells that acts as a powerful oxidant, and iNOS, a key pro-oxidant enzyme, are highly expressed and co-localized to the same cell in EOC cells [53]. These two enzymes, MPO and iNOS, work together to inhibit apoptosis, a hallmark of ovarian cancer cells. Nitric oxide, produced by iNOS, is used by MPO as a one-electron substrate to generate nitrosonium cation (NO⁺), a labile nitrosating species, resulting in a significant increase in S-nitrosylation of caspase-3, which inhibits apoptosis [53, 55, 56]. Indeed, attenuating oxidative stress by inhibiting MPO or iNOS significantly induced apoptosis in EOC cells [54]. Moreover, the remarkably higher levels of iNOS/NO, produced by EOC cells, resulted in the generation of high levels of nitrate and nitrite, powerful protein nitration agents that are known to stimulate the initiation and progression of tumor cells [53]. Under oxidative stress, where both NO and $O_2^{\bullet-}$ are elevated, MPO was reported to serve as a source of free iron which reacts with H_2O_2 and generated highly reactive hydroxyl radical (HO$^\bullet$), further increasing oxidative stress [22, 53]. Additionally, EOC cells are also character-ized by enhanced expression of NAD(P)H oxidase, a potent oxidant enzyme that is known to be the major source of $O_2^{\bullet-}$ in the cell. Such high levels of $O_2^{\bullet-}$ combined with significantly high levels of NO generates peroxynitrite, another powerful nitrosylation and nitration agent, which modifies proteins and DNA structure and function in cells [57].

Recently we have gathered compelling evidence demonstrating that talc, through alteration of the redox balance, can generate a similar pro-oxidant state in both normal ovarian epithe-lial and ovarian cancer cells. Talc and asbestos are both silicate minerals, and the carcinogenic effects of asbestos have been extensively studied and documented in the medical literature [58]. Asbestos fibers in the lung initiate an inflammatory and scarring process, and it has been proposed that ground talc, as a foreign body, might initiate a similar inflammatory response [58]. Although there is strong epidemiological evidence to suggest an association between talc use and ovarian cancer, the direct link and precise mechanisms have yet to be elucidated. We investigated the effect of talc on both oxidants and antioxidants in normal ovarian epithelial and ovarian cancer cell lines. There was a marked increase in mRNA levels of the pro-oxidant enzymes, iNOS and MPO in talc treated ovarian cancer cell lines and normal ovarian epi-thelial cells, all as compared to their control, as early as 24 hours. Additionally, there was a marked decrease in the mRNA levels of the antioxidant enzymes CAT, GPX, SOD3, but with a marked increase in GSR, and no change in GST, in talc treated ovarian cancer cell line and in normal ovarian epithelial cells, all compared to their control, as early as 24 hours (*data not pub-lished*). Thus, there is a direct effect of talc on the molecular levels of oxidant and antioxidants, elucidating a potential mechanism for the development of ovarian cancer in response to talc.

6. Biomarkers for the early detection of ovarian cancer

The discovery of MPO expression in ovarian EOC cells and tissues was surprising, as it is only expressed by cells of myeloid origin. Intriguingly, the combination of serum MPO and free iron was reported to potentially serve as biomarkers for early detection of ovarian cancer [22]. A robust detection method based on molecular profiles for ovarian cancer has not yet been developed because the disease exhibits a wide range of morphological, clinical and genetic variations during its progression. The search for non-invasive, cost-effective ovarian cancer biomarker tests has been ongoing for many years. Immunizations of mice with ovarian cancer cells has led to hybridoma validation by ELISA, while flow cytometry analysis permitted the discovery of cancer antigen (CA)-125 and mesothelin [59]. Furthermore, the screening of an array of 21,500 unknown ovarian cDNAs hybridized with labeled first-strand cDNA from ten ovarian tumors and six normal tissues led to the discovery of human epididymis protein 4 (HE4) [60]. Most interestingly, HE4 is overexpressed in 93% of serous and 100% of endometrioid

EOCs, and in 50% of clear cell carcinomas, but not in mucinous ovarian carcinomas [61]. Thus, HE4 was identified as one of the most useful biomarkers for ovarian cancer, although it lacked tissue-specificity [60, 62–64]. Secreted HE4 high levels were also detected in the serum of ovarian cancer patients [65]. Additionally, combining CA-125 and HE4 is a more accurate predictor of malignancy than either alone [66–68].

Multi-marker panels have the potential for high positive predictive values (PPVs), but careful validation with appropriate sample cohorts is mandatory and complex algorithms may be difficult to implement for routine clinical use [59]. Panels of biomarkers have been extensively investigated to improve sensitivity and specificity and have included some of the most promising reported markers such as CA72–4, M-CSF, OVX1, LPA, prostacin, osteopontin, inhibin and kallikrein [69–71]. However, most of these tests frequently require certain equipments and complex computational algorithms that may not be available in a standard immunoassay laboratory, [32]. Among postmenopausal women in the U.S., only 1 in 2500 women are reported with ovarian cancer. Due to this low prevalence of the disease, a screening method that yield a 75% sensitivity and 99.6% specificity to achieve a PPV value of 10% to be effective for the detection of all stages of ovarian cancer [72]. To date, there is no single biomarker available that met these requirements.

The established role of MPO in oxidative stress and inflammation has been a leading factor in the study of MPO as a possible marker of plaque instability and a useful clinical tool in the evaluation of patients with coronary heart disease [73]. Recent genetic studies implicated MPO in the development of lung cancer by demonstrating a striking correlation between the relative risk for development of the disease and the incidence of functionally distinct MPO polymorphisms [74]. Myeloperoxidase levels reported for various inflammatory disorders are coincidentally lower than those levels found in all stages of ovarian cancer. A previous study reported normal serum MPO and iron levels as 62 ± 11 ng/ml and 96 ± 9 µg/dl, respectively [75]. However, there was a significant increase in serum MPO and iron levels to 95 ± 20 ng/ml and 159 ± 20 µg/dl, respectively, in asthmatic individuals [75]. Although there was an increase in this reported serum iron, these levels still fell within the normal range (50 to 170 µg/dl) [22, 75]. Other studies have showed that an elevated MPO levels, reaching up to 350 ng/ml, in serum plasma, was indicative of a higher risk for cardiovascular events in patients hospitalized for chest pain [76, 77]. A recent study showed a significant correlation between MPO levels and the stage of ovarian cancer, as is the linear trend for MPO with increasing stage [22]. Similarly, there was a significant difference in the level of free iron in serum and tissues obtained from stage I as compared to combined stages II, III, and IV ovarian cancer. There was an overlap between stage I ovarian cancer and inflammation (endometriosis) serum MPO levels, however serum free iron levels were significantly higher in stage I ovarian cancer as compared to inflammation. There was no significant change in free iron levels between the healthy control group, benign gynecologic conditions group, and inflammation group [22].

Due to the overlap of MPO levels in early-stage ovarian cancer and inflammatory conditions, there is a potential for a false positive with MPO alone in patients with cardiovascular, inflammation, and/or asthmatic disorders. It has been reported that MPO heme destruction and iron release is mediated by high levels of both HOCl (a product of MPO) and oxidative stress (i.e. cancer) [22]. The free iron generated by hemoprotein destruction not only contributes to elevation of serum iron levels, but may also induce oxidative stress, which can promote lipid peroxidation, DNA strand breaks, and modification or degradation of biomolecules [78–80]. Iron reacts with H_2O_2 and catalyzes the generation of highly reactive hydroxyl radicals, which in turn further increases free iron concentrations by the Fenton and Haber–Weiss reaction [81]. Several studies from our laboratories have provided a mechanistic link between oxidative stress, MPO, higher levels of HOCl and higher free iron that could explain the observed accumulation of free iron in epithelial ovarian cancers tissues [53, 82–85]. Utilizing serum iron levels alone as a biomarker is also not sufficient for early detection of ovarian cancer due to many uncontrolled variables, i.e. dietary intake, supplements, effects of other iron-generating enzymes or factors, and more importantly they are not as specific as MPO levels. Specifically, in iron deficiency anemic patients, their free iron levels may become a confounding factor in its utilization for early detection of ovarian cancer. Thus, anemia should be ruled out to eliminate any overlap that would lead to misdiagnosis. The incorporation of iron deficiency anemic patients in a logistic regression model will help determine its overlap with early-stage ovarian cancer. Additionally, currently available clinical studies focused on either biochemical or more recently, genetic markers of iron overload have reported conflicting results regarding the use of iron levels alone for diagnosis [86–89].

Thus, the combination of serum MPO and iron levels should yield a higher power of specificity and sensitivity that should distinguish women with early-stage ovarian cancer from other disorders, specifically inflammation [22]. Additionally, combining serum MPO and iron levels with the best currently existing biomarkers through the creation of a logistic regression model may increase the overall predictive values. Collectively, there is a role for serum MPO and free iron in the pathophysiology of ovarian cancer, which thereby qualifies them to serve as biomarkers for early detection and prognosis of ovarian cancer.

7. Modulation of oxidative stress

Several studies have reported the beneficial effects of modulating the redox status of cancer cells, however few studies have been reported for ovarian cancer [90–92]. Inhibition of pro-oxidant enzymes, such as NAD(P)H oxidase, has been shown to significantly induce apoptosis of cancer cells [93, 94]. We investigated whether NAD(P)H oxidase-mediated generation of intracellular reactive ROS lead to anti-apoptotic activity and thus a growth advantage to EOC cells. Diphenyleneiodonium (DPI) has been used to inhibit ROS production mediated by NAD(P)H oxidase in various cell types [95–97]. Our results showed that NAD(P)H oxidase is over-expressed in EOC tissues and cells as compared to normal ovarian tissues and cells [52]. Indeed, high levels of NAD(P)H oxidase are known to promote tumorigenesis of NIH3T3 mouse fibroblasts and the DU-145 prostate epithelial cells [98].

Inhibition of NAD(P)H oxidase has also been reported to decrease the generation of $O_2^{\bullet-}$, H_2O_2, as well as other oxidants [93, 94]. Cancer cells are known to manifest enhanced intrinsic oxidative stress and metabolic activity that lead to mitochondrial failure [99, 100]. Indeed, it was previously reported that ovarian tumors are characterized by increased ROS levels as evident from increased $O_2^{\bullet-}$ generated from NAD(P)H oxidase as well as mitochondrial malfunction [101]. The NAD(P)H oxidase redox signaling is controlled by mitochondria, and thus loss of this control is thought to contribute to tumorigenesis [101]. Others have also shown that inhibition of NAD(P)H oxidase induced apoptosis in cancer cells [102]. Continuous ROS production by the cell and the environment further induces the inhibition of phosphorylation of AKT and subsequent suppression of AKT-mediated phosphorylation of ASK1 on Ser-83, resulting in significant decrease in apoptosis [102–104]. Furthermore, paclitaxel, a chemotherapeutic agent used in the treatment of ovarian cancer and other cancers, induced apoptosis of ovarian cancer cells by negative regulation of AKT–ASK1 phosphorylation signaling [102–104]. On the other hand, activation of AKT by ROS provided protection against apoptosis [102–104].

Data from our laboratory clearly demonstrated that treatment of EOC cells with DPI, which inhibits ROS production mediated by NAD(P)H oxidase, significantly reduced SOD3 and HIF-1α mRNA and protein levels as early as 30 minutes after treatment with a concomitant increase in apoptosis [52]. The association between increased HIF-1α expression and decreased cellular apoptosis has also been demonstrated in lung and hepatoma cancer cells [94, 105]. Overexpression of HIF-1α is thought to decrease apoptosis by the upregulation of anti-apoptotic proteins, Bcl-2 and Bcl-xL and down regulation of pro-apoptotic proteins, BAX and BAK [106]. Inhibition of HIF-1α by rapamycin increased apoptosis by decreasing the expression of apoptosis inhibitor Bcl-2 in ovarian cancer xenografts [107]. Additionally, inhibition of HIF-1α by rapamycin enhanced apoptosis through the inhibition of cell survival signals in several other cell lines [107].

Most of the NAD(P)H oxidase-generated $O_2^{\bullet-}$ is utilized to produce H_2O_2 by nonenzymatic or SOD-catalyzed reactions [108–110]. Hydrogen peroxide serves as the precursor of more toxic hydroxyl radicals and thus is extremely destructive to cells and tissues [109–111]. The expression of SOD3 was reported to increase in response to intrinsic oxidative stress in ovarian cancer cells [112]. It has been demonstrated that overexpression of the SOD3 gene significantly suppressed lung cancer metastasis as well as inhibited the growth of B16-F1 melanoma tumors in mice [113, 114]. However, in a somewhat controversial study, it has been shown that inhibition of SOD selectively induced apoptosis of leukemia and ovarian cancer cells [10].

Under hypoxic conditions, SOD3 is overexpressed and has been reported to significantly induce the expression of HIF-1α in tumors through unknown mechanisms however, steady state levels of $O_2^{\bullet-}$ and the stabilization of HIF-1α have been proposed to play a role in this mechanism [107, 115]. Therefore, inhibition of NAD(P)H oxidase and the consequent reduction of $O_2^{\bullet-}$ levels may destabilize HIF-1α, and subsequently increase apoptosis by lowering SOD3 levels. Thus, we conclude that lowering oxidative stress, possibly through the inhibition of NAD(P)H oxidase-generated $O_2^{\bullet-}$, induces apoptosis in ovarian cancer cells and may serve as a potential target for cancer therapy. This effect was attributed to the modulation of key enzymes that are central to controlling the cellular redox balance.

8. Modulation of metabolism

Cancer cells are known to favor anaerobic metabolism, even when oxygen is present and is known as the "Warburg effect" [116, 117]. Aerobic glycolysis is known to decrease ATP yield as well as increase lactate production by cancer cells [116–118]. To compensate for this decrease in

ATP, cancer cells significantly increase glucose uptake through upregulation of glucose receptors [40, 41, 118]. Increased lactate in cancer cells enhances lactic acidosis, which is significantly toxic to the surrounding tissues and can facilitate tumor growth through the stimulation of ECM degradation, angiogenesis, and metastasis [118]. Additionally, aerobic glycolysis in cancer cells activates HIF, an oxygen-sensitive transcription factor that plays an important role in initiation and maintenance of the oncogenic phenotype [118]. In this regard, HIF induces the expression of several glucose transporters and glycolysis enzymes as well as induces the expression of pyruvate dehydrogenate kinase (PDK), an enzyme that stimulates pyruvate entry into the mitochondria for oxidation [41, 118, 119]. Thus, shifting glucose metabolism in cancer cells from glycolysis to glucose oxidation may have therapeutic value [120]. Indeed, inhibiting PDK by dichloroacetate (DCA) has been reported to induce apoptosis in tumor cells and significantly decreased HIF-1α expression [40]. More importantly DCA is currently in the clinical use for the treatment of hereditary mitochondrial diseases as well as lactic acidosis [41, 121]. The use of DCA at a dose of 35 to 50 mg/kg decreased lactate levels by more than 60% [41, 122]. Dichloroacetate treatment has been shown to significantly induce apoptosis, through the stimulation of caspase-3 activity, in a dose-dependent manner in EOC cells as well as other cancers, such as glioblastoma, endometrial, prostate, and non-small cell lung cancers [40, 123]. Aerobic glycolysis is associated with resistance to apoptosis in cancer cells as many of the enzymes in the glycolysis process are known to modulate gene transcription of apoptotic proteins [40, 41, 69, 124]. Stimulation of pyruvate entry into the mitochondria by DCA, through activation of PDH and inhibition of PDK, is an ideal method to shift aerobic glycolysis to glucose oxidation as inhibiting aerobic glycolysis results in ATP depletion and necrosis, not apoptosis [41, 125].

An additional approach to induce apoptosis in cancer cells is through scavenging high levels of oxidants produced by cancer cells utilizing antioxidants [126]. Deficiency in SOD or inhibition of SOD enzyme activity causes accumulation of $O_2^{\bullet-}$ which is the precursor for several toxic free radicals that are critical to the oncogenic process [127]. Elevated levels of oxidants and free radicals are also known to induce cellular senescence and necrosis, and thus can kill tumor cells [40, 128]. The precise effect of high levels of oxidants and free radicals in cancer cells will depend on the type of cells and tissues, the site of production, and the type and concentration of oxidants [13].

9. Chemotherapy and the acquisition of chemoresistance in EOC cells

Resistance to taxanes and platinums, chemotherapy drugs in current use for ovarian cancer treatment, remains a major obstacle to a successful treatment of ovarian cancer patients [6]. Resistance to chemotherapy not only limits the use of the initial drug but also limits the use of other agents, even those with different mechanisms of action [129]. Chemotherapy drugs exert their actions by the initiation of cell death either directly through the generation of oxidative stress or as an indirect effect of exposure, as observed with several chemotherapeutic agents [130]. The development of chemoresistance to drugs is dependent on several factors that include: influx/efflux of drugs that decrease platinum accumulation in tumor cells, enhanced GSH and GST levels, upregulation of anti-apoptotic proteins such as Bcl-2, loss of tumor necrosis factor receptor ligand which induces apoptosis, increased DNA repair through up-regulation of repair

Ovarian Cancer Cells

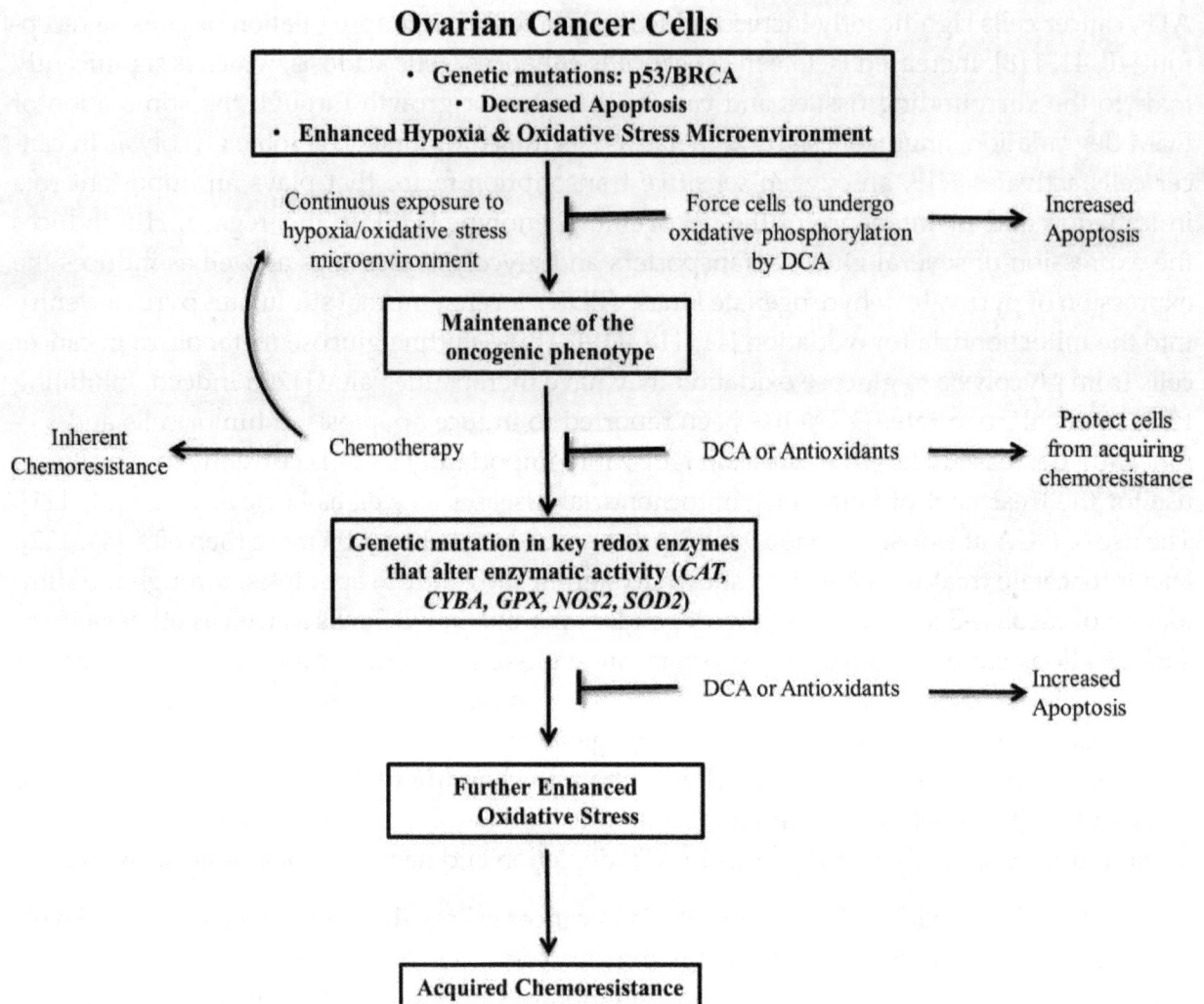

Figure 2. Summary of the role of oxidative stress in the development of sensitive and chemoresistant ovarian cancer [1].

genes, and loss of functional p53 that augments NF-κB activation [13, 131]. We have previously shown that chemoresistant EOC cells manifested increased iNOS and nitrate/nitrite levels as well as a decrease in GSR expression as compared to sensitive EOC cells, suggesting a further enhancement of the redox state in chemoresistant cells [1, 45]. Additionally, CAT, GPX, and iNOS were shown to be significantly increased while, GSR, SOD, and the NAD(P)H oxidase subunit (p22^{phox}) were decreased in chemoresistant EOC cells as compared to their sensitive counterparts [21]. These finding supports a key role for oxidative stress, not only in the development of the oncogenic phenotype, but also in the development of chemoresistance (**Figure 2**).

10. Common polymorphisms in redox enzymes are associated with ovarian cancer

A single nucleotide polymorphism (SNP) occurs as a result of gene point mutations with an estimated frequency of at least one in every 1000 base pairs that are selectively maintained and distributed in populations throughout the human genome [132]. An association between common SNPs in oxidative DNA repair genes and redox genes with human cancer susceptibility has been established [28]. Common SNPs in the redox enzymes are known to be strongly associated with an altered enzymatic activity in these enzymes, and may explain the enhanced redox state that has been linked to several malignancies, including ovarian cancer [40, 52]. Additionally, it may further explain the observation of significantly decreased apoptosis and increased survival of EOC cells [53]. It is therefore critical to determine the exact effect of common SNPs in various redox enzymes on all process involved in the development of the oncogenic phenotype [21, 46, 133, 134]. Such studies can be linked to other studies focusing on determining the effects of genes involved in carcinogen metabolism (detoxification and/or activation), redox enzymes, and DNA repair pathways [133]. Numerous SNPs associated with change of function have been identified in antioxidant enzymes including *CAT*, *GPX1*, *GSR*, and *SOD2* [21, 134]. Additionally, the association between genetic polymorphisms in genes with anti-tumor activity and those involved in the cell cycle has been reported in ovarian cancer [135, 136]. Recently, several genetic variations have been identified in genome-wide association studies (GWAS), and were found to act as low to moderate penetrant alleles, which contribute to ovarian cancer risk, as well as other diseases [23, 137].

There is now an association of specific SNPs in key oxidant and anti-oxidant enzymes with increased risk and overall survival of ovarian cancer [21, 46]. A common SNP that reduced CAT activity (rs1001179) was utilized as a significant predictor of death when present in ovarian cancer patients and was also associated with increased risk for breast cancer [21, 46, 134, 138]. This SNP is also linked to increased risk, survival, and response to adjuvant treatment of cancer patients, including ovarian [46, 139]. Another common SNP that reduced CYBA activity (rs4673) was also reported to be associated with an increased risk for ovarian cancer [21, 46]. The mutant genotype of the *CYBA* gene has been shown to both decrease and increase activity of the protein, thereby altering the generation of $O_2^{\bullet-}$ [21, 46]. Moreover, functionally distinct *MPO* polymorphisms, such as (rs2333227) have been linked to relative increased risk for development of ovarian cancer as well as other cancers [21, 44, 46]. Additional SNPs that influenced the risk of EOC have been successfully identified from the GWAS studies including rs3814113 (located at 9p22, near BNC2), rs2072590 (located at 2q31, which contains a family of HOX genes), rs2665390 (located at 3q25, intronic to TIPARP), rs10088218 (located at 8q24, 700 kb downstream of MYC), rs8170 (located at 19p13, near MERIT40), and rs9303542 (located at 17q21, intronic to SKAP1) [21, 46]. Thus, the genetic component of increased ovarian cancer risk may be attributed to SNPs that result in point mutations in the redox genes and potentially other genes [140].

11. Chemoresistance is associated with point mutations in key redox enzymes in EOC cells

To date, the acquisition of chemoresistance in ovarian cancer is not fully understood. The enhanced oxidant state reported in chemoresistant EOC cells may be linked to point mutations in key redox enzymes [21]. Chemoresistant EOC cells manifested increased levels of CAT, GPX, and iNOS and decreased levels of GSR, SOD, and NAD(P)H oxidase as compared to their sensitive counterparts [21]. Interestingly, chemoresistant EOC cells, and not their sensitive counterparts, manifested specific point mutations that corresponded to known functional SNPs, in key redox enzymes including *SOD2* (rs4880), *NOS2* (rs2297518), and *CYBA* (rs4673) [1]. However, altered enzymatic activity for CAT and GSR observed in chemoresistant EOC cells did not correspond to the specific SNP of interest in those enzymes, indicating involvement of other possible functional SNPs for those enzymes [21]. Coincidently, chemotherapy treatment induced point mutations that happen to correspond to known functional SNPs in key oxidant enzymes subsequently led to the acquisition of chemoresistance by EOC cells. Indeed, the induction of specific point mutations in *SOD2* or *GPX1* in sensitive EOC cells resulted in a decrease in the sensitivity to chemotherapy of these cells [21]. In fact, the addition of SOD to sensitive EOC cells during chemotherapy treatment synergistically increased the efficacy to chemotherapy [21].

Alternatively, the observed nucleotide switch in response to chemotherapy in EOC cells may be the result of nucleotide substitution, a process that includes transitions, replacement of one purine by the other or that of one pyrimidine by the other, or transversions, replacement of a purine by a pyrimidine or vice versa [21]. Indeed, hydroxyl radicals are known to react with DNA causing the formation of many pyrimidine and purine-derived lesions [21]. The oxidative damage to 8-Oxo-2′-deoxyguanosine, a major product of DNA oxidation, induces genetic alterations in oncogenes and tumor suppressor genes has been involved in tumor initiation and progression [21]. A GC to TA transversion has been reported in the *ras* oncogene and the *p53* tumor suppressor gene in several cancers. However, the GC to TA transversion is not unique to hydroxy-2′-deoxyguanosine, as CC to TT substitutions have been identified as signature mutations for oxidants and free radicals [21].

Moreover, the observed nucleotide switch in response to chemotherapy in EOC cells can be due to the fact that acquisition of chemoresistance generates an entirely different population of cells with a distinct genotype. Hence, chemotherapy kills the bulk of the tumor cells leaving a subtype of cancer cells with ability for repair and renewal, known as cancer stem cells (CSCs) [21]. Indeed, cancer stem cells have been isolated from various types of cancer including leukemia, breast, brain, pancreatic, prostate, ovarian and colon [21]. Interestingly, CSC populations were present in cultures of SKOV-3 EOC cells and have been shown to be chemoresistance in nature [21].

12. Further increasing pro-oxidant enzymes: potential survival mechanism

Apoptosis is a tightly regulated molecular process that removes excess or unwanted cells from organisms. Resistance to apoptosis is a key feature of cancer cells and is involved in the pathogenesis of cancer. We have previously reported that EOC cells have significantly increased levels of NO, which correlated with increased expression in iNOS [54]. We have also reported that EOC cells manifested lower apoptosis, which was markedly induced by inhibiting iNOS by L-NAME, indicating a strong link between apoptosis and NO/iNOS pathways in these cells [54]. Caspase-3 is known to play a critical role in controlling apoptosis, by participating in a cascade that is triggered in response to proapoptotic signals and culminates in cleavage of a set of proteins, resulting in disassembly of the cell [141–144]. Caspase-3 was found to be S-nitrosylated on the catalytic-site cysteine in unstimulated human lymphocyte cell lines and denitrosylated upon activation of the Fas apoptotic pathway [145]. Decreased caspase-3 S-nitrosylation was associated with an increase in intracellular caspase activity. Caspase-3 S-nitrosylation/denitrosylation is known to serve as an on/off switch regulating caspase activity during apoptosis in endothelial cells, lymphocytes and trophoblasts [146–149]. The mechanisms underlying S-nitrosothiol (SNO) formation *in vivo* are not well understood.

Myeloperoxidase typically uses H_2O_2, in combination with chloride to generate hypochlorous acid [55, 150–153]. We, and others, have demonstrated that MPO utilizes NO, produced by iNOS, as a one-electron substrate generating NO^+, a labile nitrosating species that is rapidly hydrolyzed forming nitrite as end-product [55, 56, 154, 155]. The ability of MPO to generate NO^+, from NO, led us to believe that not only does MPO play a role in S-nitrosylation of caspase-3 in EOC cells, but also highlights a possible cross-talk between iNOS and MPO. Indeed, we observed that MPO is responsible for the S-nitrosylation of caspase-3, which led to the inhibition of caspase-3 in EOC cells. Silencing MPO gene expression induced apoptosis in EOC cells through a mechanism that involved S-nitrosylation of caspase-3 by MPO.

Molecular alterations that lead to apoptosis can be inhibited by S-nitrosylation of apoptotic proteins such as caspases. Thus, S-nitrosylation conveys a key influence of NO on apoptosis signaling and may act as a key regulator for apoptosis in cancer cells. It has been known that the effects of NO on apoptosis are not only stimulatory but may also be inhibitory. These paradoxical effects of NO on apoptosis seem to be influenced by several factors. It has been suggested that biological conditions, such as the redox state, concentration, exposure time and the combination with O_2, $O_2^{\bullet-}$ and other molecules, determines the net effect of NO on apoptosis [156]. Also, NO is implicated in both apoptotic and necrotic cell death depending on the NO chemistry and the cellular biological redox state [57, 156]. As described earlier, we have previously demonstrated that the EOC cell lines, SKOV-3 and MDAH-2774, manifested lower apoptosis and had significantly higher levels of NO due to the presence of elevated levels of iNOS [54, 157]. We have also reported significant levels of MPO expression, which was found to be co-localized with iNOS, in both EOC cell lines SKOV-3 and MDAH-2774 [53]. We have demonstrated that 65% of the invasive epithelial ovarian carcinoma specimens tested expressed MPO in the neoplastic cells. The co-localization of MPO and iNOS has been demonstrated by immunohistochemical studies in cytokine-treated human neutrophils and primary granules of activated leukocytes [158]. Both plasma levels and tissue expression of MPO in gynecologic malignancies were previously evaluated and it was found that gynecologic cancer patients had higher plasma MPO compared to control subjects [159]. Using immunostaining, it was also demonstrated that MPO expression was higher in cancer tissues compared to control [159].

We have now characterized chemoresistant EOC cells to manifest an even further increase in pro-oxidant enzymes including MPO, and NO, a surrogate for iNOS activity in conjunction with a further increase in the S-nitrosylation of caspase-3 (*data not published*) and a concurrent decrease in the level of apoptosis [21]. Thus, we hypothesized that the decrease in apoptosis observed in chemoresistant EOC cells is a consequence of a further increase in the degree of S-nitrosylation of caspase-3. Since resistance to apoptosis is a hallmark of tumor growth, identifying mechanisms of this resistance such as S-nitrosylation may be a key in cancer progression and the development of chemoresistance. S-nitrosylation is reversible and seemingly a specific post-translational modification that regulates the activity of several signaling proteins. S-nitrosylation of the catalytic site cysteine in caspases serves as an on/off switch regulating caspase activity during apoptosis in endothelial cells, lymphocytes, and trophoblasts [147–149]. Targeting MPO may be a potential therapeutic intervention to reverse the resistance to apoptosis in sensitive and chemoresistant EOC cells.

13. Ovarian cancer immunotherapy and oxidative stress

It is well established that tumorigenic cells generate high levels of ROS to activate proximal signaling pathways that promote proliferation, survival and metabolic adaptation while also maintaining a high level of antioxidant activity to prevent buildup of ROS to levels that could induce cell death [160]. Moreover, there is evidence that ROS can act as secondary messengers in immune cells, which can lead to hyperactivation of inflammatory responses resulting in tissue damage and pathology [160]. Ovarian cancer is considered an ideal tumorogenic cancer because ovarian cancer cells have no negative impact on immune cells [161].

Effective immunotherapy for ovarian cancer is currently the focus of several investigations and clinical trials. Current immunotherapies for cancer treatment include therapeutic vaccines, cytokines, immune modulators, immune checkpoint inhibitors, and adoptive T cell transfer [162]. The discovery of a monoclonal antibodies (such as bevacizumab) directed against VEGF have been shown to improve progression free survival compared to cytotoxic chemotherapy alone was a major outcome of these clinical trials [163]. Other monoclonal antibodies currently approved for other cancers such as trastuzumab for breast cancer or cetuximab for colon cancer exhibited limited activity in ovarian cancer [163]. Several clinical trials are ongoing for the utilization of immune checkpoint blockade in ovarian cancer immune therapy [164]. Most recently tested were the programmed death (PD)-1 inhibitors, pembrolizumab and nivolumab, which showed a consistent response rate of 10–20% in phase 2 studies and then failed to improve outcomes in confirmatory trials [164]. Ultimately, larger phase 3 studies are needed to validate these findings for checkpoint inhibitors, particularly with regard to the duration of response seen with these agents. Additionally, the direct intraperitoneal delivery of interleukin (IL)-12, a potent immunostimulatory agent, exhibited some potential therapeutic efficacy in ovarian cancer [165]. Recently, targeting folate receptor alpha, which is found to be expressed in ovarian cancer, has shown promising therapeutic value. The targeting of the folate receptor was achieved by either a blocking monoclonal antibody (farletuzumab) or antibody conjugates of folate analogs, such as vintafolide [166].

14. Summary and conclusion

Oxidative stress has been implicated in the pathogenesis of several malignancies including ovarian cancer. Epithelial ovarian cancer is characterized to manifest a persistent pro-oxidant state through alteration of the redox balance, which is further enhanced in their chemoresistant counterparts, as summarized in **Figure 2**. Forcing ovarian cancer cells to undergo oxidative phosphorylation rather than glycolysis has been shown to be beneficial for eliminating cells via apoptosis (**Figure 2**). Collectively, there is convincing evidence that indicated a causal relationship between the acquisition of chemoresistance and chemotherapy-induced genetic mutations in key redox enzymes, leading to a further enhanced oxidative stress in chemoresistant EOC cells. This concept was further confirmed by the observation that induction of point mutations in sensitive EOC cells increased their resistance to chemotherapy. Also, a combination of antioxidants with chemotherapy significantly sensitized cells to chemotherapy. Identification of targets for chemoresistance with either biomarker and/or screening potential will have a significant impact for the treatment of this disease.

Acknowledgements

Portions of this chapter contain material that was previously published and is used with permission from Elsevier, IOS Press, and the authors. Reprinted from *Gynecologic Oncology*, 145(3), Saed GM, Diamond MP, Fletcher NM, Updates of the role of oxidative stress in the pathogenesis of ovarian cancer, 2017 Jun;145(3):595-602, with permission from Elsevier, 2017, License number 4091940523932; Reprinted from *Gynecologic Oncology*, 116(2), Saed GM, Ali-Fehmi R, Jiang ZL, Fletcher NM, Diamond MP, Abu-Soud HM, Munkarah AR, Myeloperoxidase serves as a redox switch that regulates apoptosis in epithelial ovarian cancer, 2010 Feb;116(2):276-81, with permission from Elsevier, 2017, License 4091940340178; Reprinted from *Free Radical Biology and Medicine*, 102, Fletcher NM, Belotte J, Saed MG, Memaj I, Diamond MP, Morris RT, Saed GM, Specific point mutations in key redox enzymes are associated with chemoresistance in epithelial ovarian cancer, 2017 Jan;102:122-132, with permission from Elsevier, 2017, License 4091940462337; Reprinted from *Gynecologic Oncology*, 122(2), Jiang Z, Fletcher NM, Ali-Fehmi R, Diamond MP, Abu-Soud HM, Munkarah AR, Saed GM, Modulation of redox signaling promotes apoptosis in epithelial ovarian cancer cells, 2011 Aug;122(2):418-23, with permission from Elsevier, 2017, License 4091940941920; Fletcher NM1, Jiang Z, Ali-Fehmi R, Levin NK, Belotte J, Tainsky MA, Diamond MP, Abu-Soud HM, Saed GM. Myeloperoxidase and free iron levels: potential biomarkers for early detection and prognosis of ovarian cancer. Reprinted from Cancer Biomark. 2011-2012;10(6):267-75 with permission from IOS Press. The final publication is available at IOS Press through http://dx.doi.org/10.3233/CBM-2012-0255.

Author details

Ghassan M. Saed[1]*, Robert T. Morris[2] and Nicole M. Fletcher[1]

*Address all correspondence to: gsaed@med.wayne.edu

1 Wayne State University, Detroit, MI, USA

2 Karmanos Cancer Institute, Detroit, MI, USA

References

[1] Saed GM, Diamond MP, Fletcher NM. Updates of the role of oxidative stress in the pathogenesis of ovarian cancer. Gynecologic Oncology. 2017;**145**(3):595-602

[2] Rojas V et al. Molecular characterization of epithelial ovarian cancer: Implications for diagnosis and treatment. International Journal of Molecular Sciences. 2016;**17**(12)

[3] Blagden SP. Harnessing pandemonium: The clinical implications of tumor heterogeneity in ovarian cancer. Frontiers in Oncology. 2015;**5**:149

[4] Leahy Y. Are serum protein biomarkers effective in detecting ovarian cancer in its early stages? Clinical Journal of Oncology Nursing. 2009;**13**(4):443-445

[5] Zhen W et al. Increased gene-specific repair of cisplatin interstrand cross-links in cisplatin-resistant human ovarian cancer cell lines. Molecular and Cellular Biology. 1992;**12**(9):3689-3698

[6] Lee C, Macgregor P. Drug resistance and microarrays. Modern Drug Discovery. 2004:**7**(7)

[7] Lippert TH, Ruoff HJ, Volm M. Current status of methods to assess cancer drug resistance. International Journal of Medical Sciences. 2011;**8**(3):245-253

[8] Matsuo K et al. Clinical relevance of extent of extreme drug resistance in epithelial ovarian carcinoma. Gynecologic Oncology. 2010;**116**(1):61-65

[9] Taddei ML et al. Mitochondrial oxidative stress due to complex I dysfunction promotes fibroblast activation and melanoma cell invasiveness. Journal of Signal Transduction. 2012;**2012**:684592

[10] Hileman EO et al. Intrinsic oxidative stress in cancer cells: A biochemical basis for therapeutic selectivity. Cancer Chemotherapy and Pharmacology. 2004;**53**(3):209-219

[11] Toyokuni S. Oxidative stress and cancer: The role of redox regulation. Biotherapy. 1998;**11**(2-3):147-154

[12] Toyokuni S et al. Persistent oxidative stress in cancer. FEBS Letters. 1995;**358**(1):1-3

[13] Reuter S et al. Oxidative stress, inflammation, and cancer: How are they linked? Free Radical Biology & Medicine. 2010;**49**(11):1603-1616

[14] Beckman KB, Ames BN. The free radical theory of aging matures. Physiological Reviews. 1998;**78**(2):547-581

[15] Choi JY et al. Iron intake, oxidative stress-related genes (MnSOD and MPO) and prostate cancer risk in CARET cohort. Carcinogenesis. 2008;**29**(5):964-970

[16] Coussens LM, Werb Z. Inflammation and cancer. Nature. 2002;**420**(6917):860-867

[17] Finkel T, Holbrook NJ. Oxidants, oxidative stress and the biology of ageing. Nature. 2000;**408**(6809):239-247

[18] Erickson BK, Conner MG, Landen CN Jr. The role of the fallopian tube in the origin of ovarian cancer. American Journal of Obstetrics and Gynecology. 2013;**209**(5):409-414

[19] Kurman RJ, Shih Ie M. The dualistic model of ovarian carcinogenesis: Revisited, revised, and expanded. American Journal of Pathology. 2016;**186**(4):733-747

[20] Hibbs K et al. Differential gene expression in ovarian carcinoma: Identification of potential biomarkers. The American Journal of Pathology. 2004;**165**(2):397-414

[21] Fletcher NM et al. Specific point mutations in key redox enzymes are associated with chemoresistance in epithelial ovarian cancer. Free Radical Biology & Medicine. 2016;**102**:122-132

[22] Fletcher NM et al. Myeloperoxidase and free iron levels: Potential biomarkers for early detection and prognosis of ovarian cancer. Cancer Biomarkers. 2011;**10**(6):267-275

[23] Ramus SJ et al. Consortium analysis of 7 candidate SNPs for ovarian cancer. International Journal of Cancer. 2008;**123**(2):380-388

[24] Lengyel E. Ovarian cancer development and metastasis. The American Journal of Pathology. 2010;**177**(3):1053-1064

[25] Liao J et al. Ovarian cancer spheroid cells with stem cell-like properties contribute to tumor generation, metastasis and chemotherapy resistance through hypoxia-resistant metabolism. PLoS One. 2014;**9**(1) e84941

[26] Vermeersch KA et al. OVCAR-3 spheroid-derived cells display distinct metabolic profiles. PLoS One. 2015;**10**(2):e0118262

[27] Lei XG et al. Paradoxical roles of antioxidant enzymes: Basic mechanisms and health implications. Physiological Reviews. 2016;**96**(1):307-364

[28] Klaunig JE, Kamendulis LM, Hocevar BA. Oxidative stress and oxidative damage in carcinogenesis. Toxicologic Pathology. 2010;**38**(1):96-109

[29] Fruehauf JP, Meyskens FL Jr. Reactive oxygen species: A breath of life or death? Clinical Cancer Research. 2007;**13**(3):789-794

[30] Circu ML, Aw TY. Glutathione and modulation of cell apoptosis. Biochimica et Biophysica Acta. 2012;**1823**(10):1767-1777

[31] Ishikawa T, Ali-Osman F. Glutathione-associated cis-diamminedichloroplatinum(II) metabolism and ATP-dependent efflux from leukemia cells. Molecular characterization of glutathione-platinum complex and its biological significance. The Journal of Biological Chemistry. 1993;**268**(27):20116-20125

[32] Wang J, Yi J. Cancer cell killing via ROS: To increase or decrease, that is the question. Cancer Biology & Therapy. 2008;**7**(12):1875-1884

[33] Schmidt HH et al. Antioxidants in translational medicine. Antioxidants & Redox Signaling. 2015;**23**(14):1130-1143

[34] Waris G, Ahsan H. Reactive oxygen species: Role in the development of cancer and various chronic conditions. Journal of Carcinogenesis. 2006;5:14

[35] Roos WP, Thomas AD, Kaina B. DNA damage and the balance between survival and death in cancer biology. Nature Reviews. Cancer. 2016;16(1):20-33

[36] Retel J et al. Mutational specificity of oxidative DNA damage. Mutation Research. 1993; 299(3-4):165-182

[37] Westermarck J, Kahari VM. Regulation of matrix metalloproteinase expression in tumor invasion. The FASEB Journal. 1999;13(8):781-792

[38] Mazure NM et al. Oncogenic transformation and hypoxia synergistically act to modulate vascular endothelial growth factor expression. Cancer Research. 1996;56(15):3436-3440

[39] Okada F et al. Impact of oncogenes in tumor angiogenesis: Mutant K-ras up-regulation of vascular endothelial growth factor/vascular permeability factor is necessary, but not sufficient for tumorigenicity of human colorectal carcinoma cells. Proceedings of the National Academy of Sciences of the United States of America. 1998;95(7):3609-3614

[40] Saed GM et al. Dichloroacetate induces apoptosis of epithelial ovarian cancer cells through a mechanism involving modulation of oxidative stress. Reproductive Sciences. 2011;18(12):1253-1261

[41] Michelakis ED, Webster L, Mackey JR. Dichloroacetate (DCA) as a potential metabolic-targeting therapy for cancer. British Journal of Cancer. 2008;99(7):989-994

[42] Bell EL, Emerling BM, Chandel NS. Mitochondrial regulation of oxygen sensing. Mitochondrion. 2005;5(5):322-332

[43] Mansfield KD et al. Mitochondrial dysfunction resulting from loss of cytochrome c impairs cellular oxygen sensing and hypoxic HIF-alpha activation. Cell Metabolism. 2005; 1(6):393-399

[44] Castillo-Tong DC et al. Association of myeloperoxidase with ovarian cancer. Tumour Biology. 2014;35(1):141-148

[45] Belotte J et al. The role of oxidative stress in the development of cisplatin resistance in epithelial ovarian cancer. Reproductive Sciences. 2013

[46] Belotte J et al. A single nucleotide polymorphism in catalase is strongly associated with ovarian cancer survival. PLoS One. 2015;10(8):e0135739

[47] Watson J. Oxidants, antioxidants and the current incurability of metastatic cancers. Open Biology. 2013;3(1):120144

[48] Klein EA et al. Vitamin E and the risk of prostate cancer: The selenium and vitamin E cancer prevention trial (SELECT). JAMA. 2011;306(14):1549-1556

[49] Bjelakovic G et al. Mortality in randomized trials of antioxidant supplements for primary and secondary prevention: Systematic review and meta-analysis. JAMA. 2007; 297(8):842-857

[50] Sayin VI et al. Antioxidants accelerate lung cancer progression in mice. Science Translational Medicine. 2014;**6**(221) 221ra15

[51] Senthil K, Aranganathan S, Nalini N. Evidence of oxidative stress in the circulation of ovarian cancer patients. Clinica Chimica Acta. 2004;**339**(1-2):27-32

[52] Jiang Z et al. Modulation of redox signaling promotes apoptosis in epithelial ovarian cancer cells. Gynecologic Oncology. 2011;**122**(2):418-423

[53] Saed GM et al. Myeloperoxidase serves as a redox switch that regulates apoptosis in epithelial ovarian cancer. Gynecologic Oncology. 2010;**116**(2):276-281

[54] Malone JM et al. The effects of the inhibition of inducible nitric oxide synthase on angiogenesis of epithelial ovarian cancer. American Journal of Obstetrics and Gynecology. 2006;**194**(4):1110-6; discussion 1116-8

[55] Abu-Soud HM, Hazen SL. Nitric oxide is a physiological substrate for mammalian peroxidases. The Journal of Biological Chemistry. 2000;**275**(48):37524-37532

[56] Abu-Soud HM, Hazen SL. Nitric oxide modulates the catalytic activity of myeloperoxidase. The Journal of Biological Chemistry. 2000;**275**(8):5425-5430

[57] Habib S, Ali A. Biochemistry of nitric oxide. Indian Journal of Clinical Biochemistry. 2011;**26**(1):3-17

[58] Muscat JE, Huncharek MS. Perineal talc use and ovarian cancer: A critical review. European Journal of Cancer Prevention. 2008;**17**(2):139-146

[59] Sasaroli D, Coukos G, Scholler N. Beyond CA125: The coming of age of ovarian cancer biomarkers. Are we there yet? Biomarkers in Medicine. 2009;**3**(3):275-288

[60] Schummer M et al. Comparative hybridization of an array of 21,500 ovarian cDNAs for the discovery of genes overexpressed in ovarian carcinomas. Gene. 1999;**238**(2):375-385

[61] Drapkin R et al. Human epididymis protein 4 (HE4) is a secreted glycoprotein that is overexpressed by serous and endometrioid ovarian carcinomas. Cancer Research. 2005;**65**(6):2162-2169

[62] Galgano MT, Hampton GM, Frierson HF Jr. Comprehensive analysis of HE4 expression in normal and malignant human tissues. Modern Pathology. 2006;**19**(6):847-853

[63] Gilks CB et al. Distinction between serous tumors of low malignant potential and serous carcinomas based on global mRNA expression profiling. Gynecologic Oncology. 2005;**96**(3):684-694

[64] Hough CD et al. Large-scale serial analysis of gene expression reveals genes differentially expressed in ovarian cancer. Cancer Research. 2000;**60**(22):6281-6287

[65] Bouchard D et al. Proteins with whey-acidic-protein motifs and cancer. The Lancet Oncology. 2006;**7**(2):167-174

[66] Rosen DG et al. Potential markers that complement expression of CA125 in epithelial ovarian cancer. Gynecologic Oncology. 2005;**99**(2):267-277

[67] Scholler N et al. Bead-based ELISA for validation of ovarian cancer early detection markers. Clinical Cancer Research. 2006;**12**(7 Pt 1):2117-2124

[68] Moore RG et al. The use of multiple novel tumor biomarkers for the detection of ovarian carcinoma in patients with a pelvic mass. Gynecologic Oncology. 2008;**108**(2):402-408

[69] Kim JW, Dang CV. Multifaceted roles of glycolytic enzymes. Trends in Biochemical Sciences. 2005;**30**(3):142-150

[70] Menon U et al. Prospective study using the risk of ovarian cancer algorithm to screen for ovarian cancer. Journal of Clinical Oncology. 2005;**23**(31):7919-7926

[71] Xu FJ et al. OVX1 as a marker for early stage endometrial carcinoma. Cancer. 1994;**73**(7):1855-1858

[72] Havrilesky LJ et al. Evaluation of biomarker panels for early stage ovarian cancer detection and monitoring for disease recurrence. Gynecologic Oncology. 2008;**110**(3):374-382

[73] Loria V et al. Myeloperoxidase: A new biomarker of inflammation in ischemic heart disease and acute coronary syndromes. Mediators of Inflammation. 2008;**2008**:135625

[74] Dally H et al. Myeloperoxidase (MPO) genotype and lung cancer histologic types: The MPO -463 a allele is associated with reduced risk for small cell lung cancer in smokers. International Journal of Cancer. 2002;**102**(5):530-535

[75] Ekmekci OB et al. Iron, nitric oxide, and myeloperoxidase in asthmatic patients. Biochemistry (Mosc). 2004;**69**(4):462-467

[76] Baldus S et al. Myeloperoxidase serum levels predict risk in patients with acute coronary syndromes. Circulation. 2003;**108**(12):1440-1445

[77] Brennan ML et al. Prognostic value of myeloperoxidase in patients with chest pain. The New England Journal of Medicine. 2003;**349**(17):1595-1604

[78] Muscara MN et al. Wound collagen deposition in rats: Effects of an NO-NSAID and a selective COX-2 inhibitor. British Journal of Pharmacology. 2000;**129**(4):681-686

[79] Shi HP et al. The role of iNOS in wound healing. Surgery. 2001;**130**(2):225-229

[80] Witte MB, Barbul A. Role of nitric oxide in wound repair. American Journal of Surgery. 2002;**183**(4):406-412

[81] Sadrzadeh SM et al. Hemoglobin. A biologic fenton reagent. The Journal of Biological Chemistry. 1984;**259**(23):14354-14356

[82] Galijasevic S et al. Myeloperoxidase interaction with peroxynitrite: Chloride deficiency and heme depletion. Free Radical Biology & Medicine. 2009;**47**(4):431-439

[83] Maitra D et al. Melatonin can mediate its vascular protective effect by modulating free iron level by inhibiting hypochlorous acid-mediated hemoprotein heme destruction. Hypertension. 2011;**57**(5):e22 author reply e23

[84] Maitra D et al. Reaction of hemoglobin with HOCl: Mechanism of heme destruction and free iron release. Free Radical Biology & Medicine. 2011;**51**(2):374-386

[85] Maitra D et al. Mechanism of hypochlorous acid-mediated heme destruction and free iron release. Free Radical Biology & Medicine. 2011;**51**(2):364-373

[86] Bozzini C et al. Biochemical and genetic markers of iron status and the risk of coronary artery disease: An angiography-based study. Clinical Chemistry. 2002;**48**(4):622-628

[87] de Valk B, Marx JJ. Iron, atherosclerosis, and ischemic heart disease. Archives of Internal Medicine. 1999;**159**(14):1542-1548

[88] Sullivan JL. Iron and the genetics of cardiovascular disease. Circulation. 1999;**100**(12):1260-1263

[89] Niederau C. Iron overload and atherosclerosis. Hepatology. 2000;**32**(3):672-674

[90] Brault S et al. Lysophosphatidic acid induces endothelial cell death by modulating the redox environment. American Journal of Physiology. Regulatory, Integrative and Comparative Physiology. 2007;**292**(3):R1174-R1183

[91] O'Donnell BV et al. Studies on the inhibitory mechanism of iodonium compounds with special reference to neutrophil NADPH oxidase. The Biochemical Journal. 1993;**290** (Pt 1):41-49

[92] Park SE et al. Diphenyleneiodonium induces ROS-independent p53 expression and apoptosis in human RPE cells. FEBS Letters. 2007;**581**(2):180-186

[93] Boveris A, Chance B. The mitochondrial generation of hydrogen peroxide. General properties and effect of hyperbaric oxygen. The Biochemical Journal. 1973;**134**(3):707-716

[94] Volm M, Koomagi R. Hypoxia-inducible factor (HIF-1) and its relationship to apoptosis and proliferation in lung cancer. Anticancer Research. 2000;**20**(3A):1527-1533

[95] Tanaka M et al. Anti-metastatic gene therapy utilizing subcutaneous inoculation of EC-SOD gene transduced autologous fibroblast suppressed lung metastasis of meth-a cells and 3LL cells in mice. Gene Therapy. 2001;**8**(2):149-156

[96] Wheeler MD, Smutney OM, Samulski RJ. Secretion of extracellular superoxide dismutase from muscle transduced with recombinant adenovirus inhibits the growth of B16 melanomas in mice. Molecular Cancer Research. 2003;**1**(12):871-881

[97] Suliman HB, Ali M, Piantadosi CA. Superoxide dismutase-3 promotes full expression of the EPO response to hypoxia. Blood. 2004;**104**(1):43-50

[98] Arbiser JL et al. Reactive oxygen generated by Nox1 triggers the angiogenic switch. Proceedings of the National Academy of Sciences of the United States of America. 2002;**99**(2):715-720

[99] Pelicano H, Carney D, Huang P. ROS stress in cancer cells and therapeutic implications. Drug Resistance Updates. 2004;**7**(2):97-110

[100] Trachootham D, Alexandre J, Huang P. Targeting cancer cells by ROS-mediated mechanisms: A radical therapeutic approach? Nature Reviews. Drug Discovery. 2009; **8**(7):579-591

[101] Desouki MM et al. Cross talk between mitochondria and superoxide generating NADPH oxidase in breast and ovarian tumors. Cancer Biology & Therapy. 2005;**4**(12):1367-1373

[102] Mochizuki T et al. Inhibition of NADPH oxidase 4 activates apoptosis via the AKT/ apoptosis signal-regulating kinase 1 pathway in pancreatic cancer PANC-1 cells. Onco-gene. 2006;**25**(26):3699-3707

[103] Mabuchi S et al. Estrogen inhibits paclitaxel-induced apoptosis via the phosphoryla-tion of apoptosis signal-regulating kinase 1 in human ovarian cancer cell lines. Endo-crinology. 2004;**145**(1):49-58

[104] Wang X et al. Epidermal growth factor receptor-dependent Akt activation by oxida-tive stress enhances cell survival. The Journal of Biological Chemistry. 2000;**275**(19): 14624-14631

[105] Piret JP et al. CoCl2, a chemical inducer of hypoxia-inducible factor-1, and hypoxia reduce apoptotic cell death in hepatoma cell line HepG2. Annals of the New York Academy of Sciences. 2002;**973**:443-447

[106] Li Y, Trush MA. Diphenyleneiodonium, an NAD(P)H oxidase inhibitor, also potently inhibits mitochondrial reactive oxygen species production. Biochemical and Biophysical Research Communications. 1998;**253**(2):295-299

[107] Shi Y et al. Rapamycin enhances apoptosis and increases sensitivity to cisplatin in vitro. Cancer Research. 1995;**55**(9):1982-1988

[108] Scaife RM. Selective and irreversible cell cycle inhibition by diphenyleneiodonium. Molecular Cancer Therapeutics. 2005;**4**(6):876-884

[109] Goud AP et al. Reactive oxygen species and oocyte aging: Role of superoxide, hydrogen peroxide, and hypochlorous acid. Free Radical Biology & Medicine. 2008;**44**(7):1295-1304

[110] McCord JM, Fridovich I. Superoxide dismutase. An enzymic function for erythrocu-prein (hemocuprein). The Journal of Biological Chemistry. 1969;**244**(22):6049-6055

[111] Schallreuter KU et al. In vivo and in vitro evidence for hydrogen peroxide (H2O2) accumulation in the epidermis of patients with vitiligo and its successful removal by a UVB-activated pseudocatalase. The Journal of Investigative Dermatology. Symposium Proceedings. 1999;**4**(1):91-96

[112] Hu Y et al. Mitochondrial manganese-superoxide dismutase expression in ovarian can-cer: Role in cell proliferation and response to oxidative stress. The Journal of Biological Chemistry. 2005;**280**(47):39485-39492

[113] Calastretti A et al. Damaged microtubules can inactivate BCL-2 by means of the mTOR kinase. Oncogene. 2001;**20**(43):6172-6180

[114] Jiang H, Feng Y. Hypoxia-inducible factor 1alpha (HIF-1alpha) correlated with tumor growth and apoptosis in ovarian cancer. International Journal of Gynecological Cancer. 2006;**16**(Suppl 1):405-412

[115] Kaewpila S et al. Manganese superoxide dismutase modulates hypoxia-inducible factor-1 alpha induction via superoxide. Cancer Research. 2008;**68**(8):2781-2788

[116] Chen B et al. Roles of microRNA on cancer cell metabolism. Journal of Translational Medicine. 2012;**10**:228

[117] Vander Heiden MG et al. Evidence for an alternative glycolytic pathway in rapidly proliferating cells. Science. 2010;**329**(5998):1492-1499

[118] Kroemer G, Pouyssegur J. Tumor cell metabolism: cancer's Achilles' heel. Cancer Cell. 2008;**13**(6):472-482

[119] Kim JW et al. HIF-1-mediated expression of pyruvate dehydrogenase kinase: A metabolic switch required for cellular adaptation to hypoxia. Cell Metabolism. 2006;**3**(3):177-185

[120] Xie J et al. Dichloroacetate shifts the metabolism from glycolysis to glucose oxidation and exhibits synergistic growth inhibition with cisplatin in HeLa cells. International Journal of Oncology. 2011;**38**(2):409-417

[121] Stacpoole PW et al. Evaluation of long-term treatment of children with congenital lactic acidosis with dichloroacetate. Pediatrics. 2008;**121**(5):e1223-e1228

[122] Stacpoole PW. The pharmacology of dichloroacetate. Metabolism. 1989;**38**(11):1124-1144

[123] Stockwin LH et al. Sodium dichloroacetate selectively targets cells with defects in the mitochondrial ETC. International Journal of Cancer. 2010;**127**(11):2510-2519

[124] Kim JW, Dang CV. Cancer's molecular sweet tooth and the Warburg effect. Cancer Research. 2006;**66**(18):8927-8930

[125] Xu RH et al. Inhibition of glycolysis in cancer cells: A novel strategy to overcome drug resistance associated with mitochondrial respiratory defect and hypoxia. Cancer Research. 2005;**65**(2):613-621

[126] Kinnula VL, Crapo JD. Superoxide dismutases in malignant cells and human tumors. Free Radical Biology & Medicine. 2004;**36**(6):718-744

[127] Tandon R et al. Oxidative stress in patients with essential hypertension. National Medical Journal of India. 2005;**18**(6):297-299

[128] Storz P. Reactive oxygen species in tumor progression. Frontiers in Bioscience. 2005;**10**:1881-1896

[129] Kajiyama H et al. Survival benefit of taxane plus platinum in recurrent ovarian cancer with non-clear cell, non-mucinous histology. Journal of Gynecologic Oncology. 2014;**25**(1):43-50

[130] Landriscina M et al. Adaptation to oxidative stress, chemoresistance, and cell survival. Antioxidants & Redox Signaling. 2009;**11**(11):2701-2716

[131] Traverso N et al. Role of glutathione in cancer progression and chemoresistance. Oxidative Medicine and Cellular Longevity. 2013;**2013**:972913

[132] Erichsen HC, Chanock SJ. SNPs in cancer research and treatment. British Journal of Cancer. 2004;**90**(4):747-751

[133] Klaunig JE et al. Oxidative stress and oxidative damage in chemical carcinogenesis. Toxicology and Applied Pharmacology. 2011;**254**(2):86-99

[134] Forsberg L et al. A common functional C-T substitution polymorphism in the promoter region of the human catalase gene influences transcription factor binding, reporter gene transcription and is correlated to blood catalase levels. Free Radical Biology & Medicine. 2001;**30**(5):500-505

[135] Goode EL et al. Candidate gene analysis using imputed genotypes: Cell cycle single-nucleotide polymorphisms and ovarian cancer risk. Cancer Epidemiology, Biomarkers & Prevention. 2009;**18**(3):935-944

[136] Notaridou M et al. Common alleles in candidate susceptibility genes associated with risk and development of epithelial ovarian cancer. International Journal of Cancer. 2011; **128**(9):2063-2074

[137] Savas S et al. Functional nsSNPs from carcinogenesis-related genes expressed in breast tissue: Potential breast cancer risk alleles and their distribution across human populations. Human Genomics. 2006;**2**(5):287-296

[138] Quick SK et al. Effect modification by catalase genotype suggests a role for oxidative stress in the association of hormone replacement therapy with postmenopausal breast cancer risk. Cancer Epidemiology, Biomarkers & Prevention. 2008;**17**(5):1082-1087

[139] Didziapetriene J et al. Significance of blood serum catalase activity and malondialdehyde level for survival prognosis of ovarian cancer patients. Medicina (Kaunas, Lithuania). 2014;**50**(4):204-208

[140] Sellers TA et al. Association of single nucleotide polymorphisms in glycosylation genes with risk of epithelial ovarian cancer. Cancer Epidemiology, Biomarkers & Prevention. 2008;**17**(2):397-404

[141] Porter AG, Janicke RU. Emerging roles of caspase-3 in apoptosis. Cell Death and Differentiation. 1999;**6**(2):99-104

[142] Liu L, Stamler JS. NO: An inhibitor of cell death. Cell Death and Differentiation. 1999;**6**(10):937-942

[143] Dimmeler S et al. Suppression of apoptosis by nitric oxide via inhibition of interleukin-1beta-converting enzyme (ICE)-like and cysteine protease protein (CPP)-32-like proteases. The Journal of Experimental Medicine. 1997;**185**(4):601-607

[144] Thornberry NA, Lazebnik Y. Caspases: Enemies within. Science. 1998;**281**(5381):1312-1316

[145] Mannick JB et al. Fas-induced caspase denitrosylation. Science. 1999;**284**(5414):651-654

[146] Maejima Y et al. Nitric oxide inhibits myocardial apoptosis by preventing caspase-3 activity via S-nitrosylation. Journal of Molecular and Cellular Cardiology. 2005;**38**(1):163-174

[147] Rossig L et al. Nitric oxide inhibits caspase-3 by S-nitrosation in vivo. The Journal of Biological Chemistry. 1999;**274**(11):6823-6826

[148] Dash PR et al. Nitric oxide protects human extravillous trophoblast cells from apoptosis by a cyclic GMP-dependent mechanism and independently of caspase 3 nitrosylation. Experimental Cell Research. 2003;**287**(2):314-324

[149] Mannick JB et al. S-Nitrosylation of mitochondrial caspases. The Journal of Cell Biology. 2001;**154**(6):1111-1116

[150] Harrison JE, Schultz J. Studies on the chlorinating activity of myeloperoxidase. The Journal of Biological Chemistry. 1976;**251**(5):1371-1374

[151] Kettle AJ, van Dalen CJ, Winterbourn CC. Peroxynitrite and myeloperoxidase leave the same footprint in protein nitration. Redox Report. 1997;**3**(5-6):257-258

[152] Weiss SJ et al. Chlorination of taurine by human neutrophils. Evidence for hypochlorous acid generation. Journal of Clinical Investigation. 1982;**70**(3):598-607

[153] Ortiz de Montellano PR. Catalytic sites of hemoprotein peroxidases. Annual Review of Pharmacology and Toxicology. 1992;**32**:89-107

[154] Stamler JS, Singel DJ, Loscalzo J. Biochemistry of nitric oxide and its redox-activated forms. Science. 1992;**258**(5090):1898-1902

[155] Abu-Soud HM et al. Peroxidases inhibit nitric oxide (NO) dependent bronchodilation: Development of a model describing NO-peroxidase interactions. Biochemistry. 2001;**40**(39):11866-11875

[156] Nicotera P, Melino G. Regulation of the apoptosis-necrosis switch. Oncogene. 2004;**23**(16):2757-2765

[157] Munkarah AR et al. Effects of prostaglandin E(2) on proliferation and apoptosis of epithelial ovarian cancer cells. Journal of the Society for Gynecologic Investigation. 2002;**9**(3):168-173

[158] Evans TJ et al. Cytokine-treated human neutrophils contain inducible nitric oxide synthase that produces nitration of ingested bacteria. Proceedings of the National Academy of Sciences of the United States of America. 1996;**93**(18):9553-9558

[159] Song M, Santanam N. Increased myeloperoxidase and lipid peroxide-modified protein in gynecological malignancies. Antioxidants & Redox Signaling. 2001;**3**(6):1139-1146

[160] Schieber M, Chandel NS. ROS function in redox signaling and oxidative stress. Current Biology. 2014;**24**(10):R453-R462

[161] Kandalaft LE et al. Immunotherapy for ovarian cancer: what's next? Journal of Clinical Oncology. 2011;**29**(7):925-933

[162] De Felice F et al. Immunotherapy of ovarian cancer: The role of checkpoint inhibitors. Journal of Immunology Research. 2015;**2015**:191832

[163] Zand B, Coleman RL, Sood AK. Targeting angiogenesis in gynecologic cancers. Hematology/Oncology Clinics of North America. 2012;**26**(3):543-563 viii

[164] Chester C et al. Immunotherapeutic approaches to ovarian cancer treatment. Journal of Immunotherapy Cancer. 2015;**3**:7

[165] Alvarez RD et al. A phase II trial of intraperitoneal EGEN-001, an IL-12 plasmid formulated with PEG-PEI-cholesterol lipopolymer in the treatment of persistent or recurrent epithelial ovarian, fallopian tube or primary peritoneal cancer: A gynecologic oncology group study. Gynecologic Oncology. 2014;**133**(3):433-438

[166] Marchetti C et al. Targeted drug delivery via folate receptors in recurrent ovarian cancer: A review. Oncology Targets Therapy. 2014;**7**:1223-1236

8

Ubiquitin Signaling in Ovarian Cancer: From Potential to Challenges

Sumegha Mitra

Abstract

Ubiquitin proteasome system (UPS) is an emerging arena in cancer intervention. Dysregulation of various UPS components has been implicated with many cancers, and this knowledge is starting to be exploited for its role in cancer initiation, progression, and therapeutics. UPS regulates both protein turnover and non-proteolytic regulatory function of the proteins involved in cell cycle, signal transduction, DNA repair, histone modification, and transcription. In addition, chromosomal aberrations and genomic alterations often present in the cancer cell genomes lead to excess of conformationally challenged aggregation-prone proteins and proteotoxic stress that make cancer cells more dependent on UPS-mediated protein degradation than normal cells. This proposition is the basis of the clinical use of proteasome inhibitor, Bortezomib, to treat multiple myeloma and mantle cell lymphoma targeting cancer cells and mostly sparing the normal cells. This chapter provides an overview of various components of UPS which are implicated in cancer and regulate ubiquitin-mediated oncogenic signaling in ovarian cancer.

Keywords: ovarian cancer, mutant p53, ubiquitin, proteasomes, deubiquitinating enzymes

1. Introduction

Ovarian cancer is the most lethal gynecologic malignancy with a high case-to-fatality ratio [1]. According to American Cancer Society, approximately 22,440 new cases of ovarian cancer will be diagnosed in the year 2017 and about 14,080 women in the United States will die from this deadly disease [2]. About 90% of ovarian carcinomas are heterogeneous epithelial neoplasms with distinctive biology and clinicopathologic features at cellular and molecular levels [1, 3]. The clinical management of ovarian cancer has addressed this heterogeneity and classified ovarian cancer into high-grade and low-grade serous, endometrioid, clear cell, and mucinous subtypes based on the histology, tissue of origin, prognosis, and genetic alterations that deregulate specific signaling pathways in these tumor cells [4, 5] (**Figure 1**). Of these, high-grade serous ovarian cancer (HGSOC) is the most prevalent and lethal subtype of ovarian cancer. It accounts for 70–80% of ovarian cancer deaths [1]. The low *five-year survival rate* of HGSOC patients is attributed to the late detection of extensively metastasized disease, especially to omentum, which is the primary site of ovarian cancer metastasis. Moreover, about 80–90% of HGSOC patients eventually develop chemo-resistant tumors, after an initial positive response to cytoreductive surgery and chemotherapy, which are important prognosticators of the survival of HGSOC patients [1, 3]. The initiation and development of HGSOC is known to proceed through the early acquisition of genetic alterations in the tumor suppressor gene *TP53* [3, 6]. About 96% of HGSOC patients carry gain-of-function (GOF) mutations in *TP53* gene [3]. It is believed that *TP53* mutations lead to the precursor lesions in fallopian tube fimbria, which develop into serous tubal intraepithelial carcinoma (STIC) and ultimately to HGSOC [7, 8]. The reduced risk of ovarian cancer in BRCA1 mutation carriers after salpingo-oophorectomy supports the theory of HGSOC origin from STIC [9]. Mutant p53 orchestrates a distinct pro-tumorigenic signaling network and confer chemo-resistance through transcription-dependent and independent mechanisms in cancer cells. A recent study in triple-negative breast cancer cells revealed the role of mutant p53-proteasome axis in regulating global effects on cancer cell's protein homeostasis, inhibiting tumor suppressive pathways or turning on the oncogenic signaling in cancer cells [10]. A growing number of evidences suggest the role of ubiquitin signaling in tumor progression and growth. This chapter discusses the role of ubiquitin-mediated signaling in ovarian cancer pathogenesis. The different components of ubiquitin proteasome system, which are involved in this regulation, will be highlighted.

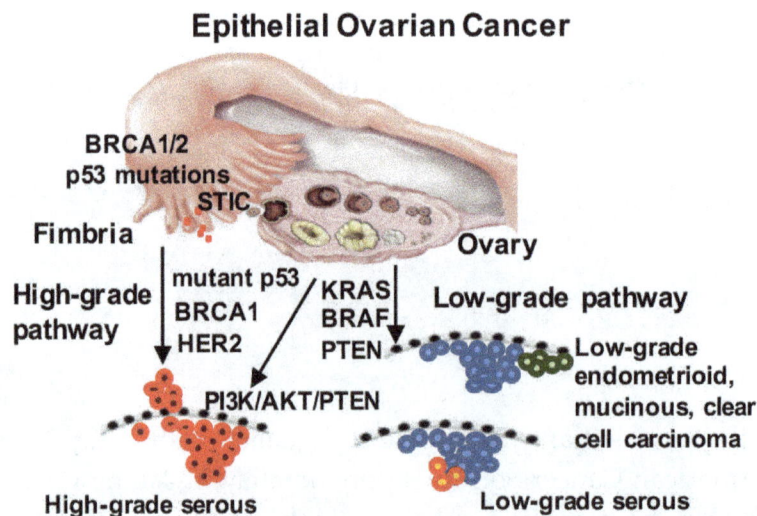

Epithelial Ovarian Cancer

Figure 1. A schematic representation of molecular drivers of low- and high-grade ovarian cancer initiation and progression. Low-grade tumors are low malignant potential (LMP) tumors associated with KRAS or BRAF mutation and loss of PTEN. High-grade serous tumors frequently have mutated *TP53* gene as well as activated members of PI3K/ Akt pathway. Highly invasive tumors originate from the fallopian tube precursor lesion, STIC, and spread to the ovary and other peritoneal surfaces. Genotoxic stresses in BRCA1/2 carriers predispose them to ovarian cancer.

1.1. Conceptual overview of ubiquitin modifications

Protein ubiquitination is a dynamic multifaceted posttranslational modification (PTM), which is involved in nearly all biological functions in a eukaryotic cell. Similar to phosphorylation, it functions as a signaling device and can be activated by extracellular stimuli, DNA damage, phosphorylation, ligand-dependent receptor activation, and signal transduction. Ubiquitin is a highly conserved 76-amino acid protein, which is expressed in all cell types. It has seven lysine (Lys or K) residues, K6, K11, K27, K29, K33, K48, and K63. Each lysine residue can result in a linkage-specific ubiquitin chain of certain topology [11, 12], which when bound to the target protein (substrate) dictates the fate of the protein (**Figure 2**). For example, the most predominant K48-linked polyubiquitin chains, which have a compact conformation, lead to the proteasomal degradation of the bound substrate. By contrast, the second most abundant K63-linked chains, which have an open conformation, are involved in non-proteolytic regulatory functions [13]. The K11-linked ubiquitin chains act as an additional proteasomal degradation signal, particularly in cell-cycle regulation [13]. The functions of the other lysine-specific ubiquitin chains remain less well characterized. K6-linked chains are shown to be upregulated with UV genotoxic stress and are known to be associated with BRCA1/BARD1 complex [14]. Similarly, K27 chains act to serve as scaffolds for protein recruitment such as p53-binding protein 1 in the DNA damage response. In addition, ubiquitin chain of mixed topology with different linkage at succeeding positions is also seen as in NF-κB signaling or in protein trafficking (**Figure 2F**) [13]. Moreover, branched ubiquitin chains of unknown function are generated when a single ubiquitin is modified with multiple molecules [12, 13]. These ubiquitin chains creating a multitude of signals with distinct cellular outcomes are referred to as "ubiquitin code" [13]. New layers of the ubiquitin code are emerging, based on findings that revealed the modification of ubiquitin chains with small ubiquitin-like (Ubl) modifier such as SUMO, phosphorylation, and acetylation [13].

Box 1. The discovery of ubiquitin-mediated protein degradation in the late 1970s by Drs. Avram Hershko, Aaron Ciechanover, and Irwin Rose was awarded 2004 Nobel Prize in Chemistry. Their study highlighted the role of protein ubiquitination in selective protein breakdown, regulating the cellular functions by modulating the levels of key enzymes, regulatory proteins and removal of abnormal proteins that arise by biosynthetic errors or post synthetic damages. Ubiquitin was first isolated from bovine thymus in 1975 by Goldstein et al. (PNAS, 1975;72:11-15) [88] and found to be covalently attached to histone 2A (Goldknopf and Busch, PNAS, 1977;74:864-868) [89]. Subsequently, Drs. Hershko, Ciechanover, and Rose in a series of biochemical studies discovered and characterized the ATP-dependent, ubiquitin-mediated protein degradation using the reticulocyte lysate system (PNAS, 1979;76:3107-3110) [90].

Ubiquitination is an orchestrated enzymatic reaction of E1 ubiquitin-activating enzyme, E2 ubiquitin-conjugating enzyme, and ubiquitin E3 ligase (E3). It is the most coordinated and conserved multistep process of covalently tagging a protein with mono- or polyubiquitin chain. The process begins with the ATP-dependent activation of ubiquitin by E1 ubiquitin-activating enzyme (E1s), which then transfers it to the active site cysteine of E2 ubiquitin-conjugating enzymes (E2s) forming a thioester linkage between ubiquitin and cysteine. Ubiquitin E3 ligases (E3s) have a central role in this process, as they recognize the specific protein substrates and facilitate the transfer of ubiquitin from the E2 onto the target protein [11, 12]. Deubiquitinating

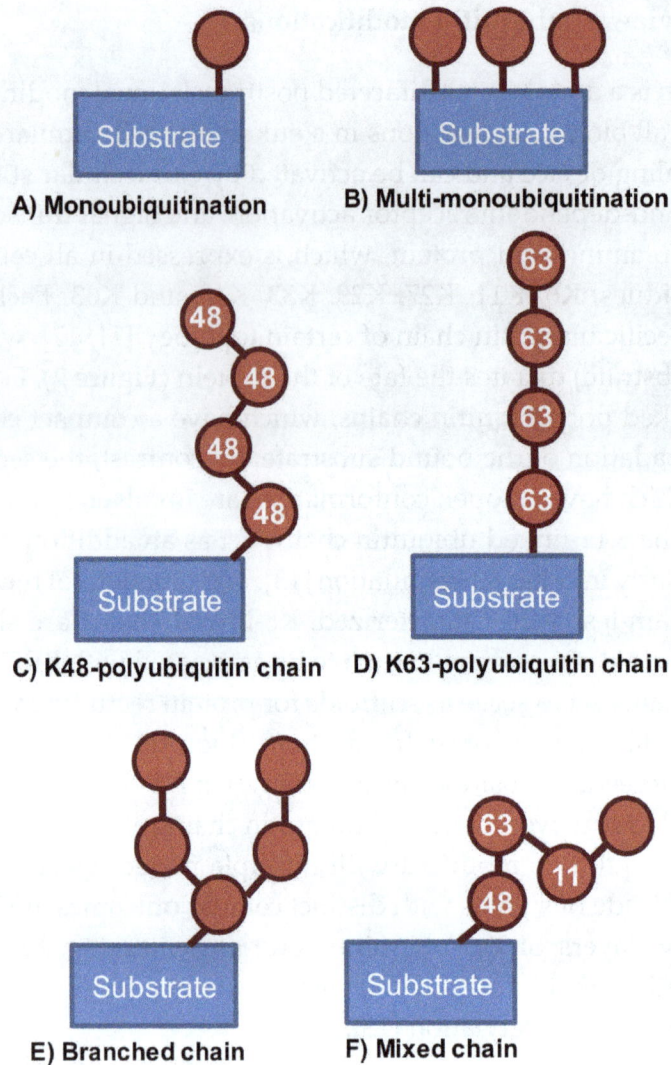

Figure 2. Linkage-specific ubiquitin chains of different topologies. Each circle represents one ubiquitin moiety. (A) Monoubiquitination, (B) multi-monoubiquitination, (C) K48-linked chain, (D) K63-linked chain, (E) branched chain, and (F) mixed chain.

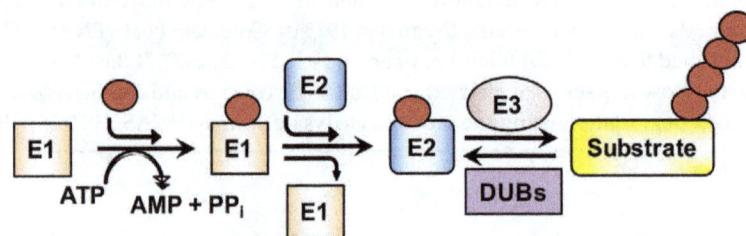

Figure 3. Enzymatic cascade of ubiquitin proteasome system. Ubiquitin is activated and conjugated to target protein by a conserved action of E1-ubiquitin-activating enzyme, E2-ubiquitin-conjugating enzyme, and E3 ubiquitin ligase.

enzymes (DUBs) are another class of enzymes, which removes or edits the ubiquitin chains attached to a protein, making this a highly reversible process and thus highlighting the dynamic regulation of ubiquitin signaling in the cell (**Figure 3**). These enzymes together with proteasomes, a cellular machinery involved in ubiquitin-mediated protein degradation, comprise the ubiquitin proteasome system (UPS). UPS plays an indispensable role in regulating ubiquitin-mediated proteolytic and non-proteolytic regulatory signaling to control cellular homeostasis, protein stability, and a wide range of signaling pathways.

2. UPS components in ovarian cancer

Ovarian cancer is characterized by multiple genetic and epigenetic abnormalities and several major (about seven) activated signaling pathways, which are directly or indirectly implicated with UPS. Moreover, several UPS components, E1s, E2s, E3s, DUBs and proteasomes are known to be deregulated or mutated in cancer (**Table 1**), suggesting their role in cancer signaling and cancer progression. This section discusses each UPS component implicated in ovarian cancer and the role of key players of each component in regulating ovarian cancer signaling (**Figure 4**).

2.1. E3 ligases

E3 ligases (E3s) are the most heterogeneous class of enzymes in UPS as they facilitate ubiquitination with exquisite spatial, temporal, and substrate specificity. There are more than 600 E3s in a human genome, indicating the precise substrate specificity of E3s [15]. E3s can be classified into three main types, RING E3s, HECT E3s, and RBR E3s depending on the presence of type-specific domains and on the mechanism of ubiquitin transfer to the substrate protein. RING E3s are the most abundant type of ubiquitin ligases. They are characterized by the presence of zinc-binding domain called Really Interesting New Gene (RING) and U-box domain. RING E3s mediate a direct transfer of ubiquitin to substrate, functioning as a scaffold to orient the ubiquitin-charged E2, whereas E3s with homologous to the E6AP carboxyl

Gene.	Role	Effect	Cancer [references]
BRCA1	E3 ligase	Mutation, loss of tumor suppressor function	Ovarian and breast cancers [19, 20]
USP13	DUB	Amplification, oncogene	Ovarian cancer [41]
Mdm2	E3 ligase	Overexpression, loss of p53 tumor suppressor function	Ovarian cancer and various malignancies [63, 64]
USP7	DUB	Overexpression, oncogene	Ovarian cancer [42]
Skp2	E3 ligase	Overexpression, loss of tumor suppressor function of p27	Ovarian, breast, and prostate cancers [76–81]
UCHL1	DUB	Overexpression or methylation, role varies with cancer	Ovarian, breast, gastric, lymphoma, lung, Esophageal squamous cell carcinoma [44–48]
FBW7	E3 ligase	Mutation, loss of tumor suppressor function	Ovarian and endometrial cancer, leukemia [71]
VHL	E3 ligase	Mutation, loss of tumor suppressor function	Clear-cell carcinoma, lung cancer [49]

Table 1. Cancer-associated alterations in UPS.

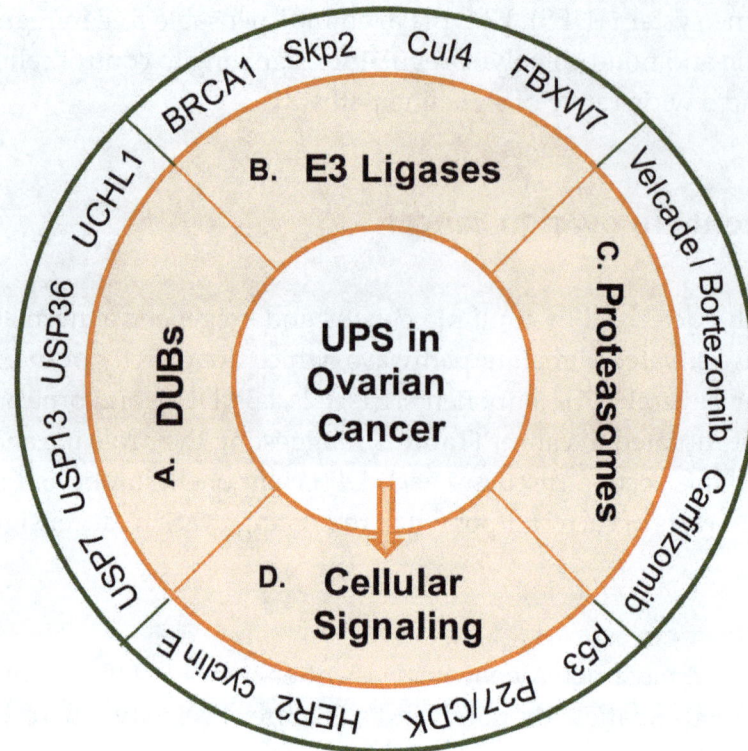

Figure 4. Key players of each UPS component involved in regulating ovarian cancer signaling. (A and B) DUBs and E3 ligases as candidate genes in ovarian cancer, (C) proteasomal activity and inhibitors in ovarian cancer, and (D) regulation of ovarian cancer oncogenic signaling by UPS.

terminus (HECT) domain transfer ubiquitin to the substrate in a two-step process—ubiquitin is first transferred to a catalytic cysteine on E3 and then to the substrate. Based on their N terminus extensions, HECTs are further classified into three subfamilies: Nedd4 family, HERC family, and other HECT that contain various domains. The RBR E3s are characterized by the presence of three RING domains, RING1 and RING2, separated by an in-between-RING (IBR) domain. RING1 recruits the ubiquitin-charged E2, RING2 possess catalytic cysteine. The IBR is called benign-catalytic domain as it lacks catalytic cysteine residue [15]. Given their cellular specificity and complexity, E3s are implicated in a number of pathophysiological conditions, which makes them an attractive therapeutic target in human diseases, including cancer [16].

2.1.1. BRCA1

The breast and ovarian cancer susceptibility gene, BRCA1, is a tumor suppressor gene [17]. Heterozygous mutations in BRCA1 gene predispose women to both familial and sporadic breast and ovarian cancers [18, 19]. Nonetheless, BRCA1 mutations are also associated with other cancers like stomach, pancreas, prostate, and colon [20]. BRCA1 acts as a hub protein, which participates in several different protein complexes to coordinate a diverse range of cellular functions including DNA repair, cell-cycle regulation, apoptosis, transcriptional regulation, and centrosome duplication to maintain genomic stability [17]. The structural analysis of BRCA1 protein suggested that it has a RING finger domain that harbors E3 ubiquitin ligase activity [14]. In addition, BRCA1 forms a heterodimer complex with BARD1, a protein with a RING finger domain [14]. BARD1 interaction stabilizes the proper conformation of BRCA1

RING domain for a potent E3 ligase activity and interaction with E2 UbcH5 [14, 21, 22]. BRCA1 E3 ligase substrate specificity is believed to depend on its phosphorylation-dependent binding to proteins containing phospho-SXXF motif such as CtIP, BACH1, and ABRA1 through a phospho-peptide recognition domain (BRCT) [23, 24]. The strong relation between BRCA1 tumor suppressor properties and E3 ligase activity is evident from the clustering of missense mutations that predispose to cancer in the Zn^{2+}-binding residues of BRCA1 RING finger domain crucial for its ubiquitin ligase activity [25]. The full range of function of BRCA1/BARD1 complex is not completely understood [18]. One of the most important functions of BRCA1 is to repair DNA double-strand breaks (DSBs). Following DNA damage, chromatin-associated histone H2AX phosphorylation by ATM and ATR at DNA damage site recruits an E3 ubiquitin ligase RFN8 and a phospho-module-binding mediator MDC1 at the damage site [17, 26–28]. RFN8 together with ubiquitin conjugase Ubc13, ubiquitinate histone H2A and H2B at chromatin lesions, which in turn translocate BRCA1 complex containing RAP80, a protein with ubiquitin-interacting motif (UIM), ABRA1, protein that interacts with BRCA1 BRCT domain and deubiquitinating enzyme, BRCC36 to Lys6- and Lys63-linked polyubiquitin chains at DSBs [17, 26, 29]. BRCA1 has also been implicated with the transcriptional activation of genes in response to DNA damage. The C-terminus of BRCA1 complexes with RNA polymerase II through RNA helicase, while N-terminus BRCA1/BRAD1 heterodimer binds to RNA polymerase II holoenzyme [30]. Identifying genes regulated by BRCA1 would shed a significant light on the transcriptional role of BRCA1. However, BRCA1 overexpression studies have shown induction in p53-responsive E3 ligase, mdm2, cell-cycle inhibitor, p21 and stress-response factor, and GADD45 in breast and small-cell lung cancer cell lines [31, 32]. Besides, BRCA1 also regulates G1/S, S-phase, and G2/M cell-cycle checkpoints through interactions with RAD3, ATM/ATR, and Chk1/Chk2 [26, 30, 33].

Over the last 10 years, significant information has been gained about the structure, function, and unique features of BRCA gene products, BRCA1 and BRCA2, which collectively contributes to the biological response to DNA damage through homologous recombination of DNA repair and regulation of cell-cycle checkpoints. BRCA1/2-deficient cancers, including ovarian cancer, are now recognized as the target for a class of drugs known as PARP (poly ADP-ribose polymerase) inhibitors [34]. PARP detects and initiates an immediate cellular response to metabolic or radiation-induced single-strand DNA breaks (SSB). It binds to DNA and synthesizes polymeric adenosine diphosphate ribose (poly ADP-ribose or PAR), which acts as signal to other DNA-repairing enzymes. PARP inhibition directly blocks the PARP enzymatic activity and subsequently leads to PARP accumulation on DNA, a process called PARP trapping, which converts an SSB into a double-strand DNA break through the collapse of replication fork [34]. BRCA-deficient tumor cells with impaired homologous recombination repair of double-strand DNA breaks are directed toward the error-prone repair process of non-homologous end joining which leads to genetic instability and cell death. Thus, BRCA1/2-deficient ovarian cancer cells with PARP inhibition undergo synthetically lethal cell death [34]. PARP inhibitor, Olaparib manufactured by AstraZeneca, is in phase I/II clinical trials for BRCA-deficient high-grade serous ovarian cancer [34]. Olaparib-treated ovarian cancer patients with BRCA1/2 mutation had a progression-free survival of 11.2 months compared to 4.3 months of patients receiving placebo [35]. In summary, BRCA is an ideal example of E3 ubiquitin ligase playing an essential role in ovarian cancer and its intervention.

2.1.2. Cullin-RING ligases: cullin 4

Cullin-RING ubiquitin ligases (CRLs), composed of CUL1, 2, 3, 4A, 4B, 5, and 7, are the largest family of E3s that ubiquitinate a wide array of substrates involved in cell-cycle, DNA-damage response, chromatin remodeling, and gene expression. Cullin (CUL) neddylation, a process of adding ubiquitin-like protein—NEDD8 to the cullin [36], is crucial for their activation. Neddylation is catalyzed by NEDD8-activating enzyme E1 (NAE), NEDD8-conjugating enzyme E2 (UBC12), and NEDD8-E3 ligase. The genome-wide analysis of human cancers revealed *CUL4A* amplification in 20% of the basal-like breast cancer subtype, characterized as "triple negative," and CUL4A levels were associated with aggressive growth and poor prognosis. Dysregulation of CUL4A in multiple tumor types leads to the hypothesis that CUL4A plays a role in promoting oncogenesis [36]. High CUL4A expression and activity in ovarian cancer is implicated with cancer cell proliferation and survival. NEDD8-activating enzyme inhibitor, MLN4924, which blocks cullin neddylation activation, is reported to induce cell-cycle arrest, apoptosis, and tumor cell growth in epithelial ovarian cancer cells. In addition, MLN4924 sensitized ovarian cancer cells to chemotherapeutic drug treatments [37].

The role of Skp2 and FBXW7 in ovarian cancer signaling is discussed in the next section.

2.2. Deubiquitinating enzymes

Reversibility is an important aspect of ubiquitin system, which is mediated by deubiquitinating enzymes or deubiquitinases (DUBs). DUBs are essential components of UPS that possess ubiquitin-isopeptidase activity and catalyze the removal of ubiquitin from the target proteins. Thus, DUBs play a crucial role in the regulation of ubiquitin-mediated regulatory and proteolytic signaling [11, 38]. DUBs activity affect the activation, recycling, localization, and turnover of multiple proteins, which in turn regulate cellular homeostasis, protein stability, and a wide range of signaling pathways [39]. DUBs also maintain ubiquitin homeostasis in the cell by generating free ubiquitin monomers, which is essential for ubiquitin-mediated regulation of cell function [38]. Consistent with this, an altered DUB expression or activity has been implicated with several diseases including cancer. Numerous DUBs have been characterized as oncogenes mediating cancer initiation and progression [11, 40]. Therefore, pharmacological interventions targeting DUB activity using small molecule inhibitors are being used as a rationale to search for novel anticancer drugs [11].

Box 2. About 98 DUBs are reported in human genome, which are mainly divided into five families based on their sequence and structural homology: Ubiquitin-specific protease (USP), ubiquitin carboxyl-terminal hydrolases (UCHs), ovarian tumor proteases (OTUs), Machado Joseph disease proteases (MJD), and JAB1/MPN/Mov34 (JAMM) metallopeptidases. Most DUBs are cysteine proteases except JAMMs, which belong to catalytic class of metalloproteases. The recent discovery of DUBs with the selectivity of cleaving extended Lys-48-linked polyubiquitin chains belongs to new family of DUBs named Mindy. The DUB-substrate specificity somewhat depends on ubiquitin chain linkage and topology; however, by large, given the complexity of ubiquitin system, it remains unknown [38].

DUBs role is evident in several cancers including Fanconi anemia (USP1), prostate cancer (USP2), adenocarcinoma (USP4), non-small-cell lung carcinoma (USP7), glioblastoma (USP15), myeloma, and leukemia (USP9x) [11, 39]. Han et al. identified the role of USP13 as the master regulator of ovarian cancer metabolism [41]. They reported the co-amplification of USP13 gene with PIK3CA (phosphatidylinositol-3-kinase catalytic subunit, α-isoform) in 29.3% of high-grade serous ovarian cancer patients and its association with poor clinical outcome. USP13 stabilized the protein levels of two key metabolic enzymes, ATP citrate lyase and oxoglutarate dehydrogenase, which in turn regulate the mitochondrial respiration, glutaminolysis, and fatty acid synthesis in ovarian cancer cells. USP13 inhibition suppressed ovarian tumor progression and sensitized the tumor cells to PI3K/AKT inhibitor [41]. Similarly, USP7 (also known as HAUSP, herpes virus-associated ubiquitin protease) plays a crucial role in ovarian cancer [42]. USP7 is a DUB for MDM2, which prevents MDM2 autoubiquitination, leading to its stabilization and consequent induction of p53 degradation. Treating an ovarian cancer xenograft model with a novel inhibitor of USP7, CDDO-Me suppressed tumor growth. CDDO-Me directly binds to USP7, which leads to a decrease in its substrate Mdm2, Mdmx protein levels [42]. USP4 overexpression is reported in invasive breast carcinoma, enhancing TGFβ signaling by stabilizing SMAD2/SMAD4 complex but not much is known about its role in ovarian cancer [11]. USP36 expression is increased in ovarian cancer cells compared to normal ovarian surface epithelium; however, further studies are needed to understand its role in ovarian cancer [43]. DUB UCHL1 (ubiquitin-carboxyl terminal hydrolase 1) plays a contradicting role in different cancers [11]; it is reported as a methylated tumor suppressor gene in ovarian cancer [44, 45], while it is overexpressed in lymphoma, esophageal squamous cell carcinoma, renal, lung cancers, and acts as an oncogene [46–48]. Under hypoxic conditions, UCHL1 is shown to deubiquitinate and stabilize HIF-1α and promote tumor metastasis [49, 50]. We for the first time identified the oncogenic overexpression of UCHL1 in high-grade serous ovarian cancer and association with poor clinical outcome (unpublished data). These studies suggest the emerging role of DUBs in ovarian cancer and the potential of DUB inhibitors in neo-adjuvant therapies for ovarian cancer.

2.3. Proteasomes

The efficient and selective degradation of cellular proteins is essential for protein quality control and maintenance of cellular homeostasis [51]. Impaired protein quality control and degradation is associated with many human diseases such as cancer, cardiovascular diseases, and aging-related pathophysiological conditions such as Alzheimer's and Parkinson's. UPS mediates targeted protein degradation under both normal and malignant conditions [52]. However, cancer cells are more dependent on UPS-mediated degradation to promote the degradation of tumor suppressors and various cell-cycle checkpoint proteins as well as to reduce proteotoxic stress accumulated due to genomic aberrations [53]. The 26S proteasome is a multi-subunit complex that contains one barrel-shaped 20S catalytic core particle (CP) and 19S regulatory particle (RP) that binds to one or both the ends of barrel-shaped CP. The active degradation of proteins is regulated by 20S CP harboring proteolytic active sites while 19S RP regulates substrate binding and target protein entry into 20S [52].

The amazing efficacy and clinical use of proteasome inhibitor Bortezomib (PS-341, Velcade) for the treatment of multiple myeloma and mantle cell lymphoma has encouraged researchers to explore the possibility of targeting other components of the UPS for cancer treatment [54]. However, Bortezomib has not demonstrated a significant activity against other solid tumors [55]. This conundrum has spurred the development of next-generation proteasome inhibitors, including MLN9708 (Millennium Pharmaceuticals), Carfilzomib and ONX0912 (Onyx Pharmaceuticals, South San Francisco, CA), and CEP18770 (Cephalon, Frazer, PA) [56]. Although these compounds target the same 20S CP, they differ in targeted active site and enzyme kinetics, resulting in activity differences based on tumor type and tumor location. Bazzaro et al. reported elevated levels of ubiquitinated proteins and 19S and 20S proteasome subunits in both low-grade and high-grade ovarian carcinoma tissues and cell lines compared to benign ovarian tumors and immortalized normal ovarian surface epithelium controls. They reported an increased sensitivity to apoptosis in proteasome inhibitor, PS-341 treated cells, and a reduced growth of ES-2 ovarian carcinoma xenograft in immunodeficient mice [57]. In a similar study, proteasome inhibitor, MG132—a peptide aldehyde—showed an enhanced sensitivity of ovarian cancer cells, SKOV3 to cisplatin both *in vitro* and *in vivo* [58]. The effect of Bortezomib on ovarian cancer cells is also supported by the increased sensitivity of Bortezomib-treated chemoresistant ovarian cancer cells to TRAIL-induced apoptosis [59]. Together, these results indicate the essential role of proteasomes in mediating prosurvival signaling in cancer, which may also be due to altered proteasome composition resulting in an enhanced proteasomal activity [52].

3. UPS in ovarian cancer cellular signaling

Several important factors that are implicated in the molecular pathogenesis of ovarian cancer are known to be regulated by UPS, highlighting its significance in disease progression. Some of these factors are discussed subsequently.

3.1. Tumor suppressor p53 and Mdm2

Tumor suppressor protein p53 is a multifunctional sequence-specific transcription factor that plays a key role in cellular stress response. Abrogating p53 function is a key event in human cancers, leading to the deregulation of cell cycle, genetic instability, resistance to stress signals, and resulting in cancer development [60]. Due to its growth inhibitory properties, p53 is maintained at low levels in the normal cells. The E3 ubiquitin ligase Mdm2 promotes p53 ubiquitination and subsequent proteasomal degradation [61]. In addition, E4 ubiquitin ligase p300/CBP promotes polyubiquitination of p53 to accelerate its degradation by proteasomes [61]. Although Mdm2 is the predominant E3 ligase for p53, several other E3 ligases have been identified that can promote the degradation of p53, including C-terminus of HSP70-interacting protein (CHIP), murine double minute 4 (MdmX), and p53-induced protein with a RING H2 domain (Pirh2) [60]. In addition to proteolytic ubiquitination, p53 mono-ubiquitination mediates p53 nuclear export and activity [62]. Thus, UPS plays a crucial role in maintaining and regulating p53 functions.

Several cancers, including invasive breast cancer, pediatric rhabdomyosarcoma, and soft-tissue sarcoma, exploit Mdm2-p53 pathway to maintain low p53 levels under genotoxic or oxidative-stressed environment of cancer cell. Thus, Mdm2 gene amplification and overexpression have been reported in many cancers [63]. In addition, the expression and activity of Usp7, a deubiquitinating enzyme for Mdm2, is increased in several cancers including breast and ovarian cancer, which prevents Mdm2 ubiquitination and promotes its stability. Reduced tumor growth was seen in an ovarian cancer xenograft model treated with Usp7 inhibitor [42]. On the other hand, when p53 acquires gain-of-function (GOF) mutations as in the case of nearly half of the cancers, it gains oncogenic functions and loses its wild-type tumor suppressor properties. Thus, in these cancer cells, several mechanisms stabilize mutant p53 through its activation or by inhibition of its degradation by disrupting Mdm2 and mutant p53 binding. Several splice variants of Mdm2 are reported in cancer, which lack a p53-binding domain and thus stabilizes mutant p53 expression [63]. In addition, GOF mutation-induced conformational changes in mutant p53 allow the binding of Hsp90 (heat shock protein 90) to mutant p53, which prevents Mdm2 binding and Mdm2-mediated degradation of mutant p53 [60]. It is now well established that elevated mutant p53 levels correlate with more aggressive tumors and poor prognosis. About 96% of high-grade serous ovarian cancer patients have GOF p53 mutations, which orchestrate a distinct pro-tumorigenic transcription and oncogenic programs. Knowledge of a UPS component responsible for mutant p53 stabilization, which could be chemically manipulated, will be useful in HGSOC. Nonetheless, Mdm2 is a great therapeutic target and prognostic factor for ovarian cancer with wild-type p53, such as clear-cell carcinomas [64].

3.2. Cyclin E

Genomic alterations in cell-cycle regulatory genes have been reported in almost every human carcinoma. Cyclins are the crucial regulators of cell-cycle progression [65]. A periodic increase in cyclin levels and their timed interplay with cyclin-dependent kinases (CDKs) is essential for the proper progression of cell cycle [65]. Their levels are regulated by a combination of transcription and ubiquitin-mediated degradation [18, 66]. About 30% of high-grade serous ovarian cancer patients have amplification of the CCNE1 gene, which encodes for G1/S-specific cyclin E. Cyclin E-CDK2 interactions commit the cell to S-phase genome duplication [3]. Aberrant accumulation and overabundance of cyclin E leads to premature entry of the cell into S-phase, resulting in chromosome instability and tumor formation [67]. Cyclin E amplification is likely to be an early event in the development of high-grade serous ovarian cancer [3]. This subclass of patients has no apparent defect in homologous recombination as seen in patients with BRCA1 and BRCA2 mutations with defect in DNA repair pathways [3]. The overexpression of cyclin E is an indicator of poor overall survival of ovarian cancer patients. Cyclin E protein levels are maintained by a multi-subunit SCF ubiquitin ligase, which mediates its ubiquitination and degradation [68]. Cyclin E auto-phosphorylation after its association with CDK2 is recognized by the SCF-associated F-box protein 7 (FBXW7), which binds to cyclin E and facilitates its ubiquitination and degradation [68, 69]. More than 30% of human cancers have a deleted FBXW7 gene located on chromosome 4q32. FBXW7 also regulates mTOR, Myc, and Notch1 degradation, depending upon the type of tumor [70, 71]. FBXW7 is known to be mutated in breast and ovarian cancer cell lines with high cyclin E levels [3]. The loss of cyclin E or CDK2 results in cell-cycle arrest or apoptosis in HGSOC cell lines [3], suggesting cyclin E inhibition as a novel therapeutic approach in ovarian cancer patients.

3.3. P27, a cyclin-dependent kinase inhibitor

Similar to cell-cycle regulatory proteins, cell-cycle inhibitors are frequently altered in cancer [72, 73]. p27^{Kip1} inhibits cell-cycle G1 phase by interacting with CDK2/cyclin A or CDK2/cyclin E complexes [73, 74]. Low levels of p27^{Kip1} protein are associated with tumor progression and growth resulting in poor prognosis of ovarian and breast cancer patients [74–76]. The evaluation of subcellular localization of p27^{Kip1} in tissue microarray of late-stage ovarian cancer patients revealed that patients with nuclear-only expression of p27^{Kip1} had a better overall survival than those with negative expression or cytoplasmic localization of the marker (p-value = 0.0002; n = 355) [77]. p27^{Kip1} level is an important prognostic marker of malignant transformation. Genetically altered mice with p27^{Kip1} haploinsufficiency are predisposed to cancer [78]. p27^{Kip1} protein levels are regulated by SCF E3 ligase-associated protein Skp2. Skp2 binds to p27^{Kip1} and mediates its ubiquitination and subsequent proteasomal degradation [79, 80]. Skp2 levels in different cancers correlate with tumor grade and inversely correlate with p27^{Kip1} levels and cancer prognosis. Skp2 levels were upregulated in ovarian cancer patients and were associated with advanced FIGO stage III and IV and high grade of the tumor [81]. Skp2 levels were also associated with downregulation of both p27 and p21 in these patients, suggesting an important role of Skp2- p27^{Kip1} pathway in ovarian cancer pathogenesis. A strong negative correlation between Skp2 levels and FOXO3a (r = −0.743; p < 0.05) in immunohistochemical analysis of ovarian cancer patients indicates that it is another potential target of Skp2 in ovarian cancer [82]. These findings and Skp2 overexpression or amplification in serous ovarian cancer characterize it as an oncogene and its inhibition a plausible approach in ovarian cancer management.

3.4. The epidermal growth factor receptor (also known as HER or ERBB) family

The EGFR family of receptor tyrosine kinases plays an important role in the pathogenesis of several cancers [83]. The four members: EGFR, HER2, HER3, and HER4 (or ERBB1–4), of EGFR family structurally consist of an extracellular ligand-binding domain, a single transmembrane-spanning region, and an intracellular tyrosine kinase domain. More than 30 ligands have been identified that bind to the EGFR family receptors, including EGF- and EGF-like ligands, transforming growth factor (TGF)-α, and heregulins (HRGs) [83]. The activated EGFR receptors undergo C-terminal phosphorylation of cytoplasmic tyrosine residues after receptor dimerization to mediate cell regulatory signaling. E3 ubiquitin ligase CBL binds to EGFR receptor at specific phosphotyrosine residues and mediates its ubiquitination subsequent internalization in clatherin-coated endosomes, which then lead to lysosome-mediated degradation of EGFR [84].

Amplifications and overexpression of various EGFR family members, including EGFR, Her2, and ErbB3, have been reported in epithelial ovarian cancer. Attenuated ubiquitination and HER2 gene amplification favor the formation of EGFR/HER2 heterodimers that recruit CBL to a lesser degree, thus stabilizing and recycling the receptor to cell surface [85]. BRCA1 mutations are known to be associated with an increased EGFR expression in serous ovarian cancer patients. EGFR expression was not only increased in BRCA1 mutated cancer tissues but was also high in BRCA1-mutated normal tissues compared to respective control tissues. These results were confirmed by knocking down BRCA1 in ovarian cancer cells [86]. However, inhibitors targeting this pathway have little effect on cancer cells as a single agent due to the presence of alternative pathways affecting the cancer phenotype, particularly the activation of the PI3K/Akt/mTOR and mitogen-activated protein kinases (MAPKs) pathway [83], suggesting a combined use of EGFR and PI3K inhibitors in ovarian cancer [87].

4. Concluding remarks

It is now well known that UPS not only mediates protein degradation but is also involved in the extensive regulation of cellular functions and signaling. A large number of studies in various cancers have uncovered the diverse and intricate role of ubiquitin in oncogenic signaling. The alterations in the genes involved in UPS support its role in cancer development and progression. However, the lack of information on DUBs specificity and multiple targets of E3s raise a question on the use of DUBs or E3s inhibitors in cancer treatment. One possible way forward is to characterize the cancer-specific and tissue-specific expression of DUBs as certain DUBs are predominantly expressed in certain tissues and cancer, suggesting the cancer-specific use of a DUB inhibitor. Moreover, most DUBs studied thus far appear to regulate a small number of targets. It is also possible that only a fraction of ubiquitinated proteins are regulated by a specific DUB family. Similarly, the E3s can be manipulated in cancer if their role is characterized in cancer-specific aberrant molecular signaling. Moreover, further characterization of mutations in DUBs or E3s in cancer patients can be used for cancer screening. In addition, proteasomes carry a great potential in cancer treatment. Although Bortezomib did not show promising results against solid tumors, the advent of next-generation proteasome inhibitors opens new possibilities. Currently, five different types of next-generation proteasome inhibitors are in phase I or phase IIb clinical trials. Moreover, understanding the regulation of proteasomal activity by altered proteasome composition may open novel ways to target proteasomes in cancer.

Compared to breast cancer, ovarian cancer is a rare but far more lethal cancer. It is estimated that 69% of all patients with ovarian carcinoma will succumb to their disease as compared with 19% of those with breast cancer [1]. Ovarian cancer heterogeneity is represented by several genetic (BRCA1/2), epigenetic, and signaling (p53, CDK/p27, CCNE1) alterations, and various UPS components are implicated in these ovarian cancer-specific alterations. Several studies have established a link between UPS and ovarian cancer. However, further studies are needed to identify potential inhibitors for proteasome-based or E3s/DUBs-based therapies in ovarian cancer, which can be taken to clinical trials.

Acknowledgements

The author acknowledges the support of the Indiana University School of Medicine, Biomedical Research Grant, Showalter Research Grant, and Ovarian Cancer Research Fund Alliance.

Abbreviations

CUL4A	Cullin 4A gene
DUBs	deubiquitinating enzymes
E1	E1 ubiquitin-activating enzyme
E2	E2 ubiquitin-conjugating enzymes
E3	ubiquitin E3 ligases
EGFR	epidermal growth factor receptor
GOF	gain-of-function
HER2	human epidermal growth factor receptor 2
HGSOC	high-grade serous ovarian cance.
K	lysine
Lys	lysine
Mdm2	murine double minute 2
OSE	ovarian surface epithelium
PTM	posttranslational modification
STIC	serous tubal intraepithelial carcinoma

Author details

Sumegha Mitra[1,2]*

*Address all correspondence to: mitras@indiana.edu

1 Department of Obstetrics and Gynecology, Indiana University School of Medicine, Indianapolis, IN, USA

2 Indiana University Melvin and Bren Simon Cancer Center, Indianapolis, IN, USA

References

[1] Lengyel E. Ovarian cancer development and metastasis. The American Journal of Pathology. 2010;**177**(3):1053-1064

[2] Siegel RL, Miller KD, Jemal A. Cancer statistics, 2017. CA: A Cancer Journal for Clinicians. 2017;**67**(1):7-30

[3] Bowtell DD et al. Rethinking ovarian cancer II: Reducing mortality from high-grade serous ovarian cancer. Nature Reviews. Cancer. 2015;**15**(11):668-679

[4] Bast Jr RC, Hennessy B, Mills GB. The biology of ovarian cancer: New opportunities for translation. Nature Reviews. Cancer. 2009;**9**(6):415-428

[5] Cho KR, ShihIe M. Ovarian cancer. Annual Review of Pathology. 2009;**4**:287-313

[6] Cancer Genome Atlas Research Network. Integrated genomic analyses of ovarian carcinoma. Nature. 2011;**474**(7353):609-615

[7] Perets R, Drapkin R. It's totally tubular....riding the new wave of ovarian cancer research. Cancer Research. 2016;**76**(1):10-17

[8] Eddie SL et al. Tumorigenesis and peritoneal colonization from fallopian tube epithelium. Oncotarget. 2015;**6**(24):20500-20512

[9] Kauff ND et al. Risk-reducing salpingo-oophorectomy for the prevention of BRCA1- and BRCA2-associated breast and gynecologic cancer: A multicenter, prospective study. Journal of Clinical Oncology. 2008;**26**(8):1331-1337

[10] Walerych D et al. Proteasome machinery is instrumental in a common gain-of-function program of the p53 missense mutants in cancer. Nature Cell Biology. 2016;**18**(8):897-909

[11] Gallo LH, Ko J, Donoghue DJ. The importance of regulatory ubiquitination in cancer and metastasis. Cell Cycle. 2017;**16**(7):634-648

[12] Pickart CM. Mechanisms underlying ubiquitination. Annual Review of Biochemistry. 2001;**70**:503-533

[13] Swatek KN, Komander D. Ubiquitin modifications. Cell Research. 2016;**26**(4):399-422

[14] Wu-Baer F et al. The BRCA1/BARD1 heterodimer assembles polyubiquitin chains through an unconventional linkage involving lysine residue K6 of ubiquitin. The Journal of Biological Chemistry. 2003;**278**(37):34743-34746

[15] Metzger MB, Hristova VA, Weissman AM. HECT and RING finger families of E3 ubiquitin ligases at a glance. Journal of Cell Science. 2012;**125**(Pt 3):531-537

[16] Kirkin V, Dikic I. Ubiquitin networks in cancer. Current Opinion in Genetics & Development. 2011;**21**(1):21-28

[17] Wu W et al. The ubiquitin E3 ligase activity of BRCA1 and its biological functions. Cell Division. 2008;**3**:1

[18] Mani A, Gelmann EP. The ubiquitin-proteasome pathway and its role in cancer. Journal of Clinical Oncology. 2005;**23**(21):4776-4789

[19] Weberpals JI, Clark-Knowles KV, Vanderhyden BC. Sporadic epithelial ovarian cancer: Clinical relevance of BRCA1 inhibition in the DNA damage and repair pathway. Journal of Clinical Oncology. 2008;**26**(19):3259-3267

[20] Friedenson B. BRCA1 and BRCA2 pathways and the risk of cancers other than breast or ovarian. MedGenMed. 2005;**7**(2):60

[21] Nishikawa H et al. Mass spectrometric and mutational analyses reveal Lys-6-linked polyubiquitin chains catalyzed by BRCA1-BARD1 ubiquitin ligase. The Journal of Biological Chemistry. 2004;**279**(6):3916-3924

[22] Brzovic PS et al. Binding and recognition in the assembly of an active BRCA1/BARD1 ubiquitin-ligase complex. Proceedings of the National Academy of Sciences of the United States of America. 2003;**100**(10):5646-5651

[23] Manke IA et al. BRCT repeats as phosphopeptide-binding modules involved in protein targeting. Science. 2003;**302**(5645):636-639

[24] Yu X et al. BRCA1 ubiquitinates its phosphorylation-dependent binding partner CtIP. Genes & Development. 2006;**20**(13):1721-1726

[25] Brzovic PS et al. BRCA1 RING domain cancer-predisposing mutations. Structural consequences and effects on protein-protein interactions. The Journal of Biological Chemistry. 2001;**276**(44):41399-41406

[26] Wu J, Lu LY, Yu X. The role of BRCA1 in DNA damage response. Protein & Cell. 2010;**1**(2):117-123

[27] Burma S et al. ATM phosphorylates histone H2AX in response to DNA double-strand breaks. The Journal of Biological Chemistry. 2001;**276**(45):42462-42467

[28] Stucki M et al. MDC1 directly binds phosphorylated histone H2AX to regulate cellular responses to DNA double-strand breaks. Cell. 2005;**123**(7):1213-1226

[29] Wu J et al. Histone ubiquitination associates with BRCA1-dependent DNA damage response. Molecular and Cellular Biology. 2009;**29**(3):849-860

[30] Yoshida K, Miki Y. Role of BRCA1 and BRCA2 as regulators of DNA repair, transcription, and cell cycle in response to DNA damage. Cancer Science. 2004;**95**(11):866-871

[31] Nadeau G et al. BRCA1 can stimulate gene transcription by a unique mechanism. EMBO Reports. 2000;**1**(3):260-265

[32] MacLachlan TK, Takimoto R, El-Deiry WS. BRCA1 directs a selective p53-dependent transcriptional response towards growth arrest and DNA repair targets. Molecular and Cellular Biology. 2002;**22**(12):4280-4292

[33] Deng CX. BRCA1: Cell cycle checkpoint, genetic instability, DNA damage response and cancer evolution. Nucleic Acids Research. 2006;**34**(5):1416-1426

[34] Walsh CS. Two decades beyond BRCA1/2: Homologous recombination, hereditary cancer risk and a target for ovarian cancer therapy. Gynecologic Oncology. 2015;**137**(2):343-350

[35] Ledermann J et al. Olaparib maintenance therapy in patients with platinum-sensitive relapsed serous ovarian cancer: A preplanned retrospective analysis of outcomes by BRCA status in a randomised phase 2 trial. The Lancet Oncology. 2014;**15**(8):852-861

[36] Lee J, Zhou P. Cullins and cancer. Genes & Cancer. 2010;**1**(7):690-699

[37] Pan WW et al. Ubiquitin E3 ligase CRL4(CDT2/DCAF2) as a potential chemotherapeutic target for ovarian surface epithelial cancer. The Journal of Biological Chemistry. 2013;**288**(41):29680-29691

[38] Fraile JM et al. Deubiquitinases in cancer: New functions and therapeutic options. Oncogene. 2012;**31**(19):2373-2388

[39] D'Arcy P, Linder S. Molecular pathways: Translational potential of deubiquitinases as drug targets. Clinical Cancer Research. 2014;**20**(15):3908-3914

[40] Luise C et al. An atlas of altered expression of deubiquitinating enzymes in human cancer. PLoS One. 2011;**6**(1):e15891

[41] Han C et al. Amplification of USP13 drives ovarian cancer metabolism. Nature Communications. 2016;**7**:13525

[42] Qin D et al. CDDO-Me reveals USP7 as a novel target in ovarian cancer cells. Oncotarget. 2016;**7**(47):77096-77109

[43] Li J et al. Differential display identifies overexpression of the USP36 gene, encoding a deubiquitinating enzyme, in ovarian cancer. International Journal of Medical Sciences. 2008;**5**(3):133-142

[44] Brait M et al. Association of promoter methylation of VGF and PGP9.5 with ovarian cancer progression. PLoS One. 2013;**8**(9):e70878

[45] Okochi-Takada E et al. Silencing of the UCHL1 gene in human colorectal and ovarian cancers. International Journal of Cancer. 2006;**119**(6):1338-1344

[46] Hussain S et al. The de-ubiquitinase UCH-L1 is an oncogene that drives the development of lymphoma in vivo by deregulating PHLPP1 and Akt signaling. Leukemia. 2010;**24**(9):1641-1655

[47] Kim HJ et al. Ubiquitin C-terminal hydrolase-L1 is a key regulator of tumor cell invasion and metastasis. Oncogene. 2009;**28**(1):117-127

[48] Takase T et al. PGP9.5 overexpression in esophageal squamous cell carcinoma. Hepato-Gastroenterology. 2003;**50**(53):1278-1280

[49] Rankin EB, Giaccia AJ. Hypoxic control of metastasis. Science. 2016;**352**(6282):175-180

[50] Goto Y et al. UCHL1 provides diagnostic and antimetastatic strategies due to its deubiquitinating effect on HIF-1alpha. Nature Communications. 2015;**6**:6153

[51] Lecker SH, Goldberg AL, Mitch WE. Protein degradation by the ubiquitin-proteasome pathway in normal and disease states. Journal of the American Society of Nephrology. 2006;**17**(7):1807-1819

[52] Padmanabhan A, Vuong SA, Hochstrasser M. Assembly of an evolutionarily conserved alternative proteasome isoform in human cells. Cell Reports. 2016;**14**(12):2962-2974

[53] Deshaies RJ. Proteotoxic crisis, the ubiquitin-proteasome system, and cancer therapy. BMC Biology. 2014;**12**:94

[54] Eldridge AG, O'Brien T. Therapeutic strategies within the ubiquitin proteasome system. Cell Death and Differentiation. 2010;**17**(1):4-13

[55] Sterz J et al. The potential of proteasome inhibitors in cancer therapy. Expert Opinion on Investigational Drugs. 2008;**17**(6):879-895

[56] Micel LN et al. Role of ubiquitin ligases and the proteasome in oncogenesis: Novel targets for anticancer therapies. Journal of Clinical Oncology. 2013;**31**(9):1231-1238

[57] Bazzaro M et al. Ubiquitin-proteasome system stress sensitizes ovarian cancer to proteasome inhibitor-induced apoptosis. Cancer Research. 2006;**66**(7):3754-3763

[58] Guo N, Peng Z, Zhang J. Proteasome inhibitor MG132 enhances sensitivity to cisplatin on ovarian carcinoma cells in vitro and in vivo. International Journal of Gynecological Cancer. 2016;**26**(5):839-844

[59] Saulle E et al. Proteasome inhibitors sensitize ovarian cancer cells to TRAIL induced apoptosis. Apoptosis. 2007;**12**(4):635-655

[60] Vijayakumaran R et al. Regulation of mutant p53 protein expression. Frontiers in Oncology. 2015;**5**:284

[61] Brooks CL, Gu W. p53 Regulation by ubiquitin. FEBS Letters. 2011;**585**(18):2803-2809

[62] Brooks CL, Li M, Gu W. Monoubiquitination: The signal for p53 nuclear export? Cell Cycle. 2004;**3**(4):436-438

[63] Zhao Y, Yu H, Hu W. The regulation of MDM2 oncogene and its impact on human cancers. Acta Biochimica et Biophysica Sinica (Shanghai). 2014;**46**(3):180-189

[64] Makii C et al. MDM2 is a potential therapeutic target and prognostic factor for ovarian clear cell carcinomas with wild type TP53. Oncotarget. 2016;**7**(46):75328-75338

[65] John PC, Mews M, Moore R. Cyclin/Cdk complexes: Their involvement in cell cycle progression and mitotic division. Protoplasma. 2001;**216**(3-4):119-142

[66] Udvardy A. The role of controlled proteolysis in cell-cycle regulation. European Journal of Biochemistry. 1996;**240**(2):307-313

[67] Spruck CH, Won KA, Reed SI. Deregulated cyclin E induces chromosome instability. Nature. 1999;**401**(6750):297-300

[68] Clurman BE et al. Turnover of cyclin E by the ubiquitin-proteasome pathway is regulated by cdk2 binding and cyclin phosphorylation. Genes & Development. 1996;**10**(16):1979-1990

[69] Won KA, Reed SI. Activation of cyclin E/CDK2 is coupled to site-specific autophosphorylation and ubiquitin-dependent degradation of cyclin E. The EMBO Journal. 1996;**15**(16):4182-4193

[70] Knuutila S et al. DNA copy number losses in human neoplasms. The American Journal of Pathology. 1999;**155**(3):683-694

[71] Wang Z et al. Tumor suppressor functions of FBW7 in cancer development and progression. FEBS Letters. 2012;**586**(10):1409-1418

[72] Chu IM, Hengst L, Slingerland JM. The Cdk inhibitor p27 in human cancer: Prognostic potential and relevance to anticancer therapy. Nature Reviews. Cancer. 2008;**8**(4):253-267

[73] Moller MB. P27 in cell cycle control and cancer. Leukemia & Lymphoma. 2000;**39**(1-2):19-27

[74] Zafonte BT et al. Cell-cycle dysregulation in breast cancer: Breast cancer therapies targeting the cell cycle. Frontiers in Bioscience. 2000;**5**:D938-D961

[75] Lu M et al. The prognostic of p27(kip1) in ovarian cancer: A meta-analysis. Archives of Gynecology and Obstetrics. 2016;**293**(1):169-176

[76] Hafez MM et al. SKP2/P27Kip1 pathway is associated with advanced ovarian cancer in Saudi patients. Asian Pacific Journal of Cancer Prevention. 2015;**16**(14):5807-5815

[77] Rosen DG et al. Subcellular localization of p27kip1 expression predicts poor prognosis in human ovarian cancer. Clinical Cancer Research. 2005;**11**(2 Pt 1):632-637

[78] Fero ML et al. The murine gene p27Kip1 is haplo-insufficient for tumour suppression. Nature. 1998;**396**(6707):177-180

[79] Carrano AC et al. SKP2 is required for ubiquitin-mediated degradation of the CDK inhibitor p27. Nature Cell Biology. 1999;**1**(4):193-199

[80] Montagnoli A et al. Ubiquitination of p27 is regulated by Cdk-dependent phosphorylation and trimeric complex formation. Genes & Development. 1999;**13**(9):1181-1189

[81] Shigemasa K et al. Skp2 overexpression is a prognostic factor in patients with ovarian adenocarcinoma. Clinical Cancer Research. 2003;**9**(5):1756-1763

[82] Lu M et al. The expression and prognosis of FOXO3a and Skp2 in human ovarian cancer. Medical Oncology. 2012;**29**(5):3409-3415

[83] Siwak DR et al. Targeting the epidermal growth factor receptor in epithelial ovarian cancer: Current knowledge and future challenges. Journal of Oncology. 2010;**2010**:568938

[84] Levkowitz G et al. c-Cbl/Sli-1 regulates endocytic sorting and ubiquitination of the epidermal growth factor receptor. Genes & Development. 1998;**12**(23):3663-3674

[85] Muthuswamy SK, Gilman M, Brugge JS. Controlled dimerization of ErbB receptors provides evidence for differential signaling by homo- and heterodimers. Molecular and Cellular Biology. 1999;**19**(10):6845-6857

[86] Li D et al. Effect of BRCA1 on epidermal growth factor receptor in ovarian cancer. Journal of Experimental & Clinical Cancer Research. 2013;**32**:102

[87] Glaysher S et al. Targeting EGFR and PI3K pathways in ovarian cancer. British Journal of Cancer. 2013;**109**(7):1786-1794

[88] Goldstein G, Scheid MS, Hammerling V, Boyse EA, Schlesinger DH, Niall HD. Isolation of a polypeptide that has lymphocyte-differentiating properties and is probably represented universally in living cells. Proceedings of the National Academy of Sciences USA. 1975;**72**:11-15

[89] Goldknopf IL, Busch H. Isopeptide linkage between nonhistone and histone 2A polypeptides of chromosomal conjugate-protein A24. Proceedings of the National Academy of Sciences USA. 1977;**74**:864-868

[90] Hershko A, Ciechanover A, Heller H, Haas AL, Rose IA. Proposed role of ATP in protein breakdown: Conjugation of proteins with multiple chains of the polypeptide of ATP-dependent proteolysis. Proceedings of the National Academy of Sciences USA. 1980;**77**:1783-1786

9

Signaling Pathways Related to Nerve Growth Factor and miRNAs in Epithelial Ovarian Cancer

Carolina Vera, Rocío Retamales-Ortega,
Maritza Garrido, Margarita Vega and
Carmen Romero

Abstract

Epithelial ovarian cancer (EOC) is a disease that causes 140,000 deaths every year. Nerve growth factor (NGF) and its high affinity receptor TRKA play important roles in follicular maturation, follicle-stimulating hormone (FSH) receptor acquisition and ovulation in normal ovary. Also, NGF has many roles in EOC cells: increasing survival, proliferation, cyclooxigenase-2 (COX-2), vascular endothelial growth factor (VEGF) and metalloproteinase ADAM17 expression. Besides, NGF inhibits calreticulin translocation from the endoplasmic reticulum to cell surface, possibly diminishing the efficacy of immunogenic therapies in EOC. Additionally, NGF acts as an angiogenic factor by a direct stimulation of migration, differentiation and proliferation of endothelial cells. Among the numerous factors actually described to be important in many types of cancer, including EOC, are the microRNAs (miRs). Indeed, it has been found that miR-143 is downregulate in EOC, which correlates with an increase of COX-2; concomitantly, NGF increases COX-2 as mentioned. Furthermore, NGF increases miR-222 and its target is the metalloproteinase inhibitor TIMP3, increasing the ADAM17 function. Also, NGF increases cMYC transcription factor in EOC, which decreases miR-23 levels regulating proteins involved in cell cycle and tumor growth. Therefore, NGF/TRKA signaling pathways alter the expression of many proteins and deregulate miRs in EOC, leading to the progression of this cancer.

Keywords: epithelial ovarian cancer, nerve growth factor, vascular endothelial growth factor, ciclooxigenasa-2, prostaglandin-E2, calreticulin, c-MYC, DAM17, microRNAs

1. Introduction

Ovarian cancer is a deadly disease that causes around 225,000 new cases and 140,000 deaths every year, remaining a major health problem worldwide [1]. Moreover, epithelial ovarian cancer (EOC) is more common in elderly women who are no longer experiencing reproductive cycles [1]. This cancer is characterized by the non-specificity of its symptoms and the lack of efficacy for therapies at advanced stages. Therefore, EOC is diagnosed at late stages and has a low overall 5-year survival below 45% [2].

A key process for EOC growth and metastasis is angiogenesis, the formation of new blood vessels from pre-existing vasculature. It is a complex process regulated by the balance between pro- and anti-angiogenic factors [3]. In the normal reproductive ovary, angiogenesis is a physiological process that occurs during every cycle in a controlled manner [4]. In cancer, pro-angiogenic factors are overexpressed and angiogenic regulation is lost. Among these factors, neurotrophins have an important role in controlling angiogenesis in the normal and neoplastic ovary, being also implicated in the regulation of other physiological and pathological processes [5]. The roles of neurotrophins in the normal ovary and in EOC are discussed in the next sections.

2. Roles of nerve growth factor in the normal ovary and in epithelial ovarian cancer

Neurotrophins are small polypeptides that were first discovered as a growth factor on the nervous system, subsequently named nerve growth factor (NGF) [6]. Besides NGF, there are four other neurotrophins: brain-derived neurotrophic factor (BDNF), neurotrophin 3 (NT-3), neurotrophin 4/5 (NT-4/5) and neurotrophin 6 (NT-6). Besides the nervous system, most of these peptides are also found in several other systems and organs, including the ovary [7].

To induce a biological effect, neurotrophins need to interact with cell-surface receptors. All neurotrophins interact with two different types of receptors: the p75 neurotrophin receptor (p75^{NTR}) and a member of the tyrosine receptor kinase (TRK) family. All neurotrophins can bind to p75^{NTR} with low affinity, but every different TRK receptor can bind to a specific neurotrophin with high affinity [8]. The TRK family is constituted by three members: TRKA, TRKB and TRKC. NGF binds to TRKA; BDNF and NT4/5 bind to TRKB; and NT-3 binds to TRKC. Moreover, alternative splicing can generate different TRK isoforms and some of them can initiate signal transduction pathways [9]. On the other hand, p75^{NTR} and also TRK receptors can dimerize, forming either homodimers or interacting with each other (heterodimers) [10].

Nerve growth factor can induce cell survival on several systems, including the nervous, cardiovascular, immune, endocrine and reproductive systems [7]. Upon binding to TRKA, the receptor homodimerizes and autophosphorylates its tyrosine residues, inducing signaling pathways that induce trophic and anti-apoptotic effects [11]; NGF deficiency, conversely, activates apoptosis (**Figure 1**) [12]. The NGF/p75^{NTR} pathway can lead to proliferation, survival or

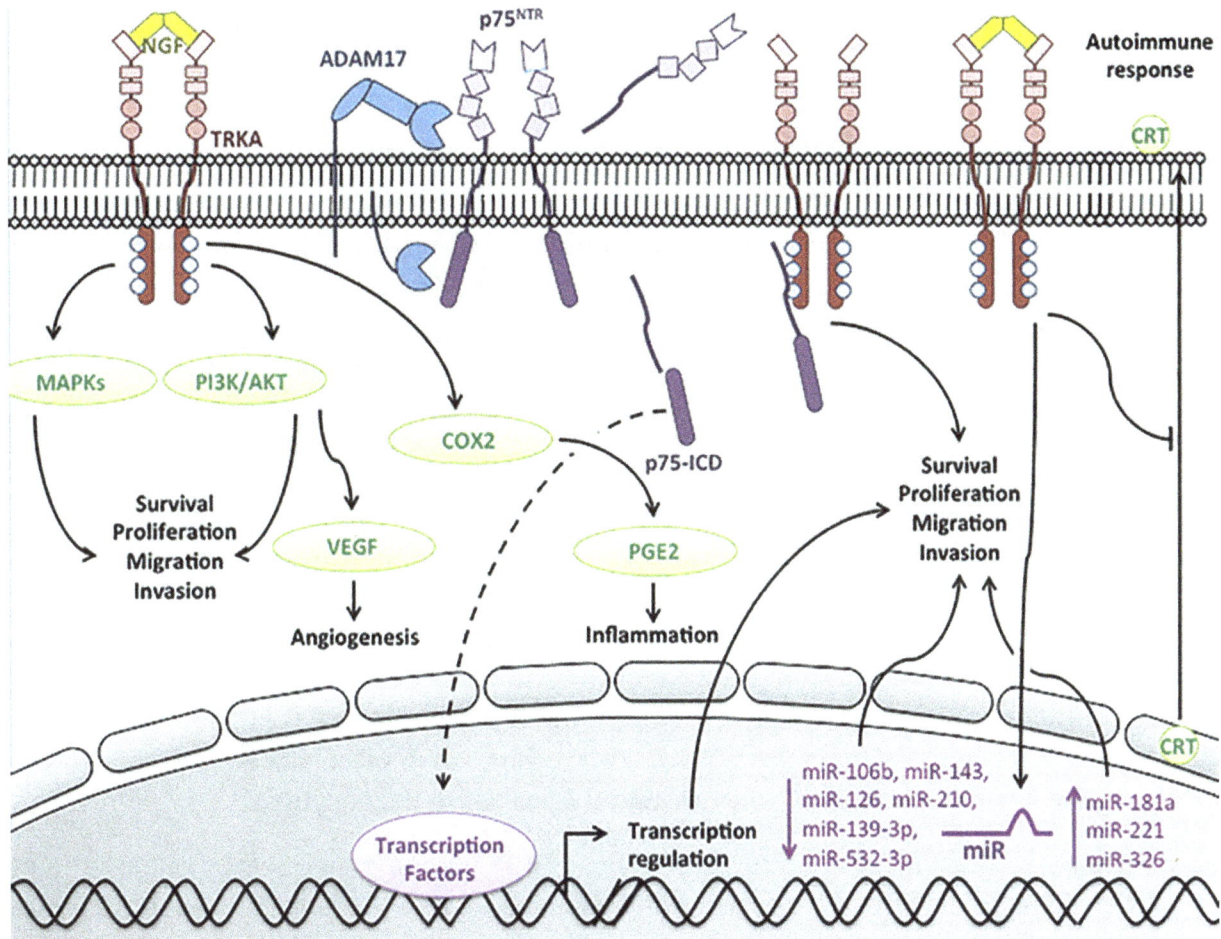

Figure 1. Several NGF-related signaling pathways are involved in epithelial ovarian cancer. NGF, a protein whose levels are elevated in EOC, activates several signaling pathways leading to carcinogenesis. Upon binding to its high affinity receptor, TRKA, NGF activates the MAPKs and PI3K/Akt signaling pathways, inducing cell survival, proliferation, migration and invasion. Through TRKA activation, NGF also increases VEGF, COX-2 and PGE 2 levels, which promotes angiogenesis and inflammation, respectively. Besides, NGF inhibits CRT translocation from the endoplasmic reticulum to the cell surface, potentially inhibiting anticancer immune responses. NGF's low affinity receptor, p75NTR, is also present in ovarian cancer cells. This receptor can be cleaved by ADAM17, a cell surface metalloproteinase, producing an intracellular domain (p75-ICD) that could be responsible for the regulation of different processes through transcription control. Furthermore, p75-ICD can interact with TRKA, increasing its activity. Several microRNAs (miRNAs) are regulated by NGF, and these miRNAs could be responsible for NGF-mediated effects.

cell death, depending on the cell context, availability of adaptors and expression of co-receptors. While NGF can trigger apoptosis through the activation of the Jun N-terminal Kinase (JNK)/c-Jun death pathway, it can also activate the canonical NFκB signaling cascade, which promotes cell survival by increasing anti-apoptotic molecules levels [13]. The receptor p75NTR can also enhance TRKA phosphorylation by increasing the TRKA ability to bind to NGF [14].

Neurotrophins are involved in normal ovarian development and functioning, regulating follicular assembly, folliculogenesis and ovulation. Concerning ovarian development, p75NTR is expressed in the stromal cells surrounding the oocytes of human fetuses previously and during follicular assembly [15]. NGF and TRKA also seem to be necessary for follicular assembly, because mutations on these genes reduce the number of primordial follicles in mice [16].

Besides, NGF increases follicle-stimulating hormone receptor (FSHR) protein levels and the ovary response to FSH, collaborating in the growth of pre-antral follicles of 2-day-old rat ovaries [17]. Neurotrophins also participate in folliculogenesis, since they are involved in the differentiation of primordial follicles into primary follicles and in the development of secondary follicles from primary follicles [18].

In humans, NGF is present in the oocyte and granulosa cells from follicles at primordial and secondary stages, suggesting that NGF is necessary for follicle maturation after the primordial stage [16]. p75^{NTR}, on the other hand, is not detected on human stromal cells after birth, but theca cells from growing follicles do express this protein [15]. Concerning TRKA, this receptor is found in granulosa cells and oocytes of neonatal mice ovaries; its expression is higher on primary follicles and diminishes with folliculogenesis [15].

In human antral follicles, both granulosa and theca cells express NGF and TRKA. Furthermore, NGF has a role in ovulation, since in human ovarian granulosa cells, NGF increases FSHR and estradiol secretion [19]. Nerve growth factor contributes to ovulation by decreasing gap junctions, stimulating the proliferation of theca cells and inducing the release of prostaglandin E2 (PGE2), which acts on granulosa cells and is necessary for successful ovulation [20, 21]. Indeed, PGE2 is a paracrine mediator of luteinizing hormone (LH), and LH induces an increase of intrafollicular levels of PGE2, controlling key molecular events of ovulation, including the facilitation of follicle rupture and the release of the oocyte [22].

Angiogenesis is a key process in the normal ovarian functioning, necessary for the growth of ovarian follicles and the development and maintenance of the corpus luteum [22]. The expression and secretion of the vascular endothelial growth factor (VEGF), an important proangiogenic molecule, is key for normal adult reproductive function, and its expression is induced by the activation of FSHR and the LH receptor (LHR) [23]. VEGF production is also stimulated by NGF in cultures of human granulosa cells through the MAPK and PI3K/AKT signaling pathways [23]. Besides, NGF can directly regulate angiogenesis by acting on endothelial cells [24]. Thus, NGF participates in normal ovarian angiogenesis through its high affinity receptor TRKA.

While NGF plays a physiological role in the ovary, regulating its development and ovulation, it can also participate in cancer-related processes, particularly through its TRKA receptor [25], as seen in **Figure 1**. In cancer cells, these pathways are linked to proliferation, survival, migration and invasiveness. Interestingly, whilst in normal epithelial ovarian cells NGF and TRKA expression is only found on a small percentage of cells, both of these proteins are present in EOC tissues [26]. The active or phosphorylated form of TRKA is highly elevated in EOC compared to normal tissues, making it a possible marker for poor prognosis [27].

The NGF/TRKA signaling pathway has also been linked to several transduction cascades that stimulate cancer progression, including VEGF production and secretion [26], the COX2/PGE2 inflammatory response [28], ADAM17 activity [29] and alterations on calreticulin (CRT) subcellular localization [30]. All the molecules mentioned above have a role in the development or progression of ovarian cancer by altering processes such as inflammation, angiogenesis, immune evasion, survival and metastasis.

Angiogenesis is a vital process necessary for solid tumors to grow, develop and metastasize [31]. Several molecules are known to promote angiogenesis, in several cancer tissues including EOC; however, VEGF is considered the main angiogenic factor [32]. Its expression is controlled by the hypoxia-inducing factor (HIF-1α), a transcription factor that is produced in cells with low oxygen levels, a condition typically found on cancer cells from solid tumors [33]. VEGF induces angiogenesis by binding to its tyrosine kinase receptors located on the surface of endothelial cells, promoting their proliferation, migration and increasing their permeability [34]. In EOC explants, NGF induces an increase of VEGF levels through TRKA activation, increasing VEGF secretion [26]. Also, the NGF-conditioned medium secreted by EOC explants and by A2780 cells (an immortalized EOC cell line) induces proliferation, migration and differentiation of human endothelial Eahy926 cells [27]. Importantly, NGF, total TRKA and p-TRKA molecules are present in endothelial cells from cancer tissues. Therefore, NGF acts on EOC cells by inducing VEGF expression, besides its direct angiogenic effect by acting on the TRKA receptor found on endothelial cells [26, 35].

Moreover, given the role of NGF in the promotion of ovulation through the increase of PGE2, this neurotrophin has been linked to pro-inflammatory responses in the ovary. Interestingly, cancer has been linked to chronic inflammation, since different inflammatory pathways are activated in tumor tissues, including pathways involving cyclooxygenase (COX) proteins [36]. PGE2 is synthesized by members of the COX family: COX-1 and COX-2 [37]. COX-2 expression is inducible by external stimuli, and several molecules found in cancer, including cytokines, growth factors, oncogenes and chemicals, can induce its expression [37]. As for PGE2, this prostaglandin induces cell growth, angiogenesis, invasiveness, inhibition of apoptosis and inflammation [38]. Importantly, non-steroidal anti-inflammatory drugs (NSAIDs), which act by selectively binding to COX-1 or COX-2 and inhibiting the arachidonic acid pathway, have preventive and inhibitory effects on carcinogenesis, highlighting the importance of COX-2 in cancer [39]. Moreover, COX-2 levels have been found to be elevated in several types of cancer, including colon, gastric, breast, pancreatic, bladder and prostate cancer [40]. Therefore, COX-2 has become a focus for cancer research as a potential therapeutic target [41].

In EOC, COX-2 levels have been found to be elevated in human ovarian cancer samples compared to normal ovaries [28]. In theca cells from bovine ovaries, NFG increases COX-2 and PGE2 levels [42] and on prostate cancer cell lines, PGE2 promotes VEGF secretion [43]. Therefore, our research group explored a possible connection between NGF, COX-2, PGE2 and VEGF. In vitro experiments on A2780 epithelial ovarian cancer cells showed that NGF induces COX-2 expression and increases PGE2 levels, suggesting that NGF could stimulate inflammatory processes [28].

Other proteins that are involved in inflammatory responses are metalloproteinases, including a disintegrin and metalloproteinase domain-containing protein 17 (ADAM17) [44]. ADAM17 is expressed in granulosa cells, being important in ovary signaling during oocyte development and follicular fate determination [45].

ADAM17 is ubiquitously expressed; it is primarily active during inflammation and in cancer tissues; therefore, ADAM17 has become another focus for cancer research [46]. In lung cancer, for instance, ADAM17 protein levels are increased, and ADAM17 inhibitors aid cancer treatment when the tumor has developed resistance mechanisms [47]. In breast cancer, ADAM17 protein levels are also overexpressed, which has been linked to tumor progression and metastasis [48]. Additionally, ADAM17 levels and activity have also been found to be elevated in colorectal, pancreatic, kidney, prostate and ovarian cancer [46].

An important ADAM17 target is TRKA, where its dimerization with p75^{NTR} favors ADAM17 activation, which in turn induces p75^{NTR} cleavage [49] through γ-secretase, resulting in a cytoplasmic fragment (p75-ICD) that can bind to the intracellular domain of TRKA, increasing TRKA signaling activity [50]. In human ovarian cancer samples, p75^{NTR} levels are lower compared to normal ovarian tissues. In A2780 cells, ADAM17 cleaves p75^{NTR}, possibly decreasing p75 anticancer effects. The p75-ICD, on the other hand, increases TRKA activation, potentially inducing pro-carcinogenic processes. Besides, NGF stimulation activates TRKA, ADAM17 and γ-secretase, reducing p75^{NTR} levels and increasing p75-CTF and p75-ICD levels, favoring cell survival [29]. Also, there is evidence that suggests that p75-ICD could act as a transcription regulator, enhancing TRKA cancer activity [51].

2.1. NGF effect on calreticulin subcellular localization: potential consequences for immunotherapy

Cancer cells are exposed to higher levels of endoplasmic reticulum (ER) stress, since they are exposed to stressful conditions such as hypoxia, nutrient deprivation and pH changes, among others [52]. In order to adjust to these changes, cancer cells activate the unfolded protein response (UPR), composed of three branches initiated by three proteins: IRE1α, PERK and ATF6 and sensors of ER stress [53]. In this context, calreticulin (CRT), a chaperone resident of the endoplasmic reticulum, plays a role in the adaptation of cancer cells to changes in the microenvironment [54]. CRT, a multifunctional, buffering and ubiquitous protein, is mainly involved in protein folding and the maintenance of calcium homeostasis; as a chaperone, CRT participates in protein folding quality control [54]. Under conditions of ER stress, calreticulin levels increase to restore the cell to homeostasis [55]. CRT protein levels are elevated in different cancer tissues, including EOC [37, 65], and while this increase could be associated with an adaptation to ER stress, CRT expression has also been linked to proliferation, metastasis, invasion and angiogenesis [56]. Moreover, in EOC cells, NGF induces an increase of CRT levels, which could be associated with the acquirement of carcinogenic properties [30, 57].

Importantly, despite the pro-carcinogenic effects of CRT, when this protein is found in the cell surface it can induce an anti-immune response against cancer cells [58]. In human ovarian cancer cells, our research group found that mitoxantrone, a direct ER stress inducer, can trigger CRT translocation from the ER to the cell surface [30]. Previous studies have shown that ER stress is a necessary step for CRT transport to the cell surface, and concordantly, in EOC cells, CRT translocation was accompanied by activation of the UPR protein PERK and its substrate eIF2α [59].

Interestingly, several reports show that NGF can inhibit the effects of ER stress, which could hinder cells' ability to translocate CRT from the ER to the cell surface [60–62]. Indeed, when A2780 cells were incubated with both NGF and mitoxantrone, CRT levels on the cell surface were diminished compared to cells stimulated with mitoxantrone alone [30]. Therefore, an anticancer immune therapy based on drugs that induce CRT translocation from the ER to the cell surface could have limited efficiency in ovarian cancer patients, since NGF levels inhibit CRT translocation.

As described above in EOC, NGF is involved in many processes such as cellular survival, proliferation, angiogenesis and response to therapy. NGF could be regulating these processes through microRNA modulation; therefore, it is important to describe the role of microRNAs in EOC and its relation with NGF.

3. Role of microRNAs (miRs) in the progression of ovarian cancer and their relation with nerve growth factor

New targets of NGF and its receptor TRKA include various microRNAs (miRs). Since the 1990s, deregulation of miRs has become important in several pathological processes, including several types of cancer [63]. Currently, miRs could be used as new biomarkers and/or for therapy in various diseases [64]. Particularly in ovarian cancer some miRs are downregulated or upregulated [65], and NGF and its receptor TRKA could be implicated in the deregulation of some miRs.

MicroRNAs are the biggest family of non-coding RNAs; they are ~22-nucleotides (nts) long and regulate mRNAs post-transcriptionally [66]. The first step on miR biogenesis is the synthesis of a long primary miR (pri-miR) by an RNA polymerase II. Then, the pri-miR is cleaved, producing a pre-miR [67] that is transported to the cytoplasm to be enzymatically cleaved in its loop structure, releasing a double-strand miR called duplex [68]. This duplex has two strands, one called "mature" or "guide" miR and the other named "passenger", which is released and degraded [69]. Mature miR has ~22 nts and binds to the three-prime untranslated region (3'-UTR) of a target mRNA in order to regulate protein expression. This regulation depends on miR-mRNA complementary: total complementarity of miR with its mRNA target is a signal to cleave or degrade the mRNA. On the other hand, partial complementarily induces deadenylation of the mRNA target (facilitating its degradation) or inhibition of its translation [70]. In normal cells, microRNAs have an important role maintaining their normal functioning; however, a deregulation in their expression can lead to cellular alterations. Most studies concerning miR roles in pathologies evaluate whether there are changes on miR expression; therefore, miR targets are still being described. Regarding these targets, one miR has several targets, meaning that one miR can be involved in the development of different pathologies.

Cancer development involves miR deregulation. Cancer-related miRs are divided in two groups: oncogenic (oncomiR) and tumor suppressor (oncosuppressor) miRs; oncomirs regulate the mRNA of tumor suppressor genes, while oncosuppressors control the mRNA of oncogenes. Both of these types of miRs are normally in equilibrium; however, during carcinogenesis, they exhibit a deregulation on their expression [71]. One miR can regulate the same mRNA targets in different types of cancer, which makes them an attractive target for the development of new therapies.

Besides their potential as therapeutic targets, currently, miRs' profiles are being described in order to obtain more accurate and reliable biomarkers for cancer development and/or progression [64]; in EOC, several miRs have been found to be upregulated [72].

Interestingly, it has been found that eight miRs could be regulating 89% of the miR-associated genes [73]. Thus, to produce a more accurate clinical diagnosis, it would be beneficial to have miR profiles as biological markers.

EOC development and progression is regulated by several miRs. OncomiRs and tumor suppressor miRs modulate different processes of the hallmarks of cancer, such as proliferation, angiogenesis, migration, invasion, survival and apoptosis, among others (**Table 1** summarizes the most important miRs involved in different cancers, including EOC).

As discussed above, NGF is overexpressed in EOC and it has a significant role in the progression of this disease [35]. Interestingly, studies show that NGF could regulate the expression of some miRs. Most of these studies have been done in PC12 cells: in these cells, NGF stimulation increases the expression of several miRs [74].

Importantly, in EOC, miR-143 is downregulated [75], which is correlated with an increase of COX-2 levels [76]. As stated in the previous section, NGF increases COX-2 levels [28]. It also decreases the expression of miR-143 in PC12 cells [74]. Therefore, in EOC, the NGF-mediated COX-2 increase could be regulated through miR-143. Another miR regulated by NGF is miR-222 [77], which targets a metalloproteinase inhibitor (TIMP3) [78]. TIMP3 inhibits ADAM17 function [79]; then, NGF could increase miR-222 in order to decrease TIMP3 levels, allowing the ADAM17 activity. Consequently, NGF regulation of miR-143 and miR-222 could be important for EOC development, through the regulation of COX-2 levels and ADAM17 activity, respectively (summarized in **Table 2**).

miR	Regulation	Cancer	Targets	References
Let-7 family	↓	Lung, hepatocellular, breast and ovarian	RAS, HMGA2, cyclin D2, c-myc	[83–86]
miR-17-92	↑	Myeloma, breast, gastric and colon cancer	BIM, E2F1 PTEN	[85, 87–89]
miR-21	↑	Oral, colon, breast, glioma, ovarian and cervical cancer	PTEN, DKK2, PDCD4, TGFbR2	[85, 90–93]
miR-23a/b	↓	Colon, pancreatic and ovarian cancer	MAP3K1, Cyclin G1, RRAS2, TGFβR2	[72, 82, 94, 95]
miR-122	↓	Hepatocellular cancer	Wnt1, TCF4, Cyclin G1, B-catenin	[84, 96]
miR-143	↓	Gastric cancer	COX2	[97]
miR-125 family	↑	Renal cell carcinoma, endometrial and breast cancer	ERBB2, P53INP1, HDAC5	[85, 98–100]
	↓	Ovarian cancer	SET	[101]

One miR can be deregulated in different types of cancer; simultaneously, several miRs can be deregulated in one type of cancer. Some examples are described in the table, including oncomiRs and tumor suppressor miRs. miRs can have a dual role. A few of their mRNA targets are also depicted.

Table 1. List of miRs and some of their targets de-regulated in cancer.

NGF-related miR	Regulation	Cancer	References
miR-92a	↑	Neuroblastoma	[102]
miR-21	↑	Pheocromocitoma	[103]
miR-221/222	↑	Pheocromocitoma	[77]
miR-23b	↓	Ovarian cancer	[80]
miR-143	↓	Pheocromocitoma	[75, 76]

NGF stimulation regulates miRs in these cancers through the upregulation of several miRs, including miR-92a, miR-21 and miR-221/222, while it downregulates other miRs, such as miR-23b and miR-143.

Table 2. List of miRs regulated by NGF.

Besides, in EOC, an increase of NGF levels induces the expression of c-MYC transcription factor [80], and c-MYC downregulates the miR-23b expression [81]. This miR levels decrease in EOC, and we described that after NGF stimulation, EOC cells diminish miR-23b levels [80]. Therefore, in this cancer, NGF could reduce miR-23b levels through c-Myc. miR-23b targets cell cycle and tumor growth proteins, regulating cyclin-G1 [82] and SP-1 transcription factor [81], respectively.

4. Conclusion

Solid scientific evidences indicate that NGF has important roles in the progression of EOC by promoting the expression or activation of several proteins involved in the different carcinogenic processes, including cell proliferation, angiogenesis and in therapy resistance. For instance, NGF interaction with its TRKA receptor can activate AKT and ERK signaling, promoting cell proliferation and survival. TRKA activation by NGF also increases COX-2 and PGE2 levels, contributing to inflammatory processes, which are important to cancer progression. Besides, NGF can act on the ADAM17 metalloproteinase, which cuts the p75^{NTR} receptor in EOC cells, leaving an intracellular fragment that can activate transcription and that can interact with TRKA, increasing its carcinogenic effects. Furthermore, NGF could modulate the immune response, since it can reduce CRT translocation from the endoplasmic reticulum to the cell membrane, reducing cancer cells' recognition by immune cells.

Additionally, it is relevant to point out that recent reports describe how NGF regulates the expression of different miRs, which in turn could affect the translation of protein participants of the abovementioned processes. Some examples include miR-143, whose levels are downregulated EOC and correlate with an increase of COX-2 levels. Another miR regulated by NGF is miR-222, which targets the metalloproteinase inhibitor TIMP3, an ADAM17 inhibitor. Furthermore, NGF stimulation reduces miR-23b levels through c-Myc, targeting the cell cycle and tumor growth proteins. Therefore, there is evidence to suggest that NGF-dependent miR regulation could lead to tumor development. Nevertheless, further studies are needed to confirm NGF's role in EOC; therefore, it is important to evaluate new miRs associated with EOC. These findings could result in new biomarkers used for diagnosis or target molecules that could allow the development of new therapies.

Abbreviations

ADAM17	a disintegrin and metalloproteinase domain-containing protein 17
COX	cyclooxygenase
CRT	calreticulin
EOC	epithelial ovarian cancer
ER	endoplasmic reticulum
FSH	follicle-stimulating hormone
FSHR	follicle-stimulating hormone receptor
LH	luteinizing hormone
LHR	luteinizing hormone receptor
miR	micro-RNA
NGF	nerve growth factor
Nts	nucleotides
p75NTR	p75 neurotrophin receptor
PGE2	prostaglandin E2
TRK	tyrosine receptor kinase
VEGF	vascular endothelial growth factor

Author details

Carolina Vera[1], Rocío Retamales-Ortega[1], Maritza Garrido[1], Margarita Vega[1,2] and Carmen Romero[1,2,3*]

*Address all correspondence to: cromero@hcuch.cl

1 Laboratory of Endocrinology and Reproductive Biology, Clinical Hospital University of Chile, Santiago, Chile

2 Department of Obstetrics and Gynecology, Clinical Hospital, Faculty of Medicine, University of Chile, Santiago, Chile

3 Advanced Center for Chronic Diseases (ACCDiS), Santiago, Chile

References

[1] Soerjomataram I, Lortet-Tieulent J, Parkin DM, Ferlay J, Mathers C, Forman D, et al. Global burden of cancer in 2008: A systematic analysis of disability-adjusted life-years in 12 world regions. Lancet. 2012;**380**:1840-1850. DOI: 10.1016/S0140-6736(12)60919-2

[2] Lowe KA, Chia VM, Taylor A, O'Malley C, Kelsh M, Mohamed M, et al. An international assessment of ovarian cancer incidence and mortality. Gynecologic Oncology. 2013;**130**:107-114. DOI: 10.1016/j.ygyno.2013.03.026

[3] Iruela-Arispe ML, Dvorak HF. Angiogenesis: A dynamic balance of stimulators and inhibitors. Thrombosis and Haemostasis. 1997;**78**:672-677

[4] Suzuki T, Sasano H, Takaya R, Fukaya T, Yajima A, Nagura H. Cyclic changes of vasculature and vascular phenotypes in normal human ovaries. Human Reproduction. 1998;**13**:953-959. DOI: 10.1093/humrep/13.4.953

[5] Carmeliet P. Angiogenesis in health and disease: Therapeutic opportunities. Nature Medicine. 2003;**9**:653-660. DOI: 10.1038/nm0603-653

[6] Mobley WC, Schenker A, Shooter EM. Characterization and isolation of proteolytically modified nerve growth factor. Biochemistry. 1976;**15**:5543-5552

[7] Sariola H. The neurotrophic factors in non-neuronal tissues. Cellular and Molecular Life Sciences. 2001;**58**:1061-1066. DOI: 10.1007/PL00000921

[8] Friedman WJ, Greene LA. Neurotrophin signaling via Trks and p75. Experimental Cell Research. 1999;**253**:131-142. DOI: 10.1006/excr.1999.4705

[9] Patapoutian A, Reichardt LF. Trk receptors: Mediators of neurotrophin action. Current Opinion in Neurobiology. 2001;**11**:272-280. DOI: 10.1016/S0959-4388(00)00208-7

[10] Bibel M, Hoppe E, Barde YA. Biochemical and functional interactions between the neurotrophin receptors trk and p75(NTR). The EMBO Journal. 1999;**18**:616-622. DOI: 10.1093/emboj/18.3.616

[11] Tessarollo L. Pleiotropic functions of neurotrophins in development. Cytokine & Growth Factor Reviews. 1998;**9**:125-137. DOI: 10.1016/S1359-6101(98)00003-3

[12] Yuan J, Yankner BA. Apoptosis in the nervous system. Nature. 2000;**407**:802-809. DOI: 10.1038/35037739

[13] Underwood CK, Coulson EJ. The p75 neurotrophin receptor. The International Journal of Biochemistry & Cell Biology. 2008;**40**:1664-1668. DOI: 10.1016/j.biocel.2007.06.010

[14] Lee FS, Kim AH, Khursigara G, Chao MV. The uniqueness of being a neurotrophin receptor. Current Opinion in Neurobiology. 2001;**11**:281-286. DOI: 10.1016/S0959-4388 (00)00209-9

[15]   Anderson RA, Robinson LLL, Brooks J, Spears N. Neurotropins and their receptors are expressed in the human fetal ovary. The Journal of Clinical Endocrinology and Metabolism. 2002;**87**:890-897

[16]   Dissen GA, Romero C, Hirshfield AN, Ojeda SR. Nerve growth factor is required for early follicular development in the mammalian ovary. Endocrinology. 2001;**142**:2078-2086. DOI: 10.1210/endo.142.5.8126

[17]   Romero C, Paredes A, Dissen GA, Ojeda SR. Nerve growth factor induces the expression of functional FSH receptors in newly formed follicles of the rat ovary. Endocrinology. 2002;**143**:1485-1494. DOI: 10.1210/endo.143.4.8711

[18]   Chaves RN, Alves AM, Lima LF, Matos HM, Rodrigues AP, Figueiredo JR. Role of nerve growth factor (NGF) and its receptors in folliculogenesis. Zygote. 2013;**21**(2):187-197. DOI: 10.1017/S0967199412000111

[19]   Salas C, Julio-Pieper M, Valladares M, Pommer R, Vega M, Mastronardi C, et al. Nerve growth factor-dependent activation of trkA receptors in the human ovary results in synthesis of follicle-stimulating hormone receptors and estrogen secretion. The Journal of Clinical Endocrinology and Metabolism. 2006;**91**:2396-2403. DOI: 10.1210/jc.2005-1925

[20]   Tsafriri A, Lindner HR, Zor U, Lamprecht SA. Physiological role of prostaglandins in the induction of ovulation. Prostaglandins. 1972;**2**:1-10. DOI: 10.1016/0090-6980(72)90024-X

[21]   Ben-Ami I, Freimann S, Armon L, Dantes A, Strassburger D, Friedler S, et al. PGE2 up-regulates EGF-like growth factor biosynthesis in human granulosa cells: New insights into the coordination between PGE2 and LH in ovulation. Molecular Human Reproduction. 2006;**12**:593-599. DOI: 10.1093/molehr/gal068

[22]   Reynolds LP, Grazul-Bilska AT, Redmer DA. Angiogenesis in the corpus luteum. Endocrine. 2000;**12**:1-9. DOI: 10.1385/ENDO:12:1:1

[23]   Geva E, Jaffe RB. Role of vascular endothelial growth factor in ovarian physiology and pathology. Fertility and Sterility. 2000;**74**:429-438. DOI: 10.1016/S0002-9440(10)65669-6

[24]   Julio-Pieper M, Lara HE, Bravo JA, Romero C. Effects of nerve growth factor (NGF) on blood vessels area and expression of the angiogenic factors VEGF and TGFbeta1 in the rat ovary. Reproductive Biology and Endocrinology. 2006;**4**:57. DOI: 10.1186/1477-7827-4-57

[25]   Nico B, Mangieri D, Benagiano V, Crivellato E, Ribatti D. Nerve growth factor as an angiogenic factor. Microvascular Research. 2008;**75**:135-141. DOI: 10.1016/j.mvr.2007.07.004

[26]   Campos X, Muñoz Y, Selman A, Yazigi R, Moyano L, Weinstein-Oppenheimer C, et al. Nerve growth factor and its high-affinity receptor trkA participate in the control of vascular endothelial growth factor expression in epithelial ovarian cancer. Gynecologic Oncology. 2007;**104**:168-175. DOI: 10.1016/j.ygyno.2006.07.007

[27]   Tapia V, Gabler F, Muñoz M, Yazigi R, Paredes A, Selman A, et al. Tyrosine kinase A receptor (trkA): A potential marker in epithelial ovarian cancer. Gynecologic Oncology. 2011;**121**:13-23. DOI: 10.1016/j.ygyno.2010.12.341

[28] Romero C, Hurtado I, Garrido M, Selman A, Vega M. The expression of coclooxigenase-2 is increased by nerve growth factor in epithelial ovarian cancer. In: 24th Bienn. Congr. Eur. Assoc. Cancer Res; Manchester, United Kingdom. 2016

[29] Romero C, Vallejos C, Gabler F, Selman A, Vega M. Activation of TRKA receptor by nerve growth factor induces shedding of p75 receptor related with progression of epithelial ovarian cancer. In: 23rd Bienn. Congr. Eur. Assoc. Cancer Res; Munich, Germany. 2014. pp. 5119-5120

[30] Vera CA, Oróstica L, Gabler F, Ferreira A, Selman A, Vega M, et al. The nerve growth factor alters calreticulin translocation from the endoplasmic reticulum to the cell surface and its signaling pathway in epithelial ovarian cancer cells. International Journal of Oncology. 2017;**50**:1261-1270. DOI: 10.3892/ijo.2017.3892

[31] Folkman J. What is the evidence that tumors are angiogenesis dependent? Journal of the National Cancer Institute. 1990;**82**:4-6

[32] Carmeliet P. VEGF as a key mediator of angiogenesis in cancer. Oncology. 2005;**69**(Suppl 3): 4-10. DOI: 10.1159/000088478

[33] Ryan HE, Lo J, Johnson RS. HIF-1 alpha is required for solid tumor formation and embryonic vascularization. The EMBO Journal. 1998;**17**:3005-3015. DOI: 10.1093/emboj/17.11.3005

[34] Olsson A-K, Dimberg A, Kreuger J, Claesson-Welsh L. VEGF receptor signalling—In control of vascular function. Nature Reviews. Molecular Cell Biology. 2006;**7**:359-371. DOI: 10.1038/nrm1911

[35] Vera C, Tapia V, Vega M, Romero C. Role of nerve growth factor and its TRKA receptor in normal ovarian and epithelial ovarian cancer angiogenesis. Journal of Ovarian Research. 2014;**7**:82. DOI: 10.1186/s13048-014-0082-6

[36] Colotta F, Allavena P, Sica A, Garlanda C, Mantovani A. Cancer-related inflammation, the seventh hallmark of cancer: Links to genetic instability. Carcinogenesis. 2009;**30**:1073-1081. DOI: 10.1093/carcin/bgp127

[37] Crofford LJ. COX-1 and COX-2 tissue expression: Implications and predictions. The Journal of Rheumatology. Supplement. 1997;**49**:15-19

[38] Greenhough A, Smartt HJM, Moore AE, Roberts HR, Williams AC, Paraskeva C, et al. The COX-2/PGE2 pathway: Key roles in the hallmarks of cancer and adaptation to the tumour microenvironment. Carcinogenesis. 2009;**30**:377-386. DOI: 10.1093/carcin/bgp014

[39] Cha YI, DuBois RN. NSAIDs and cancer prevention: Targets downstream of COX-2. Annual Review of Medicine. 2007;**58**:239-252. DOI: 10.1146/annurev.med.57.121304.131253

[40] Dannenberg AJ, Altorki NK, Boyle JO, Dang C, Howe LR, Weksler BB, et al. Cyclooxygenase 2: A pharmacological target for the prevention of cancer. The Lancet Oncology. 2001;**2**:544-551. DOI: 10.1016/S1470-2045(01)00488-0

[41] Ghosh N, Chaki R, Mandal V, Mandal SC. COX-2 as a target for cancer chemotherapy. Pharmacological Reports. n.d.;**62**:233-244

[42] Dissen GA, Parrott JA, Skinner MK, Hill DF, Costa ME, Ojeda SR. Direct effects of nerve growth factor on thecal cells from antral ovarian follicles. Endocrinology. 2000;**141**:4736-4750. DOI: 10.1210/endo.141.12.7850

[43] Wang X, Klein RD. Prostaglandin E2 induces vascular endothelial growth factor secretion in prostate cancer cells through EP2 receptor-mediated cAMP pathway. Molecular Carcinogenesis. 2007;**46**:912-923. DOI: 10.1002/mc.20320

[44] Gooz M. ADAM-17: The enzyme that does it all. Critical Reviews in Biochemistry and Molecular Biology. 2010;**45**:146-169. DOI: 10.3109/10409231003628015

[45] Field SL, Dasgupta T, Cummings M, Orsi NM. Cytokines in ovarian folliculogenesis, oocyte maturation and luteinisation. Molecular Reproduction and Development. 2014;**81**:284-314. DOI: 10.1002/mrd.22285

[46] Duffy MJ, McKiernan E, O'Donovan N, McGowan PM. Role of ADAMs in cancer formation and progression. Clinical Cancer Research. 2009;**15**(4):1140. DOI: 10.1158/1078-0432.CCR-08-1585

[47] Zhou BBS, Peyton M, He B, Liu C, Girard L, Caudler E, et al. Targeting ADAM-mediated ligand cleavage to inhibit HER3 and EGFR pathways in non-small cell lung cancer. Cancer Cell. 2006;**10**:39-50. DOI: 10.1016/j.ccr.2006.05.024

[48] McGowan PM, Ryan BM, Hill ADK, McDermott E, O'Higgins N, Duffy MJ. ADAM-17 expression in breast cancer correlates with variables of tumor progression. Clinical Cancer Research. 2007;**13**:2335-2343. DOI: 10.1158/1078-0432.CCR-06-2092

[49] Verbeke S, Tomellini E, Dhamani F, Meignan S, Adriaenssens E, Xuefen LB. Extracellular cleavage of the p75 neurotrophin receptor is implicated in its pro-survival effect in breast cancer cells. FEBS Letters. 2013;**587**:2591-2596. DOI: 10.1016/j.febslet.2013.06.039

[50] Urra S, Escudero CA, Ramos P, Lisbona F, Allende E, Covarrubias P, et al. TrkA receptor activation by nerve growth factor induces shedding of the p75 neurotrophin receptor followed by endosomal-secretase-mediated release of the p75 intracellular domain. The Journal of Biological Chemistry. 2006;**282**:7606-7615. DOI: 10.1074/jbc.M610458200

[51] Bronfman FC. Metalloproteases and gamma-secretase: New membrane partners regulating p75 neurotrophin receptor signaling? Journal of Neurochemistry. 2007;**103**(Suppl):91-100. DOI: 10.1111/j.1471-4159.2007.04781.x

[52] Koumenis C. ER stress, hypoxia tolerance and tumor progression. Current Molecular Medicine. 2006;**6**:55-69

[53] Hotamisligil GS, Davis RJ. Cell Signaling and stress responses. Cold Spring Harbor Perspectives in Biology. 2016;**8**(10):a006072. DOI: 10.1101/cshperspect.a006072

[54] Michalak M, Groenendyk J, Szabo E, Gold LI, Opas M. Calreticulin, a multi-process calcium-buffering chaperone of the endoplasmic reticulum. The Biochemical Journal. 2009;**417**:651-666. DOI: 10.1042/BJ20081847

[55] Qiu Y, Michalak M. Transcriptional control of the calreticulin gene in health and disease. The International Journal of Biochemistry & Cell Biology. 2009;**41**:531-538. DOI: 10.1016/j.biocel.2008.06.020

[56] Chen C-N, Chang C-C, Su T-E, Hsu W-M, Jeng Y-M, Ho M-C, et al. Identification of calreticulin as a prognosis marker and angiogenic regulator in human gastric cancer. Annals of Surgical Oncology. 2009;**16**:524-533. DOI: 10.1245/s10434-008-0243-1

[57] Vera C, Tapia V, Kohan K, Gabler F, Ferreira A, Selman A, et al. Nerve growth factor induces the expression of chaperone protein calreticulin in human epithelial ovarian cells. Hormone and Metabolic Research. 2012;**44**:639-643. DOI: 10.1055/s-0032-1311633

[58] Obeid M, Tesniere A, Ghiringhelli F, Fimia GM, Apetoh L, Perfettini J-L, et al. Calreticulin exposure dictates the immunogenicity of cancer cell death. Nature Medicine. 2007;**13**:54-61. DOI: 10.1038/nm1523

[59] Wiersma VR, Michalak M, Abdullah TM, Bremer E, Eggleton P. Mechanisms of translocation of ER chaperones to the cell surface and immunomodulatory roles in cancer and autoimmunity. Frontiers in Oncology. 2015;**5**:7. DOI: 10.3389/fonc.2015.00007

[60] Wei K, Liu L, Xie F, Hao X, Luo J, Min S. Nerve growth factor protects the ischemic heart via attenuation of the endoplasmic reticulum stress induced apoptosis by activation of phosphatidylinositol 3-kinase. International Journal of Medical Sciences. 2015;**12**:83-91. DOI: 10.7150/ijms.10101

[61] Zhu S-P, Wang Z-G, Zhao Y-Z, Wu J, Shi H-X, Ye L-B, et al. Gelatin nanostructured lipid carriers incorporating nerve growth factor inhibit endoplasmic reticulum stress-induced apoptosis and improve recovery in spinal cord injury. Molecular Neurobiology. 2016;**53**:4375-4386. DOI: 10.1007/s12035-015-9372-2

[62] Shimoke K, Sasaya H, Ikeuchi T. Analysis of the role of nerve growth factor in promoting cell survival during endoplasmic reticulum stress in PC12 cells. Methods in Enzymology. 2011;**490**:53-70. DOI: 10.1016/B978-0-12-385114-7.00003-9

[63] Adams BD, Kasinski AL, Slack FJ. Aberrant regulation and function of MicroRNAs in cancer. Current Biology. 2014;**24**:R762-R776. DOI: 10.1016/j.cub.2014.06.043

[64] Heneghan HM, Miller N, Kerin MJ. MiRNAs as biomarkers and therapeutic targets in cancer. Current Opinion in Pharmacology. 2010;**10**:543-550. DOI: 10.1016/j.coph.2010.05.010

[65] Katz B, Tropé CG, Reich R, Davidson B. MicroRNAs in ovarian cancer. Human Pathology. 2015;**46**:1245-1256. DOI: 10.1016/j.humpath.2015.06.013

[66] Winter J, Jung S, Keller S, Gregory RI, Diederichs S. Many roads to maturity: microRNA biogenesis pathways and their regulation. Nature Cell Biology. 2009;**11**:228-234. DOI: 10.1038/ncb0309-228

[67] Lee Y, Jeon K, Lee JT, Kim S, Kim VN. MicroRNA maturation: Stepwise processing and subcellular localization. The EMBO Journal. 2002;**21**:4663-4670. DOI: 10.1093/emboj/cdf476

[68] Bernstein E, Caudy AA, Hammond SM, Hannon GJ. Role for a bidentate ribonuclease in the initiation step of RNA interference. Nature. 2001;**409**:363-366. DOI: 10.1038/35053110

[69] Diederichs S, Haber DA. Dual role for argonautes in microRNA processing and post-transcriptional regulation of microRNA expression. Cell. 2007;**131**:1097-1108. DOI: 10.1016/j.cell.2007.10.032

[70] Ha M, Kim VN. Regulation of microRNA biogenesis. Nature Reviews. Molecular Cell Biology. 2014;**15**:509-524. DOI: 10.1038/nrm3838

[71] Calin GA, Sevignani C, Dumitru CD, Hyslop T, Noch E, Yendamuri S, et al. Human microRNA genes are frequently located at fragile sites and genomic regions involved in cancers. Proceedings of the National Academy of Sciences of the United States of America. 2004;**101**:2999-3004. DOI: 10.1073/pnas.0307323101

[72] Iorio MV, Visone R, Di Leva G, Donati V, Petrocca F, Casalini P, et al. MicroRNA signatures in human ovarian cancer. Cancer Research. 2007;**67**:8699-8707. DOI: 10.1158/0008-5472.CAN-07-1936

[73] Kinose Y, Sawada K, Nakamura K, Kimura T. The role of microRNAs in ovarian cancer. BioMed Research International. 2014;**2014**:249393. DOI: 10.1155/2014/249393

[74] Hamada N, Fujita Y, Kojima T, Kitamoto A, Akao Y, Nozawa Y, et al. MicroRNA expression profiling of NGF-treated PC12 cells revealed a critical role for miR-221 in neuronal differentiation. Neurochemistry International. 2012;**60**:743-750. DOI: 10.1016/j.neuint.2012.03.010

[75] Wang L, He J, Xu H, Xu L, Li N. MiR-143 targets CTGF and exerts tumor-suppressing functions in epithelial ovarian cancer. American Journal of Translational Research. 2016;**8**:2716-2726

[76] Wu X. MicroRNA-143 suppresses gastric cancer cell growth and induces apoptosis by targeting COX-2. World Journal of Gastroenterology. 2013;**19**:7758. DOI: 10.3748/wjg.v19.i43.7758

[77] Terasawa K, Ichimura A, Sato F, Shimizu K, Tsujimoto G. Sustained activation of ERK1/2 by NGF induces microRNA-221 and 222 in PC12 cells. The FEBS Journal. 2009;**276**:3269-3276. DOI: 10.1111/j.1742-4658.2009.07041.x

[78] Lu Y, Roy S, Nuovo G, Ramaswamy B, Miller T, Shapiro C, et al. Anti-microRNA-222 (anti-miR-222) and -181B suppress growth of tamoxifen-resistant xenografts in mouse by targeting TIMP3 protein and modulating mitogenic signal. The Journal of Biological Chemistry. 2011;**286**:42292-42302. DOI: 10.1074/jbc.M111.270926

[79] Brew K, Nagase H. The tissue inhibitors of metalloproteinases (TIMPs): An ancient family with structural and functional diversity. Biochimica et Biophysica Acta. 2010;**1803**(1):55-71

[80] Retamales-Ortega R, Oróstica L, Vera C, Cuevas P, Hernández A, Hurtado I, et al. Role of nerve growth factor (NGF) and miRNAs in epithelial ovarian cancer. International Journal of Molecular Sciences. 2017;**18**:507. DOI: 10.3390/ijms18030507

[81] Fulciniti M, Amodio N, Bandi RL, Cagnetta A, Samur MK, Acharya C, et al. miR-23b/ SP1/c-myc forms a feed-forward loop supporting multiple myeloma cell growth. Blood Cancer Journal. 2016;**6**:e380. DOI: 10.1038/bcj.2015.106

[82] Yan J, Jiang J, Meng X, Xiu Y, Zong Z. MiR-23b targets cyclin G1 and suppresses ovarian cancer tumorigenesis and progression. Journal of Experimental & Clinical Cancer Research. 2016;**35**:1-10. DOI: 10.1186/s13046-016-0307-1

[83] Takamizawa J, Konishi H, Yanagisawa K, Tomida S, Osada H, Endoh H, et al. Reduced expression of the let-7 microRNAs in human lung cancers in association with shortened postoperative survival. Cancer Research. 2004;**64**:3753-3756

[84] Gramantieri L, Ferracin M, Fornari F, Veronese A, Sabbioni S, Liu CG, et al. Cyclin G1 is a target of miR-122a, a microRNA frequently down-regulated in human hepatocellular carcinoma. Cancer Research. 2007;**67**:6092-6099. DOI: 10.1158/0008-5472.CAN-06-4607

[85] Iorio MV, Ferracin M, Liu C-G, Veronese A, Spizzo R, Sabbioni S, et al. MicroRNA gene expression deregulation in human breast cancer. Cancer Research. 2005;**65**:7065-7070. DOI: 10.1158/0008-5472.CAN-05-1783

[86] Yang N, Kaur S, Volinia S, Greshock J, Lassus H, Hasegawa K, et al. MicroRNA microarray identifies Let-7i as a novel biomarker and therapeutic target in human epithelial ovarian cancer. Cancer Research. 2008;**68**(24):10307-10314. DOI: 10.1158/0008-5472. CAN-08-1954

[87] Pichiorri F, Suh SS, Ladetto M, Kuehl M, Palumbo T, Drandi D, Taccioli C, et al. MicroRNAs regulate critical genes associated with multiple myeloma pathogenesis. Proceedings of the National Academy of Sciences. 2008;**105**(35):12885-12890. DOI: 10.1073/pnas.0806202105

[88] Li H, Wu Q, Li T, Liu C, Xue L, Ding J, et al. The miR-17-92 cluster as a potential biomarker for the early diagnosis of gastric cancer: Evidence and literature review. Oncotarget. 2017;**8**(28):45060-45071. DOI: 10.18632/oncotarget.15023

[89] Knudsen KN, Nielsen BS, Lindebjerg J, Hansen TF, Holst R, Sørensen FB. MicroRNA-17 is the most up-regulated member of the miR-17-92 cluster during early colon cancer evolution. PLoS One. 2015;**10**(10):e0140503. DOI: 10.1371/journal.pone.0140503

[90] Yu Y, Kanwar SS, Patel BB, Oh PS, Nautiyal J, Sarkar FH, et al. MicroRNA-21 induces stemness by downregulating transforming growth factor beta receptor 2 (TGFbetaR2) in colon cancer cells. Carcinogenesis. 2012;**33**:68-76. DOI: 10.1093/carcin/bgr246

[91] Kawakita A, Yanamoto S, Yamada S, Naruse T, Takahashi H, Kawasaki G, et al. MicroRNA-21 promotes oral cancer invasion via the Wnt/beta-catenin pathway by targeting DKK2. Pathology & Oncology Research. 2014;**20**:253-261. DOI: 10.1007/s12253-013-9689-y

[92] Corsten MF, Miranda R, Kasmieh R, Krichevsky AM, Weissleder R, Shah K. MicroRNA-21 knockdown disrupts glioma growth in vivo and displays synergistic cytotoxicity with neural precursor cell delivered S-TRAIL in human gliomas. Cancer Research. 2007;**67**:8994-9000. DOI: 10.1158/0008-5472.CAN-07-1045

[93] Lui WO, Pourmand N, Patterson BK, Fire A. Patterns of known and novel small RNAs in human cervical cancer. Cancer Research. 2007;**67**:6031-6043. DOI: 10.1158/0008-5472. CAN-06-0561

[94] Listing H, Mardin WA, Wohlfromm S, Mees ST, Haier J. MiR-23a/-24-induced gene silencing results in mesothelial cell integration of pancreatic cancer. British Journal of Cancer. 2015;**112**:131-139. DOI: 10.1158/0008-5472.CAN-06-0561

[95] Zhang H, Hao Y, Yang J, Zhou Y, Li J, Yin S, et al. Genome-wide functional screening of miR-23b as a pleiotropic modulator suppressing cancer metastasis. Nature Communications. 2011;**2**:554. DOI: 10.1038/ncomms1555

[96] Xu J, Zhu X, Wu L, Yang R, Yang Z, Wang Q. MicroRNA-122 suppresses cell proliferation and induces cell apoptosis in hepatocellular carcinoma by directly targeting Wnt/beta-catenin pathway. Liver International. 2012;**32**:752-760. DOI: 10.1111/ j.1478-3231.2011.02750.x

[97] Wu XL, Cheng B, Li PY, Huan- Huang J, Zhao Q, Dan ZL. MicroRNA-143 suppresses gastric cancer cell growth and induces apoptosis by targeting COX-2. World Journal of Gastroenterology. 2013;**19**(43):7758-7765. DOI: 10.3748/wjg.v19.i43.7758

[98] Yanokura M, Banno K, Iida M, Irie H, Umene K, Masuda K. MicroRNAs in endometrial cancer: Recent advances and potential clinical applications. EXCLI Journal. 2015;**14**:190-198. DOI: 10.17179/excli2014-590

[99] Hsieh TH, Hsu CY, Tsai CF, Long CY, Wu CH, Wu DC. HDAC inhibitors target HDAC5, upregulate microRNA-125a-5p, and induce apoptosis in breast cancer cells. Molecular Therapy: The Journal of the American Society of Gene Therapy. 2015;**23**(4):656-666. DOI: 10.1038/mt.2014.247

[100] Osanto S, Qin Y, Buermans HP, Berkers J, Lerut E, Goeman JJ, et al. Genome-wide microRNA expression analysis of clear cell renal cell carcinoma by next generation deep sequencing. PLoS One. 2012;**7**(6):e38298. DOI: 10.1371/journal.pone.0038298

[101] Ying X, Wei K, Lin Z, Cui Y, Ding J, Chen Y, et al. MicroRNA-125b suppresses ovarian cancer progression via suppression of the epithelial-mesenchymal transition pathway by targeting the SET protein. Cellular Physiology and Biochemistry. 2016;**39**(2):501-510. DOI: 10.1159/000445642

[102] Liao W, Zhang H, Feng C, Wang T, Zhang Y, Tang S. Downregulation of TrkA protein expression by miRNA 92a promotes the proliferation and migration of human neuroblastoma cells. Molecular Medicine Reports. 2014;**10**:778-784. DOI: 10.3892/mmr. 2014.2235

[103] Montalban E, Mattugini N, Ciarapica R, Provenzano C, Savino M, Scagnoli F, et al. MiR-21 is an Ngf-modulated microRNA that supports Ngf signaling and regulates neuronal degeneration in PC12. Cells Neuromolecular Medicine. 2014;**16**:415-430. DOI: 10.1007/s12017-014-8292-z

10

The Past, Present and Future of Diagnostic Imaging in Ovarian Cancer

Subapriya Suppiah

Abstract

Ovarian cancers (OC) include a group of diseases with variable prognoses. While most conventional imaging techniques rely on the detection of tumour burden and distant spread to identify treatment plans, more emphasis is now being placed on screening for early detection and also for more accurate staging using molecular imaging techniques. It is generally accepted that there are some incremental benefits of using serum CA125 levels coupled with cross-sectional diagnostic imaging to aid in the diagnosis, staging and treatment planning of OC. This chapter provides a review of tests and diagnostic imaging modalities that aid in the detection and staging of OC with a particular focus on F18-Fluorodeoxyglucose positron emission tomography/computed tomography (F18-FDG PET/CT) imaging. This chapter also proposes a diagnostic algorithm for the management of ovarian cancer. F18-FDG PET/CT imaging can act as a catalyst for the development of personalised medicine by stimulating advancements in targeted therapy. In conclusion, diagnostic imaging with particular focus in molecular imaging has the potential for altering management plans, which can ultimately help improve the prognosis of ovarian cancer.

Keywords: diagnostic imaging, MRI, PET/CT, molecular imaging, adnexal mass

1. Introduction

This chapter regarding diagnostic imaging aims to guide multidisciplinary teams to decide on further investigation of ovarian cancer (OC), by proposing a diagnostic imaging algorithm (**Figure 1**) for the detection and staging of this disease [1, 2]. Furthermore, it provides a special focus on the evolving utility of molecular imaging, specifically PET/CT imaging in the management of ovarian cancer [3].

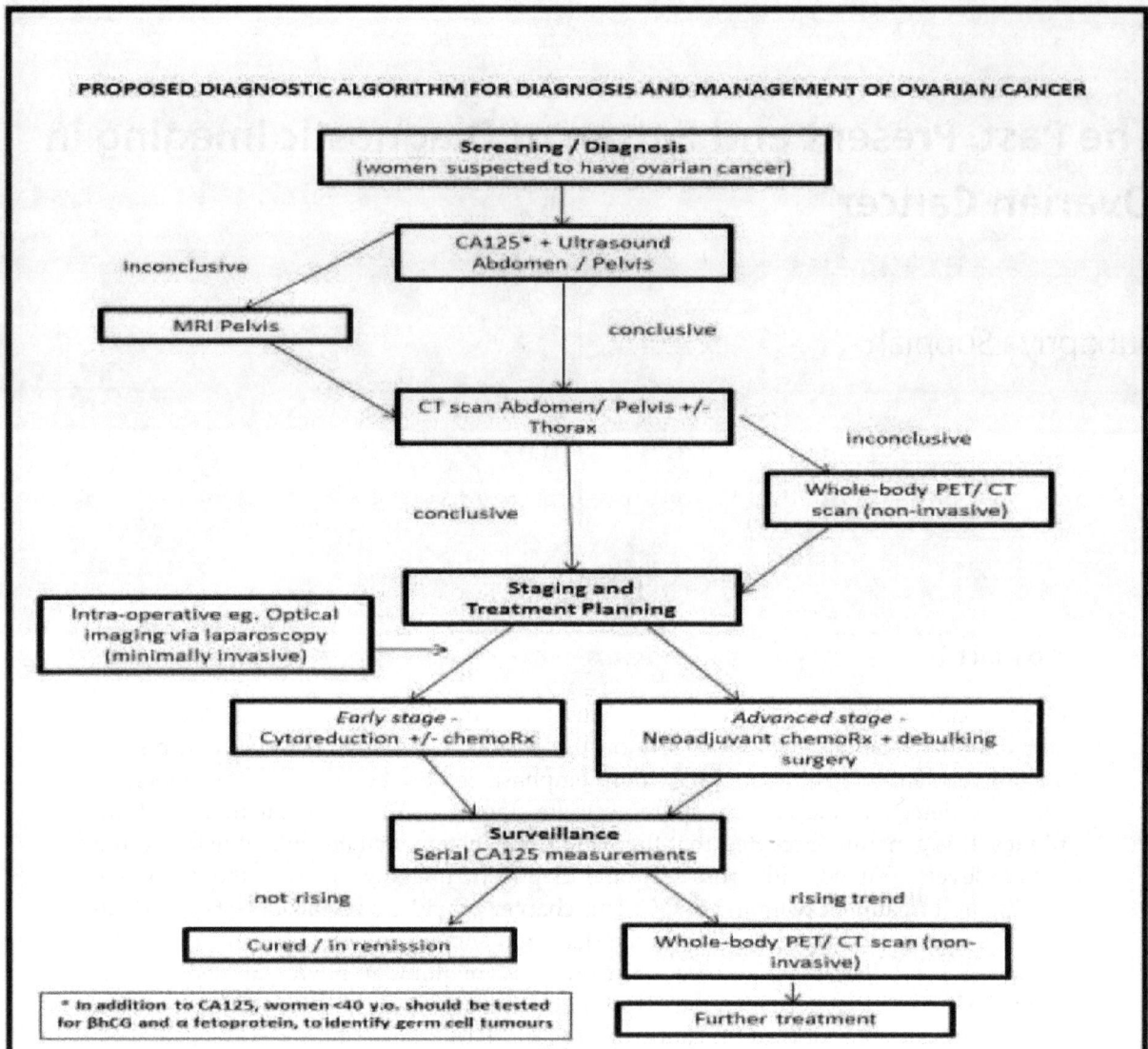

Figure 1. Diagnostic imaging algorithm for management of ovarian cancer (adapted from Suppiah et al. [1]).

Before illustrating diagnostic imaging methods for detecting OC, it is best to understand the embryology of the disease. Given that there is a remarkable morphologic and molecular heterogeneity in OC, therefore it has been postulated that ovarian cancers can be divided into Type I (indolent) and Type II (aggressive) tumours [4]. Type I is composed of low-grade serous, low-grade endometrioid, clear cell, mucinous and transitional carcinomas. These tumours are confined to the ovary at presentation and are relatively genetically stable and the majority display KRAS, BRAF and ERBB2 mutations [5]. Type II tumours include high-grade serous carcinoma (HGSC), undifferentiated carcinoma, and malignant mixed mesodermal tumours (carcinosarcoma), are highly aggressive, evolve rapidly and almost always present at an advanced stage. They display TP53 mutations in over 80% of cases and rarely harbour the mutations found in Type I tumours. Type I is suggested to be of Müllerian-type of tissues in origin, whereas Type II tumours are mesothelium in source and are suspected to originate from the Fallopian tubes [5].

Currently there is no test which is entirely distinct and suitable to be used for population screening in women with low to moderate risk of developing OC. Serum tumour marker CA125 measurement has been studied, and include single cut-off points [6] and time-series algorithms [7]. Serum CA125 coupled with conventional imaging such as ultrasound scans have been used to stratify patients who may be at a higher risk of having OC. Magnetic resonance imaging (MRI) and Computed tomography (CT) imaging are useful in further characterising lesions and staging the disease respectively. Conversely, once diagnosed, intra-operative imaging such as optical imaging and hand-held spectroscopic devices can also guide in the detection of small cancers [8].

Furthermore, the advent of newer *in vitro* cancer models to assess for ovarian cancer specific biomarkers has paved the way for the development of potential novel therapeutics [9]. The study of micro-environmental cues in the regulation of miRNAs has also generated a growing need for advancement of *in vivo* functional tests that can help determine the phenotype and physiology of ovarian cancer. Functional imaging such as positron emission tomography/computed tomography (PET/CT) using radiopharmaceuticals, namely 18F-Fluorodeoxyglucose (FDG) enables non-invasive assessment of *in vivo* cellular metabolism.

2. Multimodality diagnostic imaging

Diagnostic tests to detect epithelial ovarian cancer include using serum tumour marker levels correlated with imaging findings. Diagnostic imaging modalities that are frequently used to detect, stage and monitor treatment of ovarian cancers include ultrasound, computed tomography, magnetic resonance imaging and positron emission computed tomography.

2.1. Serum tumour marker CA125

CA125 is a protein that is found in greater concentrations in ovarian cancer tumour cells than in other cells of the human body. Therefore, a simple blood test, using a sample taken from a peripheral vein, makes it possible for it to be used as a marker to detect the presence of ovarian cancer. Nevertheless, it is non-specific for ovarian cancer, as raised levels may also be found in other malignancies, e.g., breast, lung, colon and pancreatic cancer as well as in benign conditions such as in endometriosis, pelvic inflammatory disease and ovarian cysts [10]. CA125 has a high positive predictive value (PPV) of >95%, but a low negative predictive value (NPV) ranging from 50 to 60%, for the detection of OC [11]. Some studies have advocated the use of a single CA125 level measurement, frequently quoting the value 35 IU/ml as a cut-off point to indicate the presence of malignancy [12, 13]. Levels above this have a good positive predictive value, however many actual cancers may have lower levels of CA125 and can be missed [14].

The National Institute for Health and Care Excellence (NICE) clinical guidelines recommend further tests to be done if a CA125 level of >35 IU/ml is detected in a woman suspected to have ovarian cancer [2]. Conversely, when a cut-off of 30 IU/ml is used, the test has a sensitivity of 81% and specificity of 75% [15]. In general, one of the methods for assessment of treatment response is by monitoring the CA125 levels. Moreover, longitudinal monitoring of CA125 levels can also provide additional information about survival in ovarian cancer [16].

2.2. Risk of malignancy index (RMI)

The risk of malignancy index (RMI) is a validated clinical tool that is used to assess the risk of having OC [2]. RMI combines three pre-surgical features which include serum CA125 levels using the unit IU/ml (CA125), menopausal status (M) and ultrasound score (U) for its assessment, using the formula: RMI = CA125 × M × U. The ultrasound result is scored 1 point for each of the following characteristics, namely the presence of multilocular cysts, solid areas, metastases, ascites and bilateral lesions. U = 0 (for an ultrasound score of 0), U = 1 (for an ultrasound score of 1), U = 3 (for an ultrasound score of 2–5). The menopausal status is scored as 1 = pre-menopausal and 3 = post-menopausal. The classification of 'post-menopausal' is a woman who has had no period for more than 1 year or a woman over 50 years of age and has had a hysterectomy [2].

According to the NICE guidelines, RMI scores are interpreted as low, moderate and high risk based on the total score [2]. Low-risk RMI is for scores <25 (noted in 40% of women, and the risk of cancer is <3%). Moderate-risk RMI is assigned for scores 25–250 (noted in 30% of women, and the risk of cancer is 20%), whereas scores >250 are associated with high-risk RMI (observed in 30% of women, and the risk of cancer is 75%). Women with moderate or intermediate risk are recommended to have an MRI for further evaluation of the ovarian lesion. Whereas, post-menopausal women with an RMI score of >250 should be referred to a cancer centre for further assessment and often undergo a staging computed tomography scan.

2.3. Ultrasound scan

Ultrasound (USS) is a safe, inexpensive and widely available diagnostic modality. Grey scale USS is a real-time imaging that detects the difference in the acoustic impedance (density × velocity of sound) of internal structures and can give excellent soft tissue detail for the evaluation of adnexal masses. Trans-abdominal scan (TAS) and transvaginal scan (TVS) are the first line diagnostic imaging modality for diagnosing OC. TAS utilises a low frequency (3.5–7 MHz) convex probe to characterise adnexal lesions that have grown beyond the pelvic brim. TVS uses a higher frequency (7.5–12 MHz) endocervical probe and gives better spatial resolution as it is placed closer to the ovaries; and is the first line modality of choice for small masses [16]. Nevertheless, a smaller field of view, leading to a possibility of overlooking a larger pelvic mass, is one of its limitations. Therefore, TAS is usually performed first followed by a TVS as a standard scan procedure.

In women suspected of having ovarian cancer, USS is indicated as a first line diagnostic imaging test. USS can diagnose the presence of an adnexal mass and help characterise it. The size, consistency, presence of loculations and solid component within a tumour; are some of the criteria used to characterise adnexal masses. A point to note is that an anechoic ovarian lesion detected in a postmenopausal woman should be considered as a physiological inclusion cyst, and not a pathological cyst if it was smaller than 10 mm and did not distort the ovary [17]. In certain occasions, the presence of bilateral lesions can be detected, and the pouch of Douglas is a common location for a left ovarian lesion (**Figure 2**).

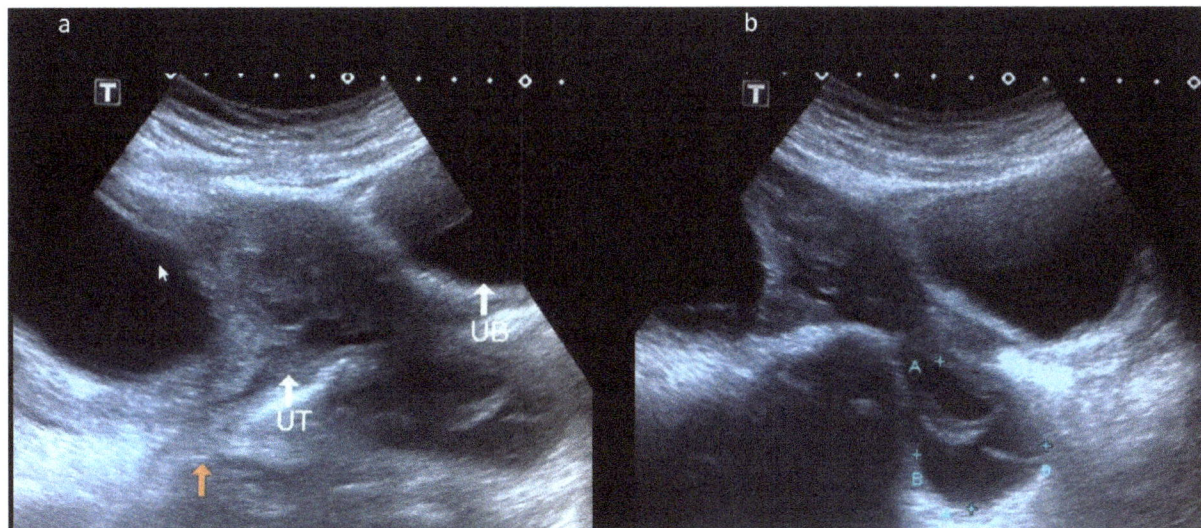

Figure 2. Grey scale ultrasound scans demonstrating suspicious bilateral large adnexal masses in a postmenopausal woman. The white arrow on the left indicates the uterus, the white arrow on the right indicates the urinary bladder and the orange arrow indicates the thick-walled right adnexal mass. Image (b) shows the dimensions of the left adnexal mass.

Figure 2a demonstrates a thick-walled, right adnexal lesion and **Figure 2b** demonstrates a multiseptated, left ovarian lesion in the pouch of Douglas.

2.4. Interpretation of ultrasound imaging

USS has improved specificity in detecting OC by the utility of simple ultrasound rules model [18]. In particular, by using the conventional technique of pattern recognition or subjective assessment by an experienced sonographer, the sensitivity and specificity were 83 and 90%. Whereas, by the technique of using the simple ultrasound rules (**Table 1**) was 92 and 96% respectively [19]. The rules comprised of five ultrasound features to predict a malignant tumour (M features) and five to predict a benign tumour (B features). These include features

Sonographic characteristics	Benign features (B features)	Malignant features (M features)
Tumour size	<100 mm	>100 mm
Loculations	Unilocular, smooth	Multilocular
Consistency	Cystic	Solid, mixed
Papillary projections	None/a few, thin	Multiple (at least 4), thick
Size of largest solid component	None/3–7 mm	Usually >7 mm
Wall	Thin, regular	Thick, irregular
Internal Doppler flow	None/minimal	Increased
Ascites	Absent	Present
Acoustic shadow	Present	Not applicable

Table 1. Sonographic characteristics of ovarian lesions based on simple ultrasound rules [18, 19].

of shape, size, solidity, and results of colour Doppler examination. Masses would be classified as malignant if one or more M features were present in the absence of a B feature. While if one or more B features were present in the absence of an M feature, the mass would be classified as benign. However, if both M features and B features were present, or if none of the features was present, the simple rules were considered inconclusive [20].

Colour Doppler can identify the presence of colour flow, within the papillary or solid components of an ovarian tumour and has good PPV for detecting malignancy. Nevertheless, the absence of colour flow in smaller lesions potentially causes falsely negative observations. False positive findings of flow can also occur in ovarian cysts in the luteal phase in premenopausal women [21].

The sensitivity and specificity of grey scale USS alone has been reported as 88% and 96% respectively; whereas, with the addition of colour Doppler as 83% and 97% respectively [22]. Although the introduction of power 3D Doppler has been able to increase the PPV of detecting malignancy; the availability of instruments and necessary expertise for interpretation has limited the use of this technique [23].

Several scoring systems have been suggested based on USS morphology of ovarian lesions to calculate and determine scores for malignancy [15, 24]. The PPV of these systems are small because the morphology of many benign lesions overlaps with that of malignant disease [21]. Rarely, certain OC are detected in large cysts, usually >7.5 cm in diameter; but do not exhibit an apparent complex morphology on ultrasound [25].

2.5. Limitations and future research in ultrasound

Recently, some experiments have been conducted to evaluate the role of contrast-enhanced USS to help further characterise ovarian tumours [26]. The meta-analysis of 10 studies revealed a pooled sensitivity of 0.89 and specificity of 0.91 respectively [27]. The limitation of ultrasound is the low sensitivity for detection of peritoneal metastasis [28]. Furthermore, screening low-risk population by transvaginal ultrasound may incidentally detect indeterminate lesions and lead to unnecessary biopsies [29]. Therefore, it should not be considered as a standalone investigation to be used to screen the general population for OC.

2.6. Computed tomography (CT) scan

Computed tomography (CT) scan utilises ionising radiation (photon beams of X-ray) to create cross sectional images of the internal organs. CT scans can give detailed information regarding tumour extent and metastatic disease (**Figure 3**). **Figure 3** is a multiplanar CT scan of a patient in axial, coronal and sagittal views, demonstrating a large ovarian cancer with intra-abdominal extension (white arrow) as well as gross ascites (black arrow) and thickened peritoneum consistent with metastasis (red arrow).

It is the preferred modality for the staging of OC and detection of recurrence because it is more widely available and less costly compared to magnetic resonance imaging (MRI) [30]. The Response Evaluation Criteria in Solid Tumours (RECIST) is often used in assessing treatment response in follow up CT scans and may be employed alone or in combination with CA125, for

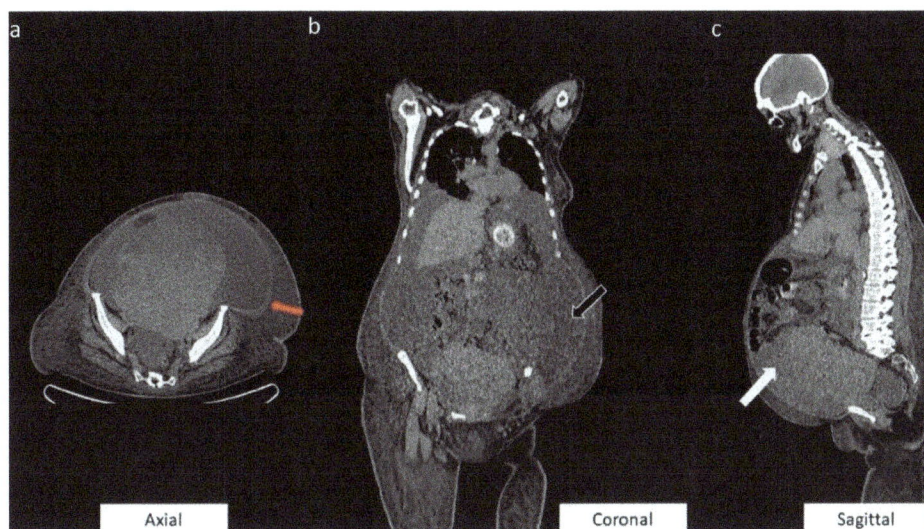

Figure 3. Multiplanar computed tomography scan demonstrating an ovarian cancer. The red arrow shows thickened peritoneum, black arrow shows gross ascites and white arrow shows a large adnexal mass.

evaluating the potential need to start or change the treatment regime [31]. Contrast-enhanced CT (CECT) studies have an added advantage compared to low dose non-enhanced CT scans, as they enable improved delineation of anatomical structures, and increased sensitivity for detection of pathological lesions [32]. Contrast-enhanced PET/CT is a more accurate imaging modality than PET using low dose CT for assessing OC recurrence [33].

Conventional CT has a limited and variable sensitivity of 40–93% and specificity of 50–98% for detection of recurrent disease [30]. Spiral CT can improve the detection of peritoneal lesions and implants, in particular in those with concurrent ascites. Obtaining a CT before secondary debulking may aid in surgical planning and to assess the feasibility of achieving maximum resectability [34].

Contrast-enhanced CT scans (CECT) can detect the involvement of specific intra-abdominal sites recognised to reduce the chances of optimal debulking. These sites include suprarenal aortic lymph nodes, disease in the root of the mesentery, portal triad disease, or bulky liver disease [35]. Conversely, multidetector CECT scans often underestimates the extent of liver surface disease and infra-renal para-aortic lymph node involvement [36]. The reliability of CT assessment is also related to improvements in imaging techniques as well as scanner equipment and this can vary across different centres [37].

2.7. Interpretation of computed tomography scans

CECT provides improved contrast resolution in delineating suspicious adnexal masses [38]. CECT is helpful in characterising benign and malignant ovarian tumours by observation of certain characteristic features (**Table 2**). It can also help differentiate OC subtypes, albeit with some overlapping features, especially the commoner subtypes such as serous tumours. Serous tumours are usually unilocular but with multiple papillary projections and often present bilaterally [39]. Furthermore, peritoneal carcinomatosis is also seen more frequently in serous adenocarcinomas [40].

CT scan characteristics	Benign	Malignant
Size	<4 cm	>4 cm
Consistency	Cystic	Mixed/Solid
Papillary projections	Absent/a few	Multiple
Wall	Thin, regular	Thick, irregular
Internal calcifications	Occasionally present	Infrequently present
Pelvic lymphadenopathy	Absent	Present
Laterality	Unilateral	Bilateral
Ascites	Absent	Present
Peritoneal involvement	Absent	Present
Distant organ metastasis	Absent	Present

Table 2. Computed tomography characteristics of adnexal masses (adapted from Suppiah et al. [38] and Jung et al. [9]).

2.8. Limitations and future research in computed tomography

The main limitation of a CT scan is its inability to detect deposits on bowel serosa, mesentery and omental regions that are smaller than 5 mm; especially in the absence of ascites. However, this can be solved by pre-surgical laparoscopic assessment. The detection of sub-diaphragmatic peritoneal deposits are also difficult, but can be aided by multiplanar reformatting of contrast-enhanced scans.

2.9. Magnetic resonance imaging (MRI)

Magnetic resonance imaging (MRI) uses a high strength magnetic field and pulsed radio-frequency waves to generate images with excellent soft tissue detail. It does not utilise ionising radiation and is relatively safe to use. It commonly involves acquiring T1-weighted, T2-weighted, fat-saturation spin echo, and usually, includes post-gadolinium contrast-enhanced T1-weighted fat-saturation sequences for the pelvic region. This protocol includes a full abdominal scan in three planes for the staging of ovarian cancer [41].

The ability of MRI to correctly stage ovarian cancer is excellent, providing a sensitivity and specificity of 98 and 88% respectively, as compared to 92 and 89% respectively for CECT [41]. MRI and CT have been noted to be more sensitive than ultrasound for detection of peritoneal metastases. The accuracy of MRI (76%) is also better than CT (57%) for detection of lymph nodes [28]. The improved soft tissue resolution achieved by MRI is able to better delineate the presence of pathological lymph nodes, both within the pelvic cavity as well as extra-pelvic spread. However, its limitations are that it is rather costly, time-consuming and often difficult to interpret due to breathing and bowel movement artefacts.

Therefore, the clinical utility of MRI is limited to evaluation of indeterminate pelvic lesions. MRI can detect haemorrhagic lesions and enhancement in papillary projections, as well as identify the fatty tissue components within individual adnexal tumours. It can delineate ovarian lesions from uterine or urinary bladder involvement. MRI is also useful in cases where CECT is relatively contraindicated such as in the pregnant woman, in a patient with, a history of dye allergy or where giving iodinated contrast material is contraindicated, e.g., in renal impairment. Hence, a non-contrast-enhanced MRI scan should be performed instead.

2.10. Interpretation of magnetic resonance imaging

MRI is able to differentiate simple ovarian cysts from malignant lesions with solid internal components. Simple cysts return a low signal in the case of T1-weighted images and a high signal in T2-weighted images, whereas malignant lesions are often heterogeneous and show marked enhancement of its solid components. MRI is best to delineate the local extent of the tumour as well as detect pelvic nodal metastases.

2.11. Limitations and future research in magnetic resonance imaging

The utility of whole-body diffusion-weighted imaging in magnetic resonance imaging (WB-DWI/MRI) has shown some promising results. Diffusion-weighted imaging measures the Brownian motion of extracellular water and thereby approximates tissue cellularity and fluid viscosity, hence malignant tumours that have increased cellularity will have restricted diffusion, thus giving lower apparent diffusion coefficient (ADC) values. Interestingly, DWI/ADC sequences have shown 94% accuracy for primary tumour characterisation which is comparable with the results of 18F-Fluorodeoxyglucose positron emission tomography/computed tomography (18F-FDG PET/CT) [42].

WB-DWI/MRI has also shown an improved accuracy of 91% for peritoneal staging compared with CT (75%) and 18F-FDG PET/CT (71%). It also has higher accuracy (87%) for detecting retroperitoneal lymphadenopathies compared to CT scans (71%) [42]. However, this study was limited by the relatively small number of cases, the discrepancy between the ratio of MRI and PET/CT cases performed as well as the relatively large number of patients who presented with advanced disease, potentially increasing the pre-test likelihood of detecting metastases.

2.12. Positron emission tomography-computed tomography (PET/CT) scan

Molecular imaging, namely Positron Emission Tomography-Computed Tomography (PET/CT) scans are indicated for the detection of recurrence of OC as even small volume disease can easily be detected. It is considered by the European Society of Medical Oncology (ESMO) as an appropriate imaging modality to help in the selection of patients for secondary debulking surgery. PET/CT can alter the management plan in metastatic ovarian cancers by detecting additional sites of disease not seen on CT scans, and identifying locations that are not amenable to cytoreduction [1].

PET/CT can assess tumour aggressiveness by demonstrating an elevated level of the injected radiopharmaceutical, e.g., 18F-Fluorodeoxyglucose (18F-FDG) that is trapped in tumour cells, as quantified by standardised uptake values (SUV) [43]. Interestingly, elevated maximum standardised uptake values (SUVmax) are frequently detected in the ovaries in the luteal phase of the menstrual cycle. This is considered as normal physiological FDG metabolism and should not be mistaken for pathology. Therefore, PET/CT scans should be scheduled right after the menstruation to minimise this observed effect in premenopausal women.

PET/CT scans are performed using a hybrid PET/CT scanner commonly using 3D lutetium oxy-orthosilicate crystals as detectors for the PET component. It is recommended that the examination include a diagnostic contrast-enhanced computed tomography (CECT) scan by the administration of low osmolar iodinated contrast media. Apart from enabling attenuation correction, and anatomical localisation; CECT is essential for performing diagnostic clinical staging [1]. Patients are instructed to fast for a minimum of 6 h before scanning, and blood glucose is checked before the scan. Subsequently, 18F-FDG will be administered and subjects are kept in a dark room for approximately 60 min to allow for uptake time. Subjects are given approximately 100 mL (2 ml/kg body weight) of iodinated contrast media during the CECT scan. Immediately after the CT, PET images acquisition will be performed over the same anatomic regions. The attenuation corrected CECT images will then be fused with PET images. The combined images will be utilised for visual interpretation, tumour size and maximum standard uptake value (SUVmax) measurements.

2.13. Interpretation of positron emission tomography-computed tomography (PET/CT) scans

Abnormal FDG hypermetabolism is analysed on the PET/CT images, starting from a survey of the maximum intensity projection (MIP) 3D image of the PET component. Regions commonly evaluated to detect nodal spread and distant metastases include the pelvic, abdominal and inguinal lymph nodes; the uterus, urinary bladder, peritoneum, omentum, bowel, liver, lungs and bones. Adnexal lesions frequently have a variable FDG uptake irrespective of their histopathological origin. For instance, mucinous carcinomas do not demonstrate avid FDG uptake compared to serous tumours [44]. It is postulated that indolent (Type I) and aggressive (Type II) ovarian cancers may arise from different cell lines [5]. Thus, Type I tumours do not demonstrate significantly elevated SUVmax values.

The sensitivity, specificity, PPV and NPV of PET/CT in detecting OC metastases are 87, 100, 81 and 100% respectively [45]. Moreover, PET/CT has improved accuracy at detecting peritoneal seeding, sub-diaphragmatic involvement, distant organ metastasis, bowel invasion and extra-abdominal lymph node involvement which has led to a reduction in the rate of second look surgery [46]. A negative PET/CT has NPV of 90% for detection of recurrence within a two-year follow-up period [2]. PET/CT scan in axial, coronal and sagittal views was able to detect bowel invasion (red arrow) in an advanced ovarian cancer disease (white arrow) (**Figure 4**). Therefore, it can aid in the decision-making for primary debulking surgery followed by platinum-based chemotherapy as opposed to treatment using neoadjuvant chemotherapy.

PET/CT is also able to demonstrate the heterogeneity of ovarian cancers. (**Figure 5**) There is moderate FDG uptake noted in serous adenocarcinomas of the ovary as seen in **Figure 5a**. Endometrioid adenocarcinomas often have multiple cystic areas within and can be associated

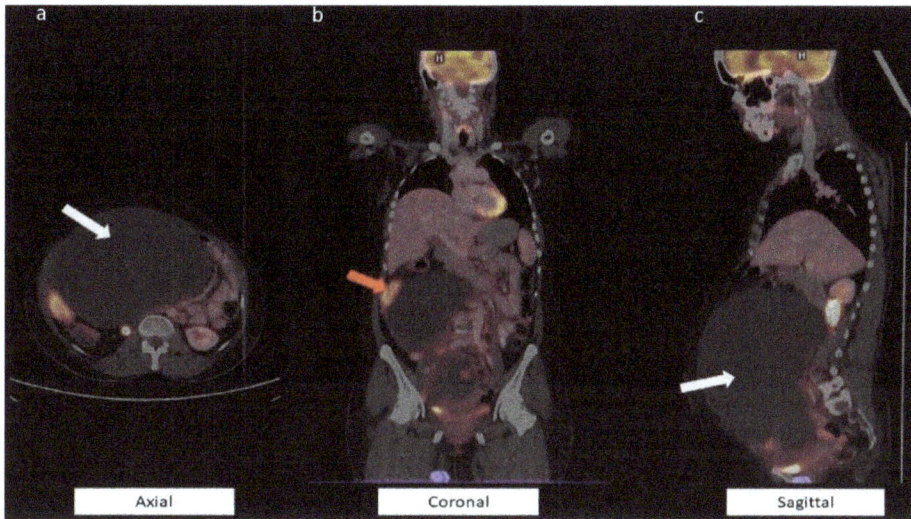

Figure 4. PET/CT scan demonstrating an advanced ovarian cancer. White arrows show a large adnexal tumour with heterogeneous FDG uptake. Red arrow shows bowel involvement.

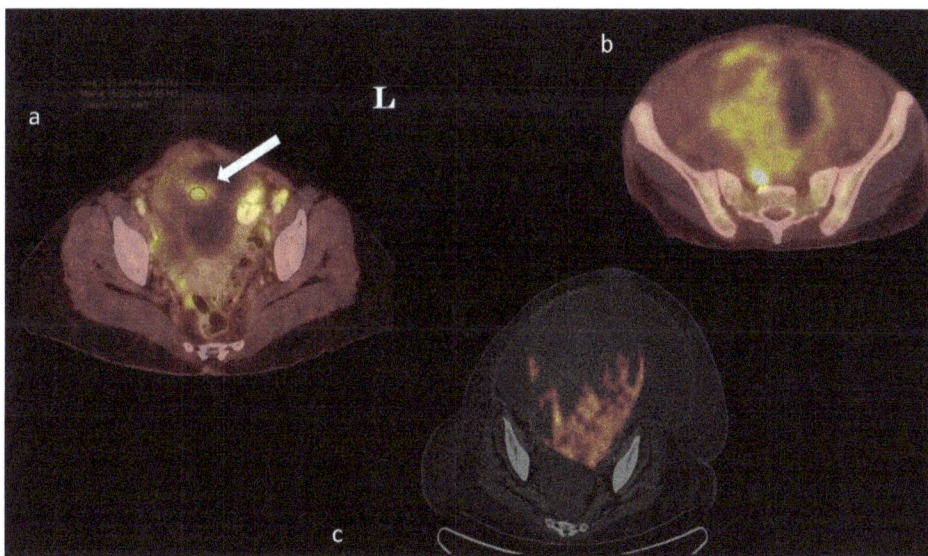

Figure 5. PET/CT scans in axial view demonstrating malignant ovarian tumours. White arrow shows markedly increased FDG uptake within the solid component of the tumour.

with internal calcifications as seen in **Figure 5b**. Mucinous adenocarcinomas often have low FDG uptake as seen in **Figure 5c** and represent a diagnostic caveat against dismissing them as benign lesions.

2.14. Limitations and future research in positron emission tomography-computed tomography (PET/CT) scans

The current theory postulates that high grade serous ovarian carcinoma (HGSC) originate from the fimbrial end of fallopian tubes [47]. It has sparked interest as to whether risk-reducing opportunistic salpingectomy could be performed to preserve fertility in a premenopausal woman with high risk of developing ovarian cancer. There is a need to explore the role of PET/CT or rather MR/PET, which may be able to detect disease at an earlier stage especially when it is still localised to the fallopian tubes.

Apart from 18F-FDG, other tracers have also been studied to assess for recurrent or residual ovarian cancer. These include 11C-Choline which can help better delineate pelvic lesions [48]; as well as 16α-18F-fluoro-17β-estradiol (FES) which have the potential to evaluate the response to hormonal therapy for ovarian cancer [44]. Another tracer also in the experimental stage, is 3′-deoxy-3′-18F-fluorothymidine (FLT) that distributes rapidly in the extracellular fluid and is phosphorylated by thymidine kinase 1(TK-1) and becomes trapped in tumours with increased cellular proliferation activity. The role of FLT PET/CT may be in assessing and predicting response to an antitumour type of therapy, where it has been shown to be superior to 18F-FDG PET/CT [49].

2.15. Other research-based imaging techniques and work in progress

Positron Emission Tomography/Magnetic Resonance (PET/MR) is an emerging technique, which uses scanners that acquire MR and PET data either simultaneously or sequentially. Simultaneous acquisition devices, some called the mMR scanners, allow for concurrent imaging of the same body region. Alternatively, sequential scanning is done using two different scanners during one examination session, and the images are fused later. PET/MR acquisition protocol for assessment of a gynaecological tumour includes whole-body Dixon and a dedicated pelvic MRI exam that includes dynamic intravenous gadolinium administration [50]. It is suitable for assessment of the loco-regional extent of a pelvic tumour and evaluates the entire body for metastases, albeit having a very long scanning time of approximately 1.0–1.5 h [50].

Additionally, PET/MRI may be a more useful modality as compared to PET/CT for the detection of miliary disseminated metastases in cases of suspected OC recurrence [2]. As evident in **Figure 6** in which PET/MRI demonstrates FDG avid uptake in the para-aortic lymph nodes (**Figure 6**). Furthermore, PET/CT potentially gives high false negative results in the case of small volume disease which predisposes it to miss low-grade tumours and early adenocarcinomas [51]. Therefore, it is recommended to be used in conjunction with transvaginal ultrasound or MRI for characterisation of adnexal masses and the detection of OC.

PET/MRI ideally has added value in oncologic imaging due to its improved soft-tissue resolution. Furthermore, sophisticated sequences such as diffusion-weighted imaging, functional MRI, and MR spectroscopy can all be incorporated with molecular imaging, giving further information but with less radiation exposure. This can provide a significant reduction in radiation dose and exposure in patients who require follow-up imaging [3].

Some other imaging techniques are performed intra-operatively, namely the sentinel node procedure (SNP). SNP is sometimes conducted in patients with a high likelihood of having an OC in whom a median laparotomy and a frozen section analysis is planned. The concept of SNP is to determine whether the OC has spread to the very first lymph node (sentinel node). If the sentinel node is negative for cancer cells, then there is a high likelihood that the cancer has not spread to other lymph nodes [52]. Blue dye and radioactive colloid are injected into either the ovaries or the ovarian ligaments to perform the SNP [53].

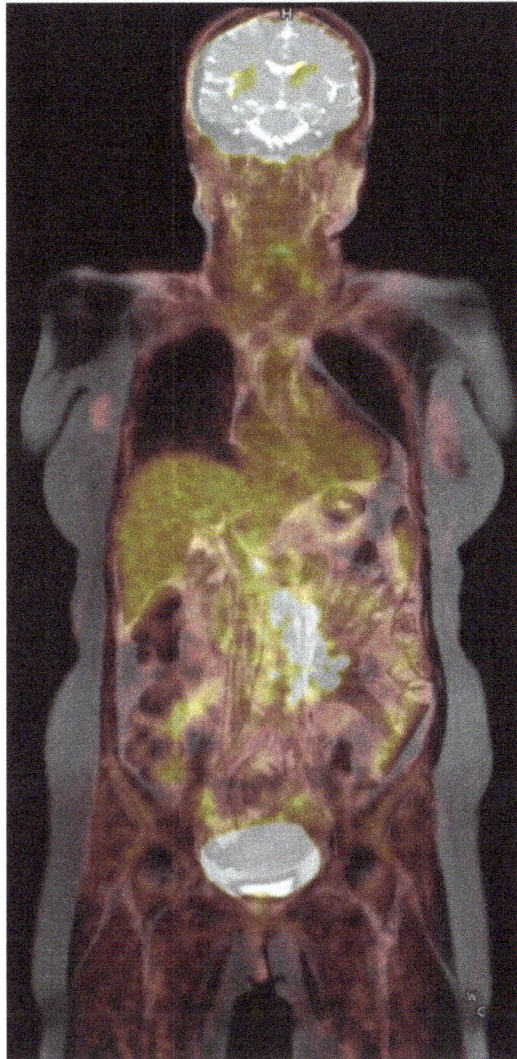

Figure 6. PET/MRI scan demonstrating recurrent ovarian cancer with para-aortic lymph nodes involvement. MRI gives good soft tissue resolution of the FDG avid lymph nodes noted at central abdomen.

After the incubation time, usually 10–15 min, the sentinel nodes can be visualised by either colorization (blue lymph nodes can be identified) and/or with a gamma probe that detects the radioactive tracer. The pathological examination of the sentinel node is an indication of the nodal status of the remaining nodes; when the sentinel node is negative, one can presume that the remaining nodes are also not involved. As a consequence, the patient may be spared from undergoing radical lymphadenectomy, and thus the morbidity associated with it.

Conventional diagnostic imaging modalities lack specificity and sensitivity in the detection of small primary and disseminated tumours in the peritoneal cavity. Using the knowledge that HER-2 receptors are overexpressed in ovarian tumours, a near infrared (NIR) optical imaging approach for detection of ovarian tumours using a HER-2 targeted nanoparticle-based imaging agent in an orthotopic mouse model of ovarian cancer has been conducted achieving improved detection of smaller lesions [54].

Furthermore, the overexpression of folate receptor-α (FR-α) in OC, has prompted the investigation of intra-operative tumour-specific fluorescence imaging. It has potential applications in patients with OC for improved intra-operative staging and more radical cytoreductive surgery [55]. Additionally, optical coherence tomography (OCT) is another emerging high-resolution imaging technique that utilises an infrared light source directed to the tissues being examined. A novel prototype intra-operative OCT system combining positron detections; namely utilising Caesium (Tl204/Cs137) sources as well as 18F-FDG have shown potential for the development of a miniaturised laparoscopic probe to detect small volume disease of OC. This can offer simultaneous functional localisation and structural imaging for improved early cancer detection [56].

3. Conclusion

In summary, ovarian cancer is a heterogeneous spectrum of disease. Early detection and accurate staging using diagnostic imaging can help improve the prognosis of this condition. Prudent selection of the appropriate imaging modality can help expedite the correct treatment being instituted for the patients (**Table 3**). Molecular imaging, particularly 18F-FDG PET/CT can be a useful non-invasive biomarker to help stage the disease and detect recurrence based on the proposed diagnostic algorithm in this chapter.

Modality	Advantage	Disadvantage
Ultrasound	• Relatively cheap • Easily available • Does not involve ionising radiation	• Operator dependent • Unable to accurately stage the disease
CT scan	• Good for staging • Readily available	• Involves ionising radiation • Has pitfalls that lead to falsely negative findings
MRI	• Excellent soft tissue detail and able to characterise the pelvic lesion • Does not involve ionising radiation	• Relatively expensive • Longer scanning time • Requires specialised skills for interpretation
PET/CT	• Excellent for staging and detection of recurrence • Good for detection of extra-abdominal metastases	• Involves ionising radiation • Prone to false positive results • Requires specialised skills for interpretation
PET/MRI	• Excellent soft tissue detail and able to improve detection of nodal and peritoneal metastases • Slightly reduced radiation dose compared to pet/CT	• Expensive • Longer scanning time • Requires specialised skills for interpretation
Intra-operative devices	• Able to detect small volume disease • Able to delineate local extent of disease in a small region of interest	• Costly • Operator dependent • Requires specialised skills for interpretation

Table 3. Comparison of the diagnostic imaging modalities for the management of ovarian cancer.

Acknowledgements

I would like to express my gratitude to the Dean of the Faculty of Medicine and Health Sciences, Universiti Putra Malaysia (UPM), Professor Dato' Dr. Abdul Jalil Nordin; and the Lead Consultant from the Nuclear Medicine Department at the Royal Liverpool and Broadgreen University Hospitals, NHS Trusts, Liverpool, the United Kingdom of Great Britain, Professor Dr. Sobhan Vinjamuri, my mentors; for their invaluable comments during preparation of this manuscript. I would also like to acknowledge Universiti Putra Malaysia research grant GP/IPM/2014/9404000 and GP/2017/9549800 that helped fund this project; and the fellowship training scholarship awarded by the International Atomic Energy Agency (IAEA) that enabled the collaboration with the United Kingdom counterparts. I would also like to thank the Director of the Centre for Diagnostic Nuclear Imaging, UPM; Associate Professor Dr. Fathinul Fikri Ahmad Saad for giving permission to use images from the centre as well as the Director General of Health, Ministry of Health Malaysia for giving permission to use images from Serdang Hospital, Malaysia.

Author details

Subapriya Suppiah

Address all correspondence to: subapriya@upm.edu.my

Centre for Diagnostic Nuclear Imaging, Universiti Putra Malaysia, Serdang, Malaysia

References

[1] Suppiah S, Asri AAA, Saad FFA, Hassan HA, CWL NM, Mahmud R, Nordin AJ. Contrast-enhanced 18F-FDG PET/CT in preoperative assessment of suspicious adnexal masses and proposed diagnostic imaging algorithm: A single centre experience in Malaysia. Malaysian Journal of Medicine and Health Sciences. 2017;**13**(1):1-8

[2] Ovarian Cancer: Recognition and Initial Management. 2011. NICE.org.uk

[3] Suppiah S, Chang WL, Hassan HA, Kaewput C, Asri AAA, Saad FFA, Nordin AJ, Vinjamuri S. Systematic review on the accuracy of positron emission tomography/computed tomography and positron emission tomography/magnetic resonance imaging in the management of ovarian cancer: Is functional information really Needed? World Journal of Nuclear Medicine. 2017;**16**(3):176-185. DOI: 10.4103/wjnm.WJNM_31_17

[4] Shih I-M, Kurman RJ. Ovarian tumorigenesis: A proposed model based on morphological and molecular genetic analysis. The American Journal of Pathology [Internet]. 2004;**164**(5):1511-1518. Available from: http://www.ncbi.nlm.nih.gov/pubmed/15111296 [cited 2017 Sept. 6]

[5] Kurman RJ, Shih IM. The origin and pathogenesis of epithelial ovarian cancer: A proposed unifying theory. The American Journal of Surgical Pathology [Internet]. 2010;

34(3):433-443. Available from: http://content.wkhealth.com/linkback/openurl?sid=WKPT LP:landingpage&an=00000478-201003000-00018 [cited 2017 Sept. 6]

[6]   Buys SS, Partridge E, Black A, Johnson CC, Lamerato L, Isaacs C, et al. Effect of screening on ovarian cancer mortality. JAMA [Internet]. 2011;**305**(22):2295. Available from: http://www.ncbi.nlm.nih.gov/pubmed/21642681 [cited 2017 Aug. 29]

[7]   Lu KH, Skates S, Hernandez MA, Bedi D, Bevers T, Leeds L, et al. A 2-stage ovarian cancer screening strategy using the Risk of Ovarian Cancer Algorithm (ROCA) identifies early-stage incident cancers and demonstrates high positive predictive value. Cancer [Internet]. 2013;**119**(19):3454-3461. Available from: http://doi.wiley.com/10.1002/cncr.28183 [cited 2017 Sept. 6]

[8]   Weissleder R, Pittet MJ. Imaging in the era of molecular oncology. Nature [Internet]. 2008;**452**(7187):580-589. NIH Public Access. Available from: http://www.ncbi.nlm.nih.gov/pubmed/18385732 [cited 2018 Jan. 15]

[9]   Mitra AK, Chiang CY, Tiwari P, Tomar S, Watters KM, Peter ME, et al. Microenvironment-induced downregulation of miR-193b drives ovarian cancer metastasis. Oncogene [Internet]. 2015;**34**(48):5923-5932. Nature Publishing Group. Available from: http://www.nature.com/doifinder/10.1038/onc.2015.43 [cited 2017 Sept. 6]

[10] Ledermann JA, Raja FA, Fotopoulou C, Gonzalez-Martin A, Colombo N, Sessa C. Newly diagnosed and relapsed epithelial ovarian carcinoma: ESMO Clinical Practice Guidelines for diagnosis, treatment and follow-up. Annals of Oncology [Internet]. 2013;**24**(Suppl. 6):vi24-vi32. Springer, Berlin,Heidelberg, New York. Available from: https://academic.oup.com/annonc/article-lookup/doi/10.1093/annonc/mdt333 [cited 2017 Sept. 6]

[11] Son H, Khan SM, Rahaman J, Cameron KL, Prasad-Hayes M, Chuang L, Machac J, Heiba S, Kostakoglu L. Role of FDG PET/CT in staging of recurrent ovarian cancer. Radiographics [Internet]. 2011;**31**:569-583. Available from: www.rsna [cited 2017 Sept. 6]

[12] Kobayashi H, Yamada Y, Sado T, Sakata M, Yoshida S, Kawaguchi R, et al. A randomized study of screening for ovarian cancer: A multicenter study in Japan. International Journal of Gynecological Cancer [Internet]. 2008;**18**(3):414-420. Available from: http://www.ncbi.nlm.nih.gov/pubmed/17645503 [cited 2017 Sept. 6]

[13] Markman M, Federico M, Liu PY, Hannigan E, Alberts D. Significance of early changes in the serum CA-125 antigen level on overall survival in advanced ovarian cancer. Gynecologic Oncology [Internet]. 2006;**103**(1):195-198. Available from: http://www.ncbi.nlm.nih.gov/pubmed/16595148 [cited 2017 Sept. 6]

[14] Beşe T, Demirkiran F, Arvas M, Oz AU, Kösebay D, Erkün E. What should be the cut-off level of serum CA125 to evaluate the disease status before second-look laparotomy in epithelial ovarian carcinoma? International Journal of Gynecological Cancer [Internet]. 1997;**7**(1):42-45. Available from: http://www.ncbi.nlm.nih.gov/pubmed/12795803 [cited 2017 Aug. 29]

[15] Jacobs I, Oram D, Fairbanks J, Turner J, Frost C, Grudzinskas JG. A risk of malignancy index incorporating CA 125, ultrasound and menopausal status for the accurate

preoperative diagnosis of ovarian cancer. British Journal of Obstetrics and Gynaecology [Internet]. 1990;**97**(10):922-929. Available from: http://www.ncbi.nlm.nih.gov/pubmed/2223684 [cited 2017 Aug. 29]

[16] Gupta D, Lammersfeld CA, Vashi PG, Braun DP. Longitudinal monitoring of CA125 levels provides additional information about survival in ovarian cancer. Journal of Ovarian Research [Internet]. 2010;**3**:22. BioMed Central. Available from: http://www.ncbi.nlm.nih.gov/pubmed/20939881 [cited 2017 Aug. 29]

[17] Menon U, Gentry-Maharaj A, Hallett R, Ryan A, Burnell M, Sharma A, et al. Sensitivity and specificity of multimodal and ultrasound screening for ovarian cancer, and stage distribution of detected cancers: results of the prevalence screen of the UK Collaborative Trial of Ovarian Cancer Screening (UKCTOCS). The Lancet Oncology [Internet]. 2009;**10**(4):327-340. Available from: http://linkinghub.elsevier.com/retrieve/pii/S1470204509700269 [cited 2017 Sept. 7]

[18] Timmerman D, Valentin L, Bourne TH, Collins WP, Verrelst H, Vergote I. Terms, definitions and measurements to describe the sonographic features of adnexal tumors: A consensus opinion from the International Ovarian Tumor Analysis (IOTA) group. Ultrasound in Obstetrics & Gynecology [Internet]. 2000;**16**(5):500-505. Blackwell Science Ltd. Available from: http://www.blackwell-synergy.com/links/doi/10.1046/j.1469-0705.2000.00287.x [cited 2017 Sept. 7]

[19] Valentin L, Hagen B, Tingulstad S, Eik-Nes S. Comparison of "pattern recognition" and logistic regression models for discrimination between benign and malignant pelvic masses: A prospective cross validation. Ultrasound in Obstetrics & Gynecology [Internet]. 2001;**18**(4):357-365. Blackwell Science Ltd. Available from: http://doi.wiley.com/10.1046/j.0960-7692.2001.00500.x [cited 2017 Sept. 7]

[20] Timmerman D, Ameye L, Fischerova D, Epstein E, Melis GB, Guerriero S, et al. Simple ultrasound rules to distinguish between benign and malignant adnexal masses before surgery: Prospective validation by IOTA group. BMJ [Internet]. 2010;**341**:c6839. Available from: http://www.ncbi.nlm.nih.gov/pubmed/21156740 [cited 2017 Sept. 7]

[21] Varras M. Benefits and limitations of ultrasonographic evaluation of uterine adnexal lesions in early detection of ovarian cancer. Clinical and Experimental Obstetrics and Gynecology [Internet]. 2004;**31**(2):85-98. Available from: http://www.ncbi.nlm.nih.gov/pubmed/15266758 [cited 2017 Sept. 7]

[22] Valentin L. Pattern recognition of pelvic masses by gray-scale ultrasound imaging: The contribution of Doppler ultrasound. Ultrasound in Obstetrics & Gynecology [Internet]. 1999;**14**(5):338-347. Blackwell Science Ltd. Available from: http://www.blackwell-synergy.com/links/doi/10.1046/j.1469-0705.1999.14050338.x [cited 2017 Sept. 7]

[23] Das PM, Bast RC Jr. Early detection of ovarian cancer. Biomarkers in Medicine [Internet]. 2008;**2**(3):291-303. NIH Public Access. Available from: http://www.ncbi.nlm.nih.gov/pubmed/20477415 [cited 2017 Aug. 29]

[24] Tingulstad S, Hagen B, Skjeldestad FE, Halvorsen T, Nustad K, Onsrud M. The risk-of-malignancy index to evaluate potential ovarian cancers in local hospitals. Obstetrics & Gynecology [Internet]. 1999;93(3):448-452. Available from: http://www.ncbi.nlm.nih.gov/pubmed/10074998 [cited 2017 Sept. 7]

[25] Brown DL, Dudiak KM, Laing FC. Adnexal masses: US characterization and reporting. Radiology [Internet]. 2010;254(2):342-354. Radiological Society of North America, Inc. Available from: http://pubs.rsna.org/doi/10.1148/radiol.09090552 [cited 2017 Sept. 7]

[26] Wang J, Lv F, Fei X, Cui Q, Wang L, Gao X, et al. Study on the characteristics of contrast-enhanced ultrasound and its utility in assessing the microvessel density in ovarian tumors or tumor-like lesions. International Journal of Biological Sciences [Internet]. 2011;7(5):600-606. Ivyspring International Publisher. Available from: http://www.ncbi.nlm.nih.gov/pubmed/21614152 [cited 2017 Sept. 7]

[27] Wu Y, Peng H, Zhao X. Diagnostic performance of contrast-enhanced ultrasound for ovarian cancer: A meta-analysis. Ultrasound in Medicine & Biology [Internet]. 2015; 41(4):967-974. Available from: http://www.ncbi.nlm.nih.gov/pubmed/25701533 [cited 2017 Sept. 7]

[28] Tempany CMC, Zou KH, Silverman SG, Brown DL, Kurtz AB, BJ MN. Staging of advanced ovarian cancer: Comparison of imaging modalities—Report from the Radiological Diagnostic Oncology Group. Radiology [Internet]. 2000;215(3):761-767. Available from: http://www.ncbi.nlm.nih.gov/pubmed/10831697 [cited 2017 Sept. 9]

[29] Partridge E, Kreimer AR, Greenlee RT, Williams C, Xu J-L, Church TR, et al. Results from four rounds of ovarian cancer screening in a randomized trial. Obstetrics & Gynecology [Internet]. 2009;113(4):775-782. Available from: http://www.pubmedcentral.nih.gov/articlerender.fcgi?artid=2728067&tool=pmcentrez&rendertype=abstract [cited 2016 Apr. 6]

[30] Marcus CS, Maxwell GL, Darcy KM, Hamilton CA, WP MG. Current approaches and challenges in managing and monitoring treatment response in ovarian cancer. Journal of Cancer [Internet]. 2014;5(1):25-30. Available from: http://www.jcancer.org/v05p0025.htm [cited 2017 Sept. 9]

[31] Eisenhauer EA. Optimal assessment of response in ovarian cancer. Annals of Oncology [Internet]. 2011;22(Suppl. 8):viii49-viii51. Available from: http://www.ncbi.nlm.nih.gov/pubmed/22180400 [cited 2017 Aug. 29]

[32] Antoch G, Freudenberg LS, Beyer T, Bockisch A, Debatin JF. To enhance or not to enhance? 18F-FDG and CT contrast agents in dual-modality 18F-FDG PET/CT. Journal of Nuclear Medicine [Internet]. 2004;45(Suppl. 1):56S-65S. Available from: http://www.ncbi.nlm.nih.gov/pubmed/14736836 [cited 2017 Sept. 9]

[33] Kitajima K, Ueno Y, Suzuki K, Kita M, Ebina Y, Yamada H, Senda M, Maeda T, Sugimura K. Low-dose non-enhanced CT versus full-dose contrast enhanced CT in integrated PET/CT scans for diagnosing ovarian cancer recurrence. European Journal of Radiology. 2012;81(11):3557-3562

[34] Funt SA, Hricak H, Abu-Rustum N, Mazumdar M, Felderman H, Chi DS. Role of CT in the management of recurrent ovarian cancer. American Journal of Roentgenology [Internet]. 2004;**182**(2):393-398. Available from: http://www.ncbi.nlm.nih.gov/pubmed/14736669 [cited 2017 Aug. 29]

[35] Eisenkop SM, Spirtos NM. What are the current surgical objectives, strategies, and technical capabilities of gynecologic oncologists treating advanced epithelial ovarian cancer? Gynecologic Oncology [Internet]. 2001;**82**(3):489-497. Available from: http://www.ncbi.nlm.nih.gov/pubmed/11520145 [cited 2017 Aug. 29]

[36] MacKintosh ML, Rahim R, Rajashanker B, Swindell R, Kirmani BH, Hunt J, et al. CT scan does not predict optimal debulking in stage III–IV epithelial ovarian cancer: A multicentre validation study. Journal of Obstetrics and Gynaecology (Lahore). 2014;**34**(5):424-428

[37] Ferrandina G, Sallustio G, Fagotti A, Vizzielli G, Paglia A, Cucci E, et al. Role of CT scan-based and clinical evaluation in the preoperative prediction of optimal cytoreduction in advanced ovarian cancer: A prospective trial. British Journal of Cancer [Internet]. 2009;**101**(7):1066-1073. Available from: http://www.ncbi.nlm.nih.gov/pubmed/19738608 [cited 2017 Aug. 29]

[38] Suppiah S, Kamal SH, Mohd Zabid A, Abu Hassan H. Characterization of adnexal masses using multidetector contrast-enhanced CT scan—Recognising common pitfalls that masquerade as ovarian cancer. Pertanika Journal of Science & Technology [Internet]. 2017;**25**(1):337-352. Available from: http://www.pertanika.upm.edu.my/ [cited 2017 Feb. 20]

[39] Jung SE, Lee JM, Rha SE, Byun JY, Jung JI, Hahn ST. CT and MR imaging of ovarian tumors with emphasis on differential diagnosis. RadioGraphics [Internet]. 2002;**22**(6):1305-1325. Radiological Society of North America. Available from: http://pubs.rsna.org/doi/10.1148/rg.226025033 [cited 2017 Aug. 29]

[40] Micci F, Haugom L, Ahlquist T, Abeler VM, Trope CG, Lothe RA, et al. Tumor spreading to the contralateral ovary in bilateral ovarian carcinoma is a late event in clonal evolution. Journal of Oncology [Internet]. 2010;**2010**:646340. Hindawi. Available from: http://www.ncbi.nlm.nih.gov/pubmed/19759843 [cited 2017 Sept. 9]

[41] Kurtz AB, Tsimikas JV, Tempany CMC, Hamper UM, Arger PH, Bree RL, et al. Diagnosis and staging of ovarian cancer: Comparative values of Doppler and conventional US, CT, and MR imaging correlated with surgery and histopathologic analysis—Report of the Radiology Diagnostic Oncology Group. Radiology [Internet]. 1999;**212**(1):19-27. Available from: http://www.ncbi.nlm.nih.gov/pubmed/10405715 [cited 2017 Sept. 10]

[42] Michielsen K, Vergote I, Op De Beeck K, Amant F, Leunen K, Moerman P, et al. Whole-body MRI with diffusion-weighted sequence for staging of patients with suspected ovarian cancer: A clinical feasibility study in comparison to CT and FDG-PET/CT. European Radiology [Internet]. 2014;**24**(4):889-901. Available from: http://www.ncbi.nlm.nih.gov/pubmed/24322510 [cited 2017 Sept. 10]

[43] Suppiah S, Fathinul Fikri AS, Mohad Azmi NH, Nordin AJ. Mapping 18F-fluorodeoxyglucose metabolism using PET/CT for the assessment of treatment response in non-small cell lung cancer patients undergoing epidermal growth factor receptor inhibitor treatment: A single-centre experience. Malaysian Journal of Medicine and Health Sciences. 2017;**13**(1):23-30

[44] Yoshida Y, Kurokawa T, Tsujikawa T, Okazawa H, Kotsuji F. Positron emission tomography in ovarian cancer: 18F–deoxy-glucose and 16alpha-18F-fluoro-17beta-estradiol PET. Journal of Ovarian Research [Internet]. 2009;**2**(1):7. BioMed Central. Available from: http://www.ncbi.nlm.nih.gov/pubmed/19527525 [cited 2017 Sept. 10]

[45] Castellucci P, Perrone AM, Picchio M, Ghi T, Farsad M, Nanni C, et al. Diagnostic accuracy of 18F-FDG PET/CT in characterizing ovarian lesions and staging ovarian cancer: Correlation with transvaginal ultrasonography, computed tomography, and histology. Nuclear Medicine Communications [Internet]. 2007;**28**(8):589-595. Available from: http://www.ncbi.nlm.nih.gov/pubmed/17625380 [cited 2017 Aug. 29]

[46] Gouhar GK, Siam S, Sadek SM, Ahmed RA. Prospective assessment of 18F-FDG PET/CT in detection of recurrent ovarian cancer. The Egyptian Journal of Radiology and Nuclear Medicine [Internet]. 2013;**44**(4):913-922. Available from: http://linkinghub.elsevier.com/retrieve/pii/S0378603X13001101 [cited 2017 Aug. 29]

[47] Reade CJ, McVey RM, Tone AA, Finlayson SJ, McAlpine JN, Fung-Kee-Fung M, et al. The fallopian tube as the origin of high grade serous ovarian cancer: Review of a paradigm shift. Journal of Obstetrics and Gynaecology Canada [Internet]. 2014;**36**(2):133-140. Available from: http://www.ncbi.nlm.nih.gov/pubmed/24518912 [cited 2017 Sept. 10]

[48] Torizuka T, Kanno T, Futatsubashi M, Okada H, Yoshikawa E, Nakamura F, et al. Imaging of gynecologic tumors: comparison of (11)C-choline PET with (18)F-FDG PET. Journal of Nuclear Medicine [Internet]. 2003;**44**(7):1051-1056. Available from: http://www.ncbi.nlm.nih.gov/pubmed/12843219 [cited 2017 Sept. 14]

[49] Richard SD, Bencherif B, Edwards RP, Elishaev E, Krivak TC, Mountz JM, et al. Noninvasive assessment of cell proliferation in ovarian cancer using [18F] 3'deoxy-3-fluoro-thymidine positron emission tomography/computed tomography imaging. Nuclear Medicine and Biology [Internet]. 2011;**38**(4):485-491. Available from: http://www.ncbi.nlm.nih.gov/pubmed/21531285 [cited 2017 Sept. 10]

[50] Lee SI, Catalano OA, Dehdashti F. Evaluation of gynecologic cancer with MR imaging, 18F-FDG PET/CT, and PET/MR imaging. Journal of Nuclear Medicine [Internet]. 2015;**56**(3):436-443. Society of Nuclear Medicine. Available from: http://www.ncbi.nlm.nih.gov/pubmed/25635136 [cited 2017 Sept. 10]

[51] Kitajima K, Murakami K, Sakamoto S, Kaji Y, Sugimura K. Present and future of FDG-PET/CT in ovarian cancer. Annals of Nuclear Medicine [Internet]. 2011;**25**(3):155-164. Available from: http://www.ncbi.nlm.nih.gov/pubmed/21113691 [cited 2017 Aug. 29]

[52] Kleppe M, Van Gorp T, Slangen BF, Kruse AJ, Brans B, Pooters IN, et al. Sentinel node in ovarian cancer: Study protocol for a phase 1 study. Trials [Internet]. 2013;**14**(1):47. Available from: http://trialsjournal.biomedcentral.com/articles/10.1186/1745-6215-14-47 [cited 2017 Aug. 29]

[53] Nyberg RH, Korkola P, Mäenpää J. Ovarian sentinel node. International Journal of Gynecological Cancer [Internet]. 2011;**21**(3):568-572. Available from: http://content.wkhealth.com/linkback/openurl?sid=WKPTLP:landingpage&an=00009577-201104000-00024 [cited 2017 Sept. 10]

[54] Satpathy M, Zielinski R, Lyakhov I, Yang L. Optical imaging of ovarian cancer using HER-2 affibody conjugated nanoparticles. Methods in Molecular Biology (Clifton, NJ) [Internet]. 2015;**1219**:171-185. Available from: http://www.ncbi.nlm.nih.gov/pubmed/25308269 [cited 2017 Sept. 10]

[55] van Dam GM, Themelis G, Crane LMA, Harlaar NJ, Pleijhuis RG, Kelder W, et al. Intraoperative tumor-specific fluorescence imaging in ovarian cancer by folate receptor-α targeting: First in-human results. Nature Medicine [Internet]. 2011;**17**(10):1315-1319. Available from: http://www.ncbi.nlm.nih.gov/pubmed/21926976 [cited 2017 Sept. 10]

[56] Gamelin J, Yang Y, Biswal N, Chen Y, Yan S, Zhang X, et al. A prototype hybrid intraoperative probe for ovarian cancer detection. Optics Express [Internet]. 2009;**17**(9):7245-7258. Available from: http://www.ncbi.nlm.nih.gov/pubmed/19399101 [cited 2017 Aug. 29]

Permissions

All chapters in this book were first published in CC&OC, by InTech Open; hereby published with permission under the Creative Commons Attribution License or equivalent. Every chapter published in this book has been scrutinized by our experts. Their significance has been extensively debated. The topics covered herein carry significant findings which will fuel the growth of the discipline. They may even be implemented as practical applications or may be referred to as a beginning point for another development.

The contributors of this book come from diverse backgrounds, making this book a truly international effort. This book will bring forth new frontiers with its revolutionizing research information and detailed analysis of the nascent developments around the world.

We would like to thank all the contributing authors for lending their expertise to make the book truly unique. They have played a crucial role in the development of this book. Without their invaluable contributions this book wouldn't have been possible. They have made vital efforts to compile up to date information on the varied aspects of this subject to make this book a valuable addition to the collection of many professionals and students.

This book was conceptualized with the vision of imparting up-to-date information and advanced data in this field. To ensure the same, a matchless editorial board was set up. Every individual on the board went through rigorous rounds of assessment to prove their worth. After which they invested a large part of their time researching and compiling the most relevant data for our readers.

The editorial board has been involved in producing this book since its inception. They have spent rigorous hours researching and exploring the diverse topics which have resulted in the successful publishing of this book. They have passed on their knowledge of decades through this book. To expedite this challenging task, the publisher supported the team at every step. A small team of assistant editors was also appointed to further simplify the editing procedure and attain best results for the readers.

Apart from the editorial board, the designing team has also invested a significant amount of their time in understanding the subject and creating the most relevant covers. They scrutinized every image to scout for the most suitable representation of the subject and create an appropriate cover for the book.

The publishing team has been an ardent support to the editorial, designing and production team. Their endless efforts to recruit the best for this project, has resulted in the accomplishment of this book. They are a veteran in the field of academics and their pool of knowledge is as vast as their experience in printing. Their expertise and guidance has proved useful at every step. Their uncompromising quality standards have made this book an exceptional effort. Their encouragement from time to time has been an inspiration for everyone.

The publisher and the editorial board hope that this book will prove to be a valuable piece of knowledge for researchers, students, practitioners and scholars across the globe.

List of Contributors

Charleen Chan
Department of Medical Oncology, Hammersmith Hospital, London, United Kingdom

Amit Samani and Jonathan Krell
Department of Medical Oncology, Hammersmith Hospital, London, United Kingdom
Department of Surgery and Cancer, Imperial College, London, United Kingdom

Atsushi Imai, Hiroyuki Kajikawa, Chinatsu Koiwai, Satsoshi Ichigo and Hiroshi Takagi
Department of Obstetrics and Gynecology, Mastunami General Hospital, Gifu, Japan

Jeff Hirst and Jennifer Crow
Department of Pathology and Laboratory Medicine, University of Kansas Medical Center, Kansas City, KS, USA

Andrew Godwin
Department of Pathology and Laboratory Medicine, University of Kansas Medical Center, Kansas City, KS, USA
University of Kansas Cancer Center, University of Kansas Medical Center, Kansas City, KS,USA

Achille Manirakiza and Fidel Rubagumya
Department of Clinical Oncology, School of Medicine, Muhimbili University of Health and Allied Sciences, Dar es Salaam, Tanzania

Sumi Sinha
Department of Radiation Oncology, University of California, San Francisco, USA

Katarina Cerne
Department of Pharmacology and Experimental Toxicology, Faculty of Medicine, University Ljubljana, Ljubljana, Slovenia

Borut Kobal
Department of Gynaecology, Division of Gynaecology and Obstetrics, University Medical Centre Ljubljana, Ljubljana, Slovenia
Department of Gynaecology and Obstetrics, Faculty of Medicine, University Ljubljana, Slovenia

Doris Barboza
Medical Institute La Floresta, Oncological Radiotherapy Service, Group GURVE, Caracas, Venezuela

Esther Arbona
Internal Medicine Infectious Disease Department, Dana–Farber Cancer Institute, Boston, USA

Ghassan M. Saed and Nicole M. Fletcher
Wayne State University, Detroit, MI, USA

Robert T. Morris
Karmanos Cancer Institute, Detroit, MI, USA

Sumegha Mitra
Department of Obstetrics and Gynecology, Indiana University School of Medicine, Indianapolis, IN, USA
Indiana University Melvin and Bren Simon Cancer Center, Indianapolis, IN, USA

Carolina Vera, Rocío Retamales-Ortega and Maritza Garrido
Laboratory of Endocrinology and Reproductive Biology, Clinical Hospital University of Chile, Santiago, Chile

Margarita Vega
Laboratory of Endocrinology and Reproductive Biology, Clinical Hospital University of Chile, Santiago, Chile
Department of Obstetrics and Gynecology, Clinical Hospital, Faculty of Medicine, University of Chile, Santiago, Chile

Carmen Romero
Laboratory of Endocrinology and Reproductive Biology, Clinical Hospital University of Chile, Santiago, Chile
Department of Obstetrics and Gynecology, Clinical Hospital, Faculty of Medicine, University of Chile, Santiago, Chile
Advanced Center for Chronic Diseases (ACCDiS), Santiago, Chile

Subapriya Suppiah
Centre for Diagnostic Nuclear Imaging, Universiti Putra Malaysia, Serdang, Malaysia

Index